Molecular Research in Human Microbiome

Molecular Research in Human Microbiome

Editor

Maria Teresa Mascellino

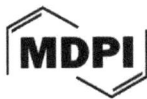

Basel • Beijing • Wuhan • Barcelona • Belgrade • Novi Sad • Cluj • Manchester

Editor
Maria Teresa Mascellino
Public Health and
Infectious Diseases
Sapienza University
Rome, Italy

Editorial Office
MDPI
St. Alban-Anlage 66
4052 Basel, Switzerland

This is a reprint of articles from the Special Issue published online in the open access journal *International Journal of Molecular Sciences* (ISSN 1422-0067) (available at: https://www.mdpi.com/journal/ijms/special_issues/Microbiome_SI).

For citation purposes, cite each article independently as indicated on the article page online and as indicated below:

Lastname, A.A.; Lastname, B.B. Article Title. *Journal Name* **Year**, *Volume Number*, Page Range.

ISBN 978-3-0365-9417-0 (Hbk)
ISBN 978-3-0365-9416-3 (PDF)
doi.org/10.3390/books978-3-0365-9416-3

© 2023 by the authors. Articles in this book are Open Access and distributed under the Creative Commons Attribution (CC BY) license. The book as a whole is distributed by MDPI under the terms and conditions of the Creative Commons Attribution-NonCommercial-NoDerivs (CC BY-NC-ND) license.

Contents

About the Editor vii

Preface ix

Maria Teresa Mascellino
Molecular Research in Human Microbiome
Reprinted from: *Int. J. Mol. Sci.* **2023**, 24, 14975, doi:10.3390/ijms241914975 1

Irina Medakina, Larisa Tsapkova, Vera Polyakova, Sergey Nikolaev, Tatyana Yanova, Natalia Dekhnich, et al.
Helicobacter pylori Antibiotic Resistance: Molecular Basis and Diagnostic Methods
Reprinted from: *Int. J. Mol. Sci.* **2023**, 24, 9433, doi:10.3390/ijms24119433 5

Kunika, Norbert Frey and Ashraf Y. Rangrez
Exploring the Involvement of Gut Microbiota in Cancer Therapy-Induced Cardiotoxicity
Reprinted from: *Int. J. Mol. Sci.* **2023**, 24, 7261, doi:10.3390/ijms24087261 21

Barbara Kneis, Stefan Wirtz, Klaus Weber, Axel Denz, Matthias Gittler, Carol Geppert, et al.
Colon Cancer Microbiome Landscaping: Differences in Right- and Left-Sided Colon Cancer and a Tumor Microbiome-Ileal Microbiome Association
Reprinted from: *Int. J. Mol. Sci.* **2023**, 24, 3265, doi:10.3390/ijms24043265 37

Raja Ganesan, Sang Jun Yoon and Ki Tae Suk
Microbiome and Metabolomics in Liver Cancer: Scientific Technology
Reprinted from: *Int. J. Mol. Sci.* **2023**, 24, 537, doi:10.3390/ijms24010537 61

Sergio Candel, Sylwia D. Tyrkalska, Fernando Pérez-Sanz, Antonio Moreno-Docón, Ángel Esteban, María L. Cayuela and Victoriano Mulero
Analysis of 16S rRNA Gene Sequence of Nasopharyngeal Exudate Reveals Changes in Key Microbial Communities Associated with Aging
Reprinted from: *Int. J. Mol. Sci.* **2023**, 24, 4127, doi:10.3390/ijms24044127 79

Aleksandra Stupak, Tomasz Geca, Anna Kwaśniewska, Radosław Mlak, Paweł Piwowarczyk, Robert Nawrot, et al.
Comparative Analysis of the Placental Microbiome in Pregnancies with Late Fetal Growth Restriction versus Physiological Pregnancies
Reprinted from: *Int. J. Mol. Sci.* **2023**, 24, 6922, doi:10.3390/ijms24086922 99

Dorota Wronka, Anna Karlik, Julia O. Misiorek and Lukasz Przybyl
What the Gut Tells the Brain—Is There a Link between Microbiota and Huntington's Disease?
Reprinted from: *Int. J. Mol. Sci.* **2023**, 24, 4477, doi:10.3390/ijms24054477 117

Francisco Dionisio, Célia P. F. Domingues, João S. Rebelo, Francisca Monteiro and Teresa Nogueira
The Impact of Non-Pathogenic Bacteria on the Spread of Virulence and Resistance Genes
Reprinted from: *Int. J. Mol. Sci.* **2023**, 24, 1967, doi:10.3390/ijms24031967 137

Giovanna Traina
The Connection between Gut and Lung Microbiota, Mast Cells, Platelets and SARS-CoV-2 in the Elderly Patient
Reprinted from: *Int. J. Mol. Sci.* **2022**, 23, 14898, doi:10.3390/ijms232314898 149

Andrea Piccioni, Federico Rosa, Federica Manca, Giulia Pignataro, Christian Zanza, Gabriele Savioli, et al.
Gut Microbiota and *Clostridium difficile*: What We Know and the New Frontiers
Reprinted from: *Int. J. Mol. Sci.* **2022**, *23*, 13323, doi:10.3390/ijms232113323 . . . . **167**

Klaudia Ustianowska, Łukasz Ustianowski, Filip Machaj, Anna Goracy, Jakub Rosik, Bartosz Szostak, et al.
The Role of the Human Microbiome in the Pathogenesis of Pain
Reprinted from: *Int. J. Mol. Sci.* **2022**, *23*, 13267, doi:10.3390/ijms232113267 . . . . **181**

About the Editor

Maria Mascellino

Maria Teresa Mascellino graduated at the age of 25 in Rome during the period of 1980 and specialized in clinical microbiology at the Sapienza University of Rome (Italy). She works as an aggregate professor in the Department of Public Health and Infectious Diseases. She was responsible for the Simple Operative Unit of Microbiology. She has published about 100 papers in reputed journals and has been serving as an editorial board member of repute for several scientific journals. She is a reviewer for important international journals and for the research projects of the Ministry of University and Scientific Research of Rome, other than being a referee at the Fund for Disease Control in Hong Kong. She teaches clinical microbiology to medical students at the University of Rome and was in charge of teaching for foreign students at Trinity College in Dublin in the years 2011–2012 and other foreign nations. Her topics of interest include the following: antibiotics, antibiotic resistance, Gram-negative bacterial infections, antimicrobial susceptibility testing, antimicrobial agents, clinical microbiology, infectious disease epidemiology, medical microbiology, pathogens, bacteria, infection control, infection diseases, microbial pathogenesis, nosocomial infections, MRSA, PCR and molecular analyses, multi-drug-resistant bacteria, COVID-19, and vaccines.

Preface

This reprint deals with the study of the human microbiome and its influence on different pathologies, especially cancer, inflammation, intestinal damage, alterations in the normal gut integrity during *Clostridioides difficile* infections (CDIs), etc.

There are a variety of microorganisms in the human body, including fungi, bacteria, and viruses, that are usually harmless to the human body, and some can even protect our health by making vitamins, decomposing food, and regulating immunity. These microorganisms form a large group called the microbiome. The aim and purpose of this topic are related to the study of the changes in the human microbiome in the occurrence of many situations, such as CDIs, microbial translocation, pain, the spread of virulence and resistance genes among microbiomes, and so on.

The reasons for writing this work are correlated with the fact that our microbiota plays a vital role in our health. In fact, it protects us against pathogens, promotes the development of our immune system, and helps metabolize various compounds. Maintaining a balanced microbial ecosystem is essential for defending our health. This scientific study is mainly addressed to health professionals dealing with cancer, pain, and, in general, human health diseases other than metabolites secreted by the microbiome and their effects on patients with neuropathic diseases. Metabolomic technologies may provide critical information about the role of gut microbiome in cancer as well as molecular investigations, such as 16S rRNA sequencing, used in a study concerning the variability of human microbiome in the nasopharyngeal site in a population at different ages.

The authors involved in this Special Issue are the following: Piccioni A. Kneis B., Kunick F., Medakina I., Ganesan R., Candel S., Stupak A., Wronka D., Traina G., Dionisio F., Ustianowska K., and their respective collaborators.

I would like to acknowledge the support of my coworkers, Dania Al Ismail for drawing up the figure and Alessandra Oliva for the bibliography.

Maria Teresa Mascellino
Editor

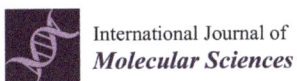

Editorial

Molecular Research in Human Microbiome

Maria Teresa Mascellino

Department of Public Health and Infectious Diseases, Sapienza University of Rome, 00185 Rome, Italy; mariateresa.mascellino@uniroma1.it

Recent evidence has shown that the human microbiome is associated with a wide range of diseases, from non-neoplastic to tumourigenesis, including cancer, inflammation, intestinal damage, etc. Thus, alterations in the normal gut integrity are present during *Clostridioides difficile* infections (CDIs) [1,2]. Some studies have also demonstrated a close relationship between gut microbiota metabolism and cerebral stroke [3]. Our microbiota plays a vital role in our health; it protects us against pathogens, promotes the development of our immune system, and helps metabolize various compounds. Maintaining a balanced microbial ecosystem is essential for protecting our health. The application of omics technology to investigate the mechanism underlying the role of gut microbiome is crucial.

The microbiome is shown to be especially involved in cancer. In this situation, most bacteria, such as salivary and fecal microbiome, other than circulating microbial DNA in blood plasma, impact various kinds of therapies (radiotherapy, chemotherapy, and immunotherapy). Kneis et al., 2023, [4] widely underlined the specificity of the microbiome in different parts of the colon (right- or left-sided colon) or in the rectal portion [4]. This situation affects the progression or outcome of cancer. The right- and left-sided colon have distinct embryological origins and different clinical and molecular characteristics. Thus, they harbor distinct niches and have different microbiome compositions. Another study has indicated that the gut microbiota may serve as a potential target in cancer therapy modulation by enhancing the effectiveness of chemotherapy or immunotherapy [5]. In this article, the role of the microbiome in cancer treatment is evaluated, speculating a potential connection between treatment-related microbial changes and cardiotoxicity. The authors investigate some bacterial families of the microbiome and their possible relationship between cancer treatment and cardiac disease. In this case, a serious consequence due to cancer treatment could be avoided, potentially reducing this fatal side effect (cardiotoxicity), focusing on a potential complex interaction among the microbiome, cancer treatment, and cardiovascular diseases.

Helicobacter pylori is involved in different ranges of infections, such as gastritis, peptic ulcer, atrophic gastritis, gastric cancer, and gastric MALT-lymphoma [6]. The establishment of a correct therapy is crucial for eradicating *H. pylori* infection. The use of empiric or tailored therapy may depend on several factors, such as concomitant diseases, number of previous antibiotic treatments, differences in bacterial virulence in individuals with positive or negative cultures, together with local antibiotic resistance patterns in real-world settings. The regional knowledge of clarithromycin and levofloxacin resistance is very important to establish an appropriate therapy in different geographical areas.

Metabolomic technologies may provide critical information about the role of gut microbiome in cancer. Liver cancer, liver cirrhosis, and emerging therapies for hepatocellular carcinoma (HCC) interact with metabolism at the cellular and systemic levels [7]. The gut microbiota, through the gut–liver axis, significantly contributes to the development of HCC. Dysbiosis, as a consequence of a poor lifestyle, can be overcome by the use of probiotics and symbiotics. Metabolomics science and scientific technologies are reported to be crucial in detecting the biomarkers of liver cancer, and they are currently being considered the new tools to fight similar pathologies.

Citation: Mascellino, M.T. Molecular Research in Human Microbiome. *Int. J. Mol. Sci.* **2023**, *24*, 14975. https://doi.org/10.3390/ijms241914975

Received: 22 September 2023
Accepted: 27 September 2023
Published: 7 October 2023

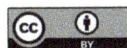

Copyright: © 2023 by the author. Licensee MDPI, Basel, Switzerland. This article is an open access article distributed under the terms and conditions of the Creative Commons Attribution (CC BY) license (https://creativecommons.org/licenses/by/4.0/).

Molecular investigations, such as 16S rRNA sequencing, were used in a study concerning the variability of human microbiome in the nasopharyngeal site in a population at different ages [8]. The variability in the nasopharyngeal microbiome is associated with patient's susceptibility to several infections, so it is thought that the nasopharynx may play an important role in health and disease.

The composition of the placental microbiome and the relative microbial characteristics were taken into account by Stupak et al. regarding their role in placental development and function in late fetal growth restriction (FGR) [9]. In this study, the microbiome of normal and FGR placentas were compared, and the bacteria present in both placentas were identified by an analysis of bacterial proteins set through proteomic and bioinformatic studies. The authors demonstrated that placental dysbiosis could be an important factor in the etiology of FGR, leading to the conclusion that placental microbiota and its metabolites may greatly affect the screening, prevention, diagnosis, and treatment of FGR.

A relationship between microbiome composition and the brain is often reported. Given that dysbiosis in the gut microbiota is involved in many neurodegenerative diseases such as Parkinson's and Alzheimer's, it could be assumed that Huntington's disease (HD) can also be induced by dysbiosis, highlighting the essential role of the intestine–brain axis in HD pathogenesis and evolution [10].

The correlation between gut with lung microbiota, mast cells, platelets, and SARS-CoV-2 was also studied [11]. It was demonstrated that an altered condition of gut microbiota, especially in elderly patients, could be an important factor and have a strong impact on lung homeostasis and COVID-19 together with the activation of mast cells and platelets, and also influence the outcome of the pathology. Changes in the microbial population of elderly people can lead to a chronic state of inflammation, which affects host–microbiome interactions and increases the weaknesses of seniors.

The relationship between gut microbiota and *Clostridioides difficile* infection (CDI) has been widely studied by many researchers from different perspectives. In Piccioni A et al.'s study, it is underlined which types of microbiota alterations are most at risk for the onset of this infection [1]. CDI is one of the greatest public health challenges worldwide as its role is crucial to the interaction with the microbiota. Other than the classic antibiotic treatment, numerous therapeutic alternative strategies have been developed against CDI, such as the use of bacteriophages, fecal microbiota transplantation, both active and passive immunization, and products of the human microbiota that counteract the occurrence of *Clostridioides difficile* infection.

A very interesting topic is the possible impact of non-pathogenic bacteria on the spread of virulence and resistance genes among microbiomes [12]. The role of the above microorganisms is underlined and evaluated in the light of virulence, drug resistance, and other kind of genes able to increase the success of pathogens during infection. Commensal bacteria, including those with drug resistance or virulence genes, could colonize and be transmitted to susceptible hosts for prolonged periods by helping pathogenic cells to receive these genes, and consequently amplify their presence among microbiomes.

Definitely, the principal and crucial role of the gut microbiome includes its relationship with pain [13]. It is well known that the microbiome may lead to different pathologies through the gut–brain axis. The disorder of this relationship is not only associated with gastrointestinal syndromes but also with different types of disease such as cancer, neurological, and cardiovascular and metabolic diseases other than inflammatory disturbances and migraine attacks. Consequently, the human microbiome may be an essential component of the pathogenesis of multiple types of pain. Probiotics, a dietary restriction of short-chain fermentable carbohydrates (low-FODMAP diet), and fecal microbiota transplantation are reported to be beneficial for reducing symptoms and pain episodes.

In summary, the articles in this Special Issue provide a great range of reviews and updates to the role of gut microbial metabolites in the maintenance of health and homeostasis within the human body, as well as to the prevention of infection and disease. The potential anti-cancer properties of different groups of gut metabolites against various cancer types play a crucial role and should be further investigated (Figure 1). Therefore, understanding the specific link between the microbiome and each type of cancer is vital for developing effective treatments.

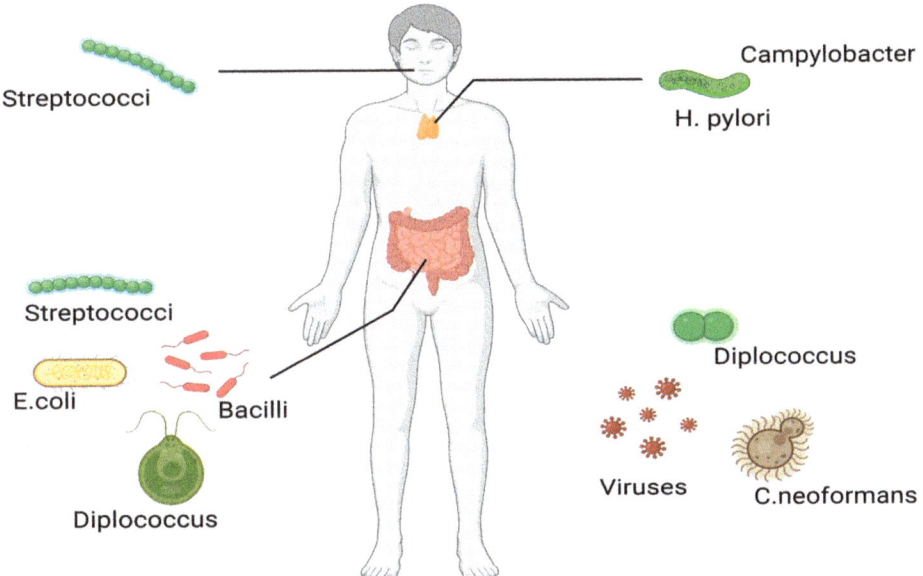

Figure 1. Human microbiomes in different parts of the body. These bacteria can affect cancer progression and the outcome of other diseases. Created with BioRender.com (accessed on 21 September 2023).

Funding: This research received no external funding.

Conflicts of Interest: The author declares no conflict of interest.

References

1. Piccioni, A.; Rosa, F.; Manca, F.; Pignataro, G.; Zanza, C.; Savioli, G.; Covino, M.; Ojetti, V.; Gasbarrini, A.; Franceschi, F.; et al. Gut Microbiota and *Clostridium difficile*: What We Know and the New Frontiers. *Int. J. Mol. Sci.* **2022**, *23*, 13323. [CrossRef] [PubMed]
2. Oliva, A.; Aversano, L.; De Angelis, M.; Mascellino, M.T.; Miele, M.C.; Morelli, S.; Battaglia, R.; Iera, J.; Bruno, G.; Corazziari, E.S.; et al. Persistent Systemic Microbial Translocation, Inflammation, and Intestinal Damage During *Clostridioides difficile* Infection. *Open Forum Infect Dis.* **2019**, *7*, ofz507. [CrossRef] [PubMed]
3. Peh, A.; O'Donnell, J.A.; Broughton, B.R.S.; Marques, F.Z. Gut Microbiota and Their Metabolites in Stroke: A Double-Edged Sword. *Stroke* **2022**, *53*, 1788–1801. [CrossRef]
4. Kneis, B.; Wirtz, S.; Weber, K.; Denz, A.; Gittler, M.; Geppert, C.; Brunner, M.; Krautz, C.; Siebenhüner, A.R.; Schierwagen, R.; et al. Colon Cancer Microbiome Landscaping: Differences in Right- and Left-Sided Colon Cancer and a Tumor Microbiome-IlealMicrobiome Association. *Int. J. Mol. Sci.* **2023**, *24*, 3265. [CrossRef] [PubMed]
5. Kunika; Frey, N.; Rangrez, A.Y. Exploring the Involvement of Gut Microbiota in CancerTherapy-Induced Cardiotoxicity. *Int. J. Mol. Sci.* **2023**, *24*, 7261. [CrossRef] [PubMed]
6. Medakina, I.; Tsapkova, L.; Polyakova, V.; Nikolaev, S.; Yanova, T.; Dekhnich, N.; Khatkov, I.; Bordin, D.; Bodunova, N. *Helicobacter pylori*: Antibiotic Resistance: Molecular Basis and Diagnostic Methods. *Int. J. Mol. Sci.* **2023**, *24*, 9433. [CrossRef] [PubMed]
7. Ganesan, R.; Yoon, S.J.; Suk, K.T. Microbiome and Metabolomics in Liver Cancer: Scientific Technology. *Int. J. Mol. Sci.* **2023**, *24*, 537. [CrossRef]
8. Candel, S.; Tyrkalska, S.D.; Pérez-Sanz, F.; Moreno-Docón, A.; Esteban, Á.; Cayuela, M.L.; Mulero, V. Analysis of 16S rRNA Gene Sequence of Nasopharyngeal Exudate Reveals Changes in Key Microbial Communities Associated with Aging. *Int. J. Mol. Sci.* **2023**, *24*, 4127. [CrossRef] [PubMed]
9. Stupak, A.; Geca, T.; Kwasniewska, A.; Mlak, R.; Piwowarczyk, P.; Nawrot, R.; Gozdzicka-Józefiak, A.; Kwasniewski, W. Comparative Analysis of the Placental Microbiome in Pregnancies with Late Fetal Growth Restriction versus Physiological Pregnancies. *Int. J. Mol. Sci.* **2023**, *24*, 6922. [CrossRef]

10. Wronka, D.; Karlik, A.; Misiorek, J.O.; Przybyl, L. What the Gut Tells the Brain—Is There a Link between Microbiota and Huntington's Disease? *Int. J. Mol. Sci.* **2023**, *24*, 4477. [CrossRef]
11. Traina, G. The Connection between Gut and Lung Microbiota, Mast Cells, Platelets and SARS-CoV-2 in the Elderly Patient. *Int. J. Mol. Sci.* **2022**, *23*, 14898. [CrossRef]
12. Dionisio, F.; Domingues, C.P.F.; Rebelo, J.S.; Monteiro, F.; Nogueira, T. The Impact of Non-Pathogenic Bacteria on the Spread of Virulence and Resistance Genes. *Int. J. Mol. Sci.* **2023**, *24*, 1967. [CrossRef]
13. Ustianowska, K.; Ustianowski, L.; Machaj, F.; Goracy, A.; Rosik, J.; Szostak, B.; Szostak, J.; Pawlik, A. The Role of the Human Microbiome in the Pathogenesis of Pain. *Int. J. Mol. Sci.* **2022**, *23*, 13267. [CrossRef] [PubMed]

Disclaimer/Publisher's Note: The statements, opinions and data contained in all publications are solely those of the individual author(s) and contributor(s) and not of MDPI and/or the editor(s). MDPI and/or the editor(s) disclaim responsibility for any injury to people or property resulting from any ideas, methods, instructions or products referred to in the content.

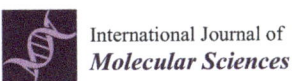

Review

Helicobacter pylori Antibiotic Resistance: Molecular Basis and Diagnostic Methods

Irina Medakina [1], Larisa Tsapkova [1,*], Vera Polyakova [1], Sergey Nikolaev [1], Tatyana Yanova [1], Natalia Dekhnich [2], Igor Khatkov [1,3], Dmitry Bordin [1,3,4] and Natalia Bodunova [1]

1. SBHI Moscow Clinical Scientific Center, 111123 Moscow, Russia
2. FSBEI HE Smolensk State Medical University of the Ministry of Health of Russia, 214019 Smolensk, Russia
3. Department of Propaedeutic of Internal Diseases and Gastroenterology, FSBEI HE Moscow State University of Medicine and Dentistry, 127473 Moscow, Russia
4. Department of General Medical Practice and Family Medicine, FSBEI HE Tver State Medical University of the Ministry of Health of Russia, 170100 Tver, Russia
* Correspondence: l.capkova@mknc.ru

Abstract: *Helicobacter pylori* is one of the most common cause of human infections. Infected patients develop chronic active gastritis in all cases, which can lead to peptic ulcer, atrophic gastritis, gastric cancer and gastric MALT-lymphoma. The prevalence of *H. pylori* infection in the population has regional characteristics and can reach 80%. Constantly increasing antibiotic resistance of *H. pylori* is a major cause of treatment failure and a major problem. According to the VI Maastricht Consensus, two main strategies for choosing eradication therapy are recommended: individualized based on evaluating sensitivity to antibacterial drugs (phenotypic or molecular genetic method) prior to their appointment, and empirical, which takes into account data on local *H. pylori* resistance to clarithromycin and monitoring effectiveness schemes in the region. Therefore, the determination of *H. pylori* resistance to antibiotics, especially clarithromycin, prior to choosing therapeutic strategy is extremely important for the implementation of these treatment regimens.

Keywords: *Helicobacter pylori*; antibiotic resistance; methods for determining *H. pylori* resistance; molecular genetic diagnostics; phenotypic methods for determining antibiotic resistance; geographical distribution of *H. pylori* antibiotic resistance

1. Introduction

Helicobacter pylori is one of the most common human infections [1–3]. Infected patients develop chronic active gastritis in all cases, which can lead to peptic ulcer, atrophic gastritis, gastric cancer and gastric MALT-lymphoma [4–7]. Eradication of *H. pylori* can prevent long-term complications, or relapses of the disease. The treatment the infection is recognized as the primary prevention of gastric cancer.

The prevalence of *H. pylori* infection in the population has geographical distribution characteristics, determined by the level of hygiene, and can reach 80% [8]. According to a meta-analysis published in 2017, the number of people infected with *H. pylori* in the Russian Federation was estimated at 78.5% [9]. At the same time, the prevalence of infection in developed countries is decreasing. Thus, a recently published study showed, that about 40% of the population in Russia is infected, while the prevalence of *H. pylori* increases with age [10].

The recently published Maastricht VI Consensus proposed two strategies for selecting eradication therapy: individualized, based on antibacterial susceptibility, and empirical, in which data regarding local resistance of *H. pylori* to clarithromycin (<15% or >15%) are taken into account when choosing a treatment regimen and monitoring the effectiveness of schemes used in the particular region [4]. Therefore, the determination of *H. pylori* resistance to antibiotics, primarily to clarithromycin, is extremely important for the implementation of these treatment strategies.

The efficacy of antibacterial drugs depends on the sensitivity of the bacteria to them. Currently, a major problem is the decreasing efficacy of therapy regimens, which is associated with the rise of antibiotic resistance in *H. pylori* strains. The prevalence of *H. pylori* resistance varies in different countries and depends on the overall frequency of antibiotic use.

The main objective of this study was to provide a comprehensive analysis of current state of research on the study of antibiotic resistance in *H. pylori*, the molecular mechanisms underlying its emergence, as well as an overview and comparison of methods used for resistance evaluation.

The structure of this article is presented in a diagram (Figure 1).

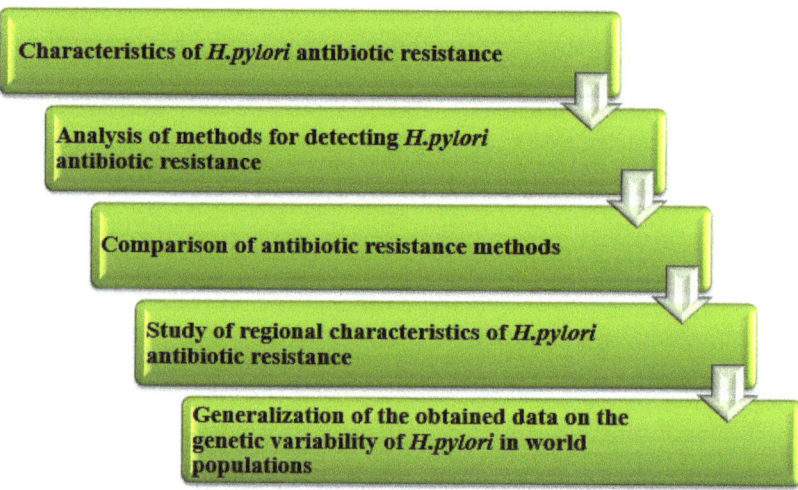

Figure 1. The structure of this article.

2. Characteristics of *H. pylori* Antibiotic Resistance

It has been previously demonstrated, that antibiotic resistance in *H. pylori* a result of mutations in its genome. Point mutations in the V domain of *23S* ribosomal RNA can change the affinity of clarithromycin for the peptidyltransferase loop and lead to resistance to clarithromycin [11–13]. The most common *23S* rRNA mutations associated with clarithromycin resistance are A2143G, A2142G, A2142C [11–13]. The sensitivity of *H. pylori* to clarithromycin is also affected by outer membrane proteins. Proteins such as HopT (BabB), HofC, and OMP31 were absent in clarithromycin-sensitive strains, and were only identified in clarithromycin-resistant strains of *H. pylori*. The mechanism of their association with antibiotic resistance is not yet to metronidazole resistance clear [11].

Mutations in the *rdxA* gene encoding oxygen-insensitive nitroreductase and in the *frxA* gene encoding flavin oxidase reductase are the main cause of resistance to metronidazole. Mutations in these genes reduce the ability of metronidazole to recover to active forms (NO^{2-}, NO_2^{2-}), which have a damaging effect on the bacterial DNA structure [14,15].

Levofloxacin is a fluoroquinolone, which acts via its interaction with DNA gyrase encoded by the *gyrA* and *gyrB* genes. DNA gyrase performs an important function: it promotes the separation of DNA strands during replication. Under the influence of levofloxacin, the process of DNA synthesis and the process of replication of a bacterial cell are disrupted. In levofloxacin-resistant strains of *H. pylori*, mutations were found in codons 87, 88, 91, 97 of the *gyrA* gene and in position 463 of the *gyrB* gene [11–13].

Amoxicillin belongs to the group of beta-lactams, interacts with penicillin-binding proteins and leads to the disruption of cell wall synthesis and destruction of *H. pylori*. Mutations that can interfere with cell wall synthesis disrupt the mechanism of action of amoxicillin: *pbp1A*, *pbp2*, *pbp3*, *hefC*, *hopC* and *hofH*. In addition, the effect of amoxicillin on *H. pylori* is further complicated by the fact that the bacterium itself produces beta-lactamases and there is a reduced membrane permeability for amoxicillin due to efflux pumps [16–18].

In a cohort of Taiwanese patients ($n = 70$) diagnosed with refractory *H. pylori* infection, 39 isolates were successfully cultured. *H. pylori* isolates were obtained from the gastric mucosa, subjected to phenotypic testing for sensitivity to amoxicillin and molecular analysis of genetic variants of the *pbp1A* amoxicillin resistance gene. 30 substitutions were identified (K352, K363, F366, G367, A369, V374, Q376, T386, F396, H409, S414, R418, F448, F473, D508, V509, T513, L530, T541, S543, T550, N561, G59 1, Y604, S615, K617, R618, F620, V622 and P623) in amoxicillin-resistant isolates. It is noted that the majority of resistant isolates carry the P623L substitution, which is potentially responsible for the development of resistance to amoxicillin. Three amino acid substitutions (D479E, D535N and S589G) were identified in all amoxicillin-resistant *H. pylori* isolates obtained from Taiwanese patients [19].

Tetracycline, an antibiotic from the tetracycline group, destroys the codon-anticodon bond at the level of the 30S ribosome subunit, which halts bacterial protein synthesis. Mutations in the *16S rRNA* of the *TET-1* gene lead to the development of resistance to tetracycline. The most common genetic alteration is the substitution of the AGA-GGA triplet (926–928) [20].

The bactericidal action of rifabutin is realized due to its interaction with DNA-dependent RNA polymerase and leads to inhibition of the process of transcription of bacterial DNA. Resistance to rifabutin arises due to mutation of the *rpoB* gene, which encodes the beta subunits of RNA polymerase [1].

Furazolidone (nitrofuran), affects the activity of bacterial oxidoreductase, thus disrupting bacterial metabolism. Mutations associated with resistance to this antibiotic have been identified in the *porD* and *oorD* genes encoding integral ferredoxin-like subunits [21].

Despite the fact that the factors ensuring the adaptation of *H. pylori* to antibiotics are already known, in particular: the effect of the efflux pump, membrane permeability, changes in outer membrane proteins, the ability to form a biofilm and mutations in number of genes, the molecular mechanisms of some remain unclear. Thus, the matter of prescribing effective therapy against *H. pylori* for patients with antibiotic resistance to several drugs remains open [1,22].

3. Methods for Detection of *H. pylori* Antibiotic Resistance

The methods used to detect antibiotic resistance are divided into phenotypic and molecular genetic. Phenotypic methods include: diffusion method (disk diffusion), serial dilution method (in agar, in broth) and combined E-test [23–28].

The method of serial dilutions (limiting dilutions) is based on the determination of a quantitative indicator characterizing the microbiological activity of an antibiotic–the minimum inhibitory concentration (MIC). To determine the MIC, concentrations of the drug prepared in advance are added to the nutrient medium, followed by inoculation and incubation of nutrient medium with the antibiotic. After incubation, bacterial growth is assessed and the active dose of the antibiotic is determined [26,27]. Depending on the concentrations to which *H. pylori* strains are sensitive, they can be divided into sensitive, moderately resistant and resistant. The dilution method using liquid nutrient media is quite convenient and it can be automated, however, due to the difficulties of cultivating *H. pylori*, this method is not convenient for large-scale application.

The disk-diffusion method is based on the diffusion of the drug from the carrier into a dense nutrient medium and suppression of the growth of the studied culture in the zone where the antibiotic concentration exceeds the minimum inhibitory concentration [28]. A paper disk is used as an antibiotic carrier in the disk diffusion method. The effect of an antibiotic is estimated by the diameter size of the growth suppression zone. The growth inhibition diameter, the lower the MIC of the antibiotic and the more active it is against the microorganism under study. Due to the presence of a sufficiently long period of time between the preparation of the medium and the start of this test, the result may be distorted due to a change in the redox potential of the medium, which makes it impossible to use this method for the study of metronidazole. It should be noted that there are no clear criteria for interpreting the results obtained from this method; therefore, at present, the disk diffusion method is not practically used.

The E-test is a type of the disk-diffusion method, where a polymer strip is used as an antibiotic carrier, on which a drug concentration gradient is applied. The activity of the antibiotic is also assessed by the inhibition zone of the microorganisms' growth–the drop-shaped zone of growth inhibition. The MIC value is assessed in the place where the zone of growth suppression is closely adjacent to the drug carrier [23–25].

Criteria for assessing the sensitivity of *H. pylori* to antimicrobial agents are shown in Table 1.

Table 1. Criteria for assessing the sensitivity of *H. pylori* to antimicrobial agents. (in accordance with EUCAST).

Antibiotic	MIC, mg/L	
	Sensitive, ≤	Resistant, >
Amoxicillin	0.25	0.125
Clarithromycin	0.25	0.5
Levofloxacin	1.0	1.0
Tetracycline	1.0	1.0
Metronidazole	8.0	8.0
Rifampicin	1.0	1.0

Molecular genetic methods for detecting antibiotic resistance include real-time polymerase chain reaction (RT-PCR), hybridization with oligonucleotide probes, analysis of restriction fragment length polymorphism (RFLP), Sanger sequencing and NGS sequencing. These methods facilitate the identification of specific mutations that lead to antibiotic resistance.

The PCR-RFLP method is based on amplification of DNA gene regions and selective cleavage of PCR products using restriction endonucleases that recognize mutation sites.

Real-time PCR is the most sensitive and specific method for the detection of infectious agents in comparison with traditional methods (phenotypic, immunological). Real-time polymerase chain reaction is a repetitive cycle of target DNA synthesis. In each cycle, the number of copies of the amplified region is doubled, which makes it possible to generate a DNA fragment bounded by a pair of selected primers in an amount sufficient for its detection using fluorescent probes in 35 cycles. By the end of the procedure, at least 10^{12} fragments should accumulate. The real-time PCR method allows both to determine the presence of a pathogen and its quantification it. Since the kinetics of amplicon accumulation directly depends on the number of the evaluated matrix copies, which allows quantitative measurements of DNA and RNA of infectious agents. To date, real-time polymerase chain reaction method is characterized by one of the lowest error rates [29]. A group of scientists led by M. Pichon conducted a study of *H. pylori* resistance to clarithromycin in stool samples using real-time PCR. Sensitivity and specificity for detecting *H. pylori* were 96.3% (95% CI, 92–98%) and 98.7% (95% CI, 97–99%), respectively [30].

Fluorescence in situ hybridization (FISH) is used to detect *H. pylori* antibiotic resistance in biopsy specimens. The method is applicable to histological preparations. The interpretation of the results is carried out using a fluorescent microscope.

The Sanger sequencing method is the analysis of the studied DNA section's nucleotide sequence of the, namely, the determination of the exact order of the nucleotides in the DNA molecule. With its help, in one working cycle, it is possible to "read" sequences up to 1000 base pairs long with a high accuracy of 98% [31].

NGS–next generation sequencing. The main advantage of the method is high performance and accuracy of the method. Modern sequencers have a capacity of more than 15 billion base pairs per run, maximum read length of more than 600 base pairs and ability to analyze up to 96 samples per run. However, this method is very expensive and requires highly qualified personnel. Therefore, its implementation into clinical practice remains problematic. It is possible that in the future, with the reduction in the cost of analysis, NGS would be implemented into routine clinical practice [32].

A significant advantage of molecular genetic methods in comparison to phenotypic methods is their automation, lower labor input, and high accuracy of results.

Hulten K.G. with a group of scientists compared molecular genetic (NGS) and phenotypic methods for determining the sensitivity of *H. pylori* to amoxicillin, clarithromycin, metronidazole, levofloxacin, tetracycline and rifabutin. The NGS analysis was aimed at studying the already known antimicrobial resistance genes *23SrRNA*, *gyrA*, *16SrRNA*, *pbp1*, *rpoB*, and *rdxA*. The study was carried out on tissue samples of the gastric mucosa fixed in formalin. The results showed that compared to the phenotypic method, the NGS method determined resistance to clarithromycin, levofloxacin, rifabutin and tetracycline with higher accuracy. However, the results for amoxicillin and metronidazole were noted to be less accurate. This fact might be attributed to the poorly understood molecular characteristics of this antibiotic resistance type. There is a possibility that genetic changes in other genes may also be associated with resistance to metronidazole and amoxicillin [33].

The results of recent study regarding the evaluation of *H. pylori* resistance to antibiotics demonstrate a close correlation between the results of NGS analysis of stool samples and gastric biopsy samples from the same patients, which indicates the suitability of feces as a biological material for molecular genetic identification of *H. pylori* antibiotic resistance [34]. Comparative characteristics of *H. pylori* antibiotic resistance research methods are presented in Table 2.

Table 2. Comparison of methods for determining the antibiotic resistance of *H. pylori*.

Method	Sensitivity/Specificity (%)	The Degree of Labor Intensity	Automation Degree	Time Cost
Diffusion method	96/99	High	Low	18–48 h
Serial dilution method	High	High	Low	16–48 h
E-test	96/99	High	Low	16–48 h
PCR method	96/99	Low	High	4–5 h
Direct sequencing	98/98	Medium	High	8–9 h
NGS	98/98	High	Medium	up to 72 h
FISH	High	Medium	High	14–20 h

Interesting findings have been reported in a review paper by Francesca Celiberto et al. on a molecular genetic study of *H. pylori* antibiotic resistance in stool samples. The authors analyzed scientific publications for the period from 1996. The results of these studies showed high sensitivity, and majority of them–high specificity, of the molecular method for determining *H. pylori* antibiotic resistance in stool samples compared to phenotypic methods and RT-PCR of gastric biopsies. Interestingly, the method proved to be more reliable in diagnosing the infection in comparison with commonly used non-invasive diagnostic methods: 13C-urease breath test and fecal antigen determination [35].

4. Regional Characteristics of *H. pylori* Resistance

H. pylori has regional resistance patterns. In Europe, resistance rates of *H. pylori* to clarithromycin are 18–21.4%, levofloxacin −11.0–16.3%, to metronidazole −39.1–56%. At the same time, in the countries of Central and Southern Europe these rates are significantly higher in comparison to the countries of Northern Europe (Figure 2) [36].

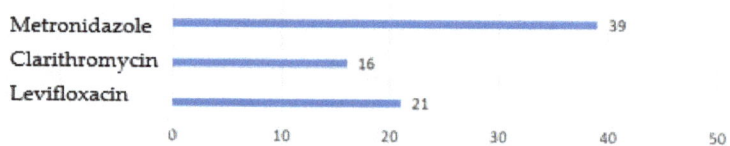

Figure 2. Antibiotic resistance rates (in %) in Europe.

There has been an increase in *H. pylori* resistance to clarithromycin, levofloxacin, and metronidazole in Europe (Figure 3).

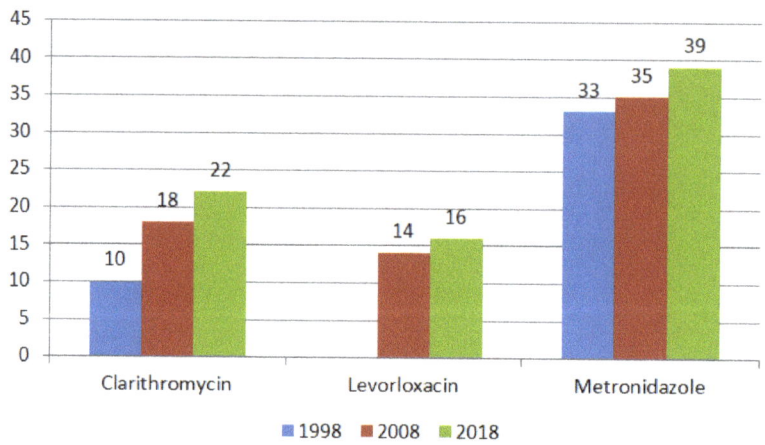

Figure 3. Dynamics of H. pylori antibiotic resistance (%) in Europe. 1998: n = 1227 (22 centers, 17 countries); 2008: n = 1893 (32 centers, 18 countries); 2018: n = 1332 (24 centers, 18 countries).

In the USA, resistance to clarithromycin has been reported at the level of 10% [37]. In China, primary *H. pylori* resistance to clarithromycin, metronidazole, and levofloxacin is estimated at 28.9%, 63.8%, and 28%, respectively. Similar rates of *H. pylori* resistance are observed in South Korea [38,39].

General rates of antibiotic resistance in Southwest China are shown in Figure 4 [40].

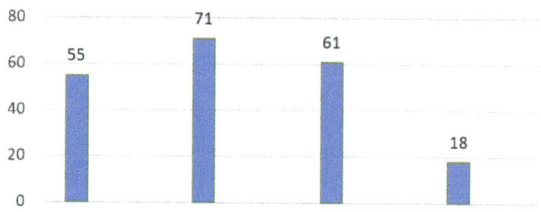

Figure 4. Antibiotic resistance rates (%) of *H. pylori* in Southwest China.

A study was conducted to investigate the changes in antibiotic resistance over time among children in southeastern China. *H. pylori* was cultured from gastric biopsies obtained from children in the time period from 2015 to 2020. Sensitivity to clarithromycin (CLA), amoxicillin (AML), metronidazole (MTZ), furazolidone (FZD), tetracycline (TET), and levofloxacin (LEV) was evaluated. Previously reported data from 2012 to 2014 was used to compare temporal trends in antibiotic resistance. A total of 1638 *H. pylori* strains (52.7%) were isolated from biopsies of 3111 children. The resistance rates to CLA, MTZ, and LEV were 32.8%, 81.7%, and 22.8%, respectively (Figure 5). Single resistance was found in 52.9% of strains, double resistance in 28.7%, and triple resistance in 9.0%. The overall resistance rate and resistance rates to CLA, MTZ, LEV, CLA + LEV, and CLA + MTZ + LEV increased linearly every year. All types of resistance, except single resistance, clearly increased from 2015 to 2017 and from 2018 to 2020 compared with 2012–2014. Double resistance to CLA + MTZ increased significantly with age. The resistance rate to CLA and triple resistance to CLA, MTZ, and LEV were higher in children with previously treated for *H. pylori* infection in comparison to the ones who did not receive any treatment. The rates of antibiotic resistance of *H. pylori* were found to be at high levels in a large cohort of children in southeastern China from 2015 to 2020 [41].

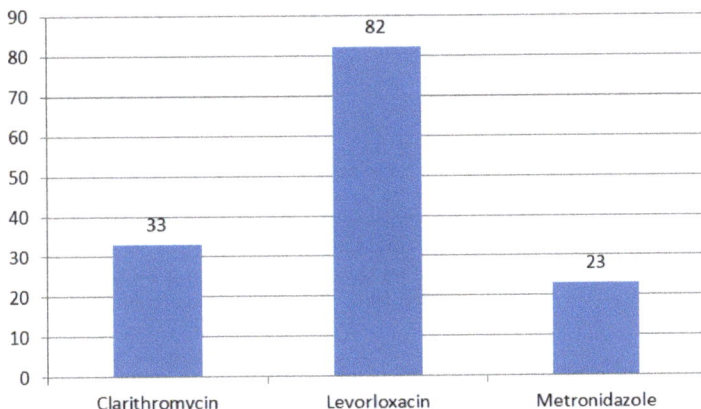

Figure 5. *H. pylori* antibiotic resistance rates (%) in children in Southeast China.

The number of *H. pylori* strains studied in Russia is limited and most studies were carried out about 10 years ago. According to a recently published meta-analysis, in Russia, the level of *H. pylori* resistance to clarithromycin is 10%, to levofloxacin—20%, metronidazole—34%, amoxicillin—1.35% and tetracycline—0.98% (95% CI) (Figure 6) [42].

Data on the low resistance of *H. pylori* to clarithromycin contradicts the data obtained from clinical practice, reflected in the European register of *H. pylori* infection management (Hp-EuReg). According to Hp-EuReg the effectiveness of classical triple therapy in Russia is only 80% with a prescription frequency of 56% [43]. Based on the data from the European registry Hp-EuReg, resistance of *H. pylori* to clarithromycin in Russia is 24%, to levofloxacin—27%, to metronidazole—29% [44].

During the revision of our article, a review paper on the evolution of *H. pylori* resistance to antibiotics by Lyudmila Boyanova was published [45]. The study included review articles on antibiotic resistance data from 14 countries, including Australia, Belgium, Bulgaria, Chile, China, Colombia, France, Italy, Iran, Russia, Spain, Taiwan, Vietnam, and the United States. The most commonly used susceptibility test in these studies was the E-test, the agar dilution method, disk diffusion whereas molecular methods were less common. Sensitivity criteria according to EUCAST and CLSI were used. The dynamics of resistance to amoxicillin, metronidazole, tetracycline, levofloxacin were evaluated. It has been shown that in some countries, such as Bulgaria, Belgium, Iran and Taiwan, there has been an increase in *H. pylori* resistance to three or more antibacterial drugs over time, in France and Spain, on the contrary, resistance levels to most antibiotics have stabilized. The absence of antibiotic resistance growth and even a decrease in resistance levels were usually associated with a decrease in the consumption of that antibiotic in the country, adherence to the latest recommendations for the treatment of *H. pylori* infections, and strict antibiotic policies in countries such as France and the United States [46,47].

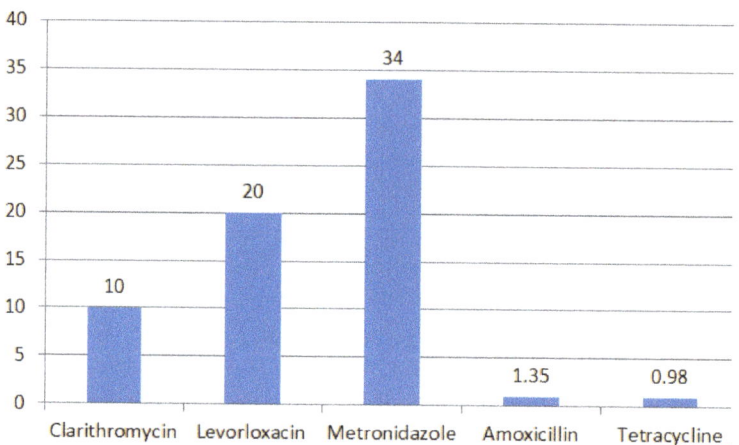

Figure 6. Antibiotic resistance rates (%) in Russia.

Table 3 presents a summary of studies regarding *H. pylori* genetic resistance in world populations. Colombia and South America are characterized by relatively high rates of *H. pylori* infection and stomach cancer. Antibiotic resistance was evaluated for 28 strains of *H. pylori* isolated from gastric biopsy samples from residents of two Colombia regions: with a high risk of gastric cancer (HGCR), and 31 strains from a region with a low risk of gastric cancer (LGCR). Mutations leading to antibiotic resistance were investigated by PCR for all isolates, and for 29 isolates whole genome sequencing was performed. None of the strains were resistant to amoxicillin, clarithromycin, or rifampin. One strain was resistant to tetracycline and had the A926G mutation in the *16S rRNA* gene. Levofloxacin resistance was observed in 12 of 59 isolates and was mainly associated with N87I/K and/or D91G/Y mutations in *gyrA*. Most of the isolates were resistant to metronidazole, and this resistance was significantly higher in the low-risk gastric cancer group (31/31) compared to the high-risk gastric cancer group (24/28). Mutations in the *rdxA* and *frxA* genes were present in almost all metronidazole-resistant strains [48].

Sequencing of the *H. pylori 23S rRNA* gene in the Iranian population showed that the most common mutations leading to antibiotic resistance to clarithromycin are the A2143G and A2142 mutations [49].

During the analysis of the *rdxA* and *frxA* gene in 12 metronidazole-resistant and 10 metronidazole-sensitive *H. pylori* strains in the Myanmar population, it was found that all twelve resistant strains had mutations in the *rdxA* gene, three of them contained mutations with a preliminary stop codon. The most common was the point substitution V175I (8/12, 66.7%), followed by S91P (5/12, 41.7%) and R16H/C (4/12, 33.3%). Mutations in the *frxA* gene were observed in 76.9% (10/13) of resistant strains, preliminary early stop codon was observed in only one strain. In the *frxA* gene, the most frequent point mutation was the L33M substitution (3/13, 23.1%) [50].

Several genetic determinants of *pbp-1* have been reported to be associated with amoxicillin resistance: S414R and N562Y [51]. Two mutations, S414R and V45I, were present in 67% of amoxicillin-resistant *H. pylori* strains [50,51].

In a study by P. Subsomwong et al. in the Myanmar population, almost all levofloxacin-resistant *H. pylori* isolates had an amino acid substitution at position 91 (Asp-91 to Asn or Tyr). Interestingly, no mutation was identified at position 87, which is associated with fluoroquinolone resistance and is found in levofloxacin-resistant *H. pylori* strains in Myanmar's neighboring Southeast Asian countries such as Indonesia, Malaysia, and Cambodia. Both mutations are also found in Chinese and Turkish populations [50].

Table 3. Evaluation of genetic resistance of *H. pylori* in world populations.

Region	Number of Samples	Specimen	Methods Used	Antibiotic Type	Gen (Mutation)	Source
Columbia, S. America	n = 59	biopsy	PCR, WGS	Amoxicillin Clarithromycin Rifampicin Tetracycline Levofloxacin Metronidazole	WT WT WT 16S rRNA (A926G) gyrA (N87I/K, 91G/Y) rdxA, frxA	[48]
Iran	n = 82	biopsy	PCR, Sequencing	Clarithromycin	23S rRNA (A2143G, A2142G)	[49]
Myanmar	n = 150	biopsy	NGS	Metronidazole Amoxicillin Levofloxacin Clarithromycin	rdxA (V175I, S91P, R16H/C), frxA (L33M) pdp1-A (V45I, S414R, V414R, D465K/D, V471H, N564Y) gyrA (D91N/G/Y, D210N, K230Q, A524V, A661T) gyrB (A584V, N679H, M676V, V614I) 23S rRNA (T248C)	[50]
South Korea	n = 144	biopsy	PCR, Sequencing	Amoxicillin	pdp1 (Val16Ile, Val45Ile, Ser414Arg, Asn562Tyr, Thr593Ala, Gly595Ser, Ala599Thr)	[51]
USA	n = 262	biopsy feces	NGS	Amoxicillin Clarithromycin Metronidazole Levofloxacin Tetracycline Rifabutin	pdp1 23S rRNA rdxA, frxA gyrA 16S rRNA rpoB	[33,34,52]
Tunisia	n = 124	biopsy	PCR	Clarithromycin	23S rRNA (2142G, 2143G)	[53]
Sudan	n = 288	biopsy	PCR	Clarithromycin	23S rRNA (A2142G, A2143G, T2182C, C2195T)	[54]
Vietnam	n = 185 n = 308	biopsy	Sequencing	Clarithromycin Amoxicillin	23S rRNA (A2142G, A2143G and other point mutations) pbp1A (366, 414,473, ins595–596)	[55] [16]
Russia	n = 15	cultures from the biopsy	Sequencing	Clarithromycin Levofloxacin	23S rRNA (2142G, 2143G) gyrA (N87I/K, 91G/Y)	[56]

Table 3. Cont.

Region	Number of Samples	Specimen	Methods Used	Antibiotic Type	Gen (Mutation)	Source
Italy	$n = 95$	feces	-	Clarithromycin Levofloxacin	23S rRNA (A2142G, A2143G) gyrA (N87I/K, 91G/Y)	[57]
China	$n = 511$	cultures from the biopsy	Sequencing	Metronidazole	rdxA (R16H/C, Y47C, A67V/T, A80T/S, V204I)	[58]
Bangladesh	$n = 133$	cultures from the biopsy	WGS	Metronidazole Amoxicillin Levofloxacin Clarithromycin	ribF (D253E), frxA, rdxA, mdaB, omp11, pbp1a (N562Y), pbp2 pbp3, pbp4 gyrA (87, 91), gyrB (A343V) 23S rRNA, infB	[59]

In a large-scale study conducted by Tal Domanovich-Asor et al., the whole genome of *H. pylori* was sequenced (WGS) with the aim of studying the bacterium's phylogeny and genetic aspects of antibiotic resistance. A total of 1040 genomes of *H. pylori* isolates were analyzed. The study focused on identifying point mutations in genes associated with bacterial antibiotic resistance (*pbp1A, 23S rRNA, gyrA, rdxA, frxA*, and *rpoB*), as well as conducting phylogenetic analysis. As a result, a significant geographic clustering of *H. pylori* genomes was identified in different regions of the world. The resistance analysis showed that the most common point mutations leading to antibiotic resistance were S589G (*pbp1A*, 48.8% of perfectly aligned sequences), A2143G (*23S rRNA*, 27.4% of perfectly aligned sequences), N87 K\I\Y (*gyrA*, 14.7% of perfectly aligned sequences), R131K (*rdxA*, 65.7% of perfectly aligned sequences), and C193S (*frxA*, 62.6% of perfectly aligned sequences). These research results provide a greater understanding of the relationship between antibiotic resistance and changes in the *H. pylori* genome. Further analyses that combine WGS and phenotypic methods will provide a deeper understanding of the relationship between mutations and resistance [60,61].

A group of scientists conducted a 6-year study on the antibiotic susceptibility of *H. pylori* in Israel. The study included 540 *H. pylori* isolates obtained from gastric biopsy specimens, that were collected from 2015 to 2020. Antibiotic resistance to amoxicillin, clarithromycin, metronidazole, levofloxacin, rifampicin, and tetracycline, was evaluated using the E-test method. Generalized linear models were used to estimate differences in gross and adjusted mean MIC values and odds ratios (ORs) for each year compared to the baseline year of 2015, for each antibiotic and for multi-resistance. The results showed the highest resistance rates to clarithromycin and metronidazole: 46.3% and 16.3%, respectively. Patients over 18 years old had higher levels of resistance to rifampicin and multi-resistance (3.3% and 14.8%, respectively) compared to those under 18 years old (0.5% and 8.4%, respectively). Resistance rates to levofloxacin, rifampicin, and multi-resistance were significantly higher among Arab patients compared to Jewish patients. This study highlights the importance of continuous monitoring of *H. pylori* antibiotic resistance for increasing eradication rates of this bacterium. Therapy for *H. pylori* infection should be revisited and updated based on data on antibiotic resistance [62].

A study on the antibiotic resistance of *H. pylori* was conducted in the Tibetan Autonomous Region of China. The study included 397 patients, from whom 153 strains of *H. pylori* were isolated. The overall resistance rates were as follows: clarithromycin (27.4%), levofloxacin (31.3%), metronidazole (86.2%), amoxicillin (15.6%), tetracycline (0%), furazolidone (0.6%), and rifampicin (73.2%). 2.0% of the *H. pylori* isolates were susceptible to all tested antibiotics, with monoresistance, dual resistance, triple resistance, quadruple resistance, and quintuple resistance rates of 18.3%, 44.4%, 18.3%, 12.4%, and 4.6%, respectively.

The resistance rates to levofloxacin (40.5%) and amoxicillin (21.5%) in strains obtained from female patients were significantly higher than those in strains obtained from male patients (21.6% and 9.5%, respectively).

The conducted study indicates a very high level of *H. pylori* antibiotic resistance in the Tibetan region of China, which suggests a high risk of developing *Helicobacter*-associated complications in these patients. The high resistance to rifampicin demonstrates the need for further research of its derivative, rifabutin [63].

A group of scientists from Portugal conducted a meta-analysis of data on *H. pylori* antibiotic resistance in this Country. The analysis included eight cross-sectional studies evaluating the resistance of *H. pylori* to antibiotics. The overall frequency of resistance was as follows: clarithromycin (CLA) 42% (95% CI: 30–54), metronidazole (MTZ) 25% (95% CI: 15–38), ciprofloxacin (CIP) 9% (95% CI: 3–18), levofloxacin (LVX) 18% (95% CI: 2–42), tetracycline (TTC) 0.2% (95% CI: 0–1), and amoxicillin (AMX) 0.1% (95% CI: 0–0.2) (Figure 7). Multiple drug resistance was also evaluated and results for global resistance rates were as follows: CLA plus MTZ 10% (20% in adults (95% CI: 15–26) compared to 6% in children (95% CI: 4–9) and 2% for CLA plus CIP (primary resistance in the pediatric group). High rates of secondary resistance were found for all antibiotics. In relation to antibiotic resistance, the findings indicate that adults exhibited higher levels of resistance to all antibiotics, with the exception of clarithromycin (CLA), which demonstrated high resistance levels in both adults and children (42% 95% CI: 14–71 and 40% 95% CI: 33–47) [64].

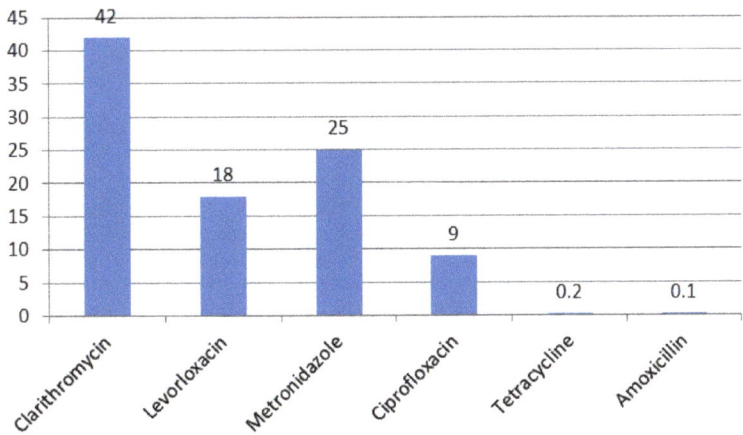

Figure 7. Antibiotic resistance rates (%) of *H. pylori* in Portugal.

A study was conducted to investigate the resistance of *H. pylori* in a cohort of children in Jordan ($n = 166$). The age of the children ranged from 10 to 14 years, with 82.7% of them not having received anti-*Helicobacter* therapy. The authors noted that the detection rate of *H. pylori* infection by rapid urease test, histological, phenotypic, and molecular genetic methods was 93.9%, 89.6%, 61.7%, and 84.3%, respectively. The resistance rates obtained by the phenotypic method were 25.9% for clarithromycin, 50% for metronidazole, and 6.9% for levofloxacin. Interestingly, mutations in the clarithromycin resistance gene were detected in 26.1% of the samples, while mutations in the levofloxacin resistance gene were found in 5.3% of the samples. The authors have concluded that real-time PCR is a valuable alternative method for the identification of *H. pylori* and determination of antibiotic susceptibility [65].

5. Conclusions

Eradication therapy is considered as the basis for the elimination of *H. pylori* infection, which leads to a cure for chronic gastritis and a decrease the risk of occurrence and recurrence of erosive and ulcerative lesions of the gastric and duodenal mucosa, prevention of the development and progression of precancerous changes in the gastric mucosa (atrophic gastritis, intestinal metaplasia) and primary prevention of gastric cancer. The main reason for the decrease in the effectiveness of eradication therapy regimens is the formation and increase in *H. pylori* resistance to antibiotics.

H. pylori antibiotic resistance is a consequence of the use of ineffective eradication therapy regimens and the widespread use of macrolides and fluoroquinolones for various indications, which leads to the development of corresponding mutations in the *H. pylori* genes. The latest Maastricht VI international consensus recommends individualized prescription of eradication regimens, taking into account antibiotic resistance, as well as empiric therapy, considering also account regional differences in resistance and therapeutic efficacy. These recommendations make it actualize the introduction and increase in the availability of methods for determining the resistance of *H. pylori* to antibiotics, both phenotypic and molecular genetics.

Further investigation of the regional peculiarities of *H. pylori* resistance to antimicrobial agents is crucial, as there are geographical differences in the distribution of bacterial resistance. Accumulation of data on regional features of *H. pylori* antibiotic resistance, assessment of its genetic determinants in combination with the diagnosis of *H. pylori* resistance before the administration anti-*Helicobacter* therapy will make it possible to contain the growth of *H. pylori* antibiotic resistance and increase effectiveness anti-*Helicobacter* therapy.

Author Contributions: All authors have read and agreed to the published version of the manuscript.

Funding: This research received no external funding.

Data Availability Statement: Not applicable.

Conflicts of Interest: The authors declare no conflict of interest.

References

1. Maev, I.V. *Helicobacter Pylori Infection: Monograph*; GEOTAR-Mediayu: Moscow, Russia, 2016; p. 256.
2. Mezmale, L.; Coelho, L.G.; Bordin, D.; Leja, M. Epidemiology of *Helicobacter pylori*. *Helicobacter* **2020**, *9*, 25. [CrossRef] [PubMed]
3. De Brito, B.B.; Da Silva, F.A.F.; Soares, A.S.; Pereira, V.A.; Santos, M.L.C.; Sampaio, M.M.; Neves, P.H.M.; De Melo, F.F. Pathogenesis and clinical management of Helicobacter pylori gastric infection. *World J. Gastroenterol.* **2019**, *25*, 5578–5589. [CrossRef] [PubMed]
4. Malfertheiner, P.; Megraud, F.; Rokkas, T.; Gisbert, J.P.; Liou, J.-M.; Schulz, C.; Gasbarrini, A.; Hunt, R.H.; Leja, M.; O'Morain, C.; et al. Management of Helicobacter pylori infection: The Maastrix VI/Florence consensus report. *Gut* **2022**, *71*, 1724–1762. [CrossRef] [PubMed]
5. Tran, V.; Saad, T.; Tesfaye, M.; Walelign, S.; Wordofa, M.; Abera, D.; Desta, K.; Tsegaye, A.; Ay, A.; Taye, B. Analysis of risk factors of Helicobacter pylori (*H. pylori*) and prediction of prevalence: Machine learning approach: Infectious diseases. *Gut* **2022**, *22*, 655. [CrossRef]
6. Noto, J.M.; Rose, K.L.; Hachey, A.J.; Delgado, A.G.; Romero-Gallo, J.; Wroblewski, L.E.; Schneider, B.G.; Shah, S.C.; Cover, T.L.; Wilson, K.T.; et al. Carcinogenic strains of *Helicobacter pylori* selectively dysregulate the stomach proteome In Vivo, which may be associated with the progression of gastric cancer. *Mol. Cell Proteom.* **2019**, *18*, 352–371. [CrossRef]
7. Elbehiry, A.; Marzouk, E.; Aldubaib, M.; Abalkhail, F.; Anagreyyah, S.; Anajirih, N.; Almuzaini, A.M.; Rawway, M.; Alfadhel, A.; Draz, A.; et al. *Helicobacter pylori* Infection: Current Status and Future Prospects on Diagnostic, Therapeutic and Control Challenges. *Antibiotics* **2023**, *12*, 191. [CrossRef]
8. Kotilea, K.; Bontems, P.; Touati, E. Epidemiology, diagnosis and risk factors of *Helicobacter pylori* infection. *Adv. Exp. Med. Biol.* **2019**, *11*, 17–33. [CrossRef]
9. Hooi, J.K.Y.; Lai, W.Y.; Ng, W.K.; Suen, M.M.Y.; Underwood, F.E.; Tanyingoh, D.; Malfertheiner, P.; Graham, D.Y.; Wong, V.W.S.; Wu, J.C.Y. Prevalence of *Helicobacter pylori* Infection: Systematic Review and Meta-Analysis. *Gastroenterology* **2019**, *8*, 420–429. [CrossRef]
10. Bordin, D.; Morozov, S.; Plavnik, R.; Bakulina, N.; Voynovan, I.; Skibo, I.; Isakov, V.; Bakulin, I.; Andreev, D.; Maev, I. *Helicobacter pylori* infection prevalence in ambulatory settings in 2017–2019 in Russia: The data of real-world national multicenter trial. *Helicobacter* **2022**, *27*, 5. [CrossRef]
11. Puah, S.M.; Goh, K.L.; Ng, H.K.; Chua, K.H. The current state of resistance of Helicobacter pylori to clarithromycin and levofloxacin in Malaysia—Results of a molecular study. *PeerJ* **2021**, *1*, 12. [CrossRef]
12. Li, Y.; Lv, T.; He, C.; Wang, H.; Cram, D.S.; Zhou, L.; Zhang, J.; Jiang, W. Evaluation of multiplex ARMS-PCR for detection of *Helicobacter pylori* mutations conferring resistance to clarithromycin and levofloxacin. *Gut Pathog.* **2020**, *7*, 10–12. [CrossRef] [PubMed]

13. Ziver-Sarp, T.; Yuksel-Mayda, P.; Saribas, S.; Demiryas, S.; Gareayaghi, N.; Ergin, S.; Tasci, I.; Ozbey, D.; Bal, K.; Erzin, Y. Point mutations at *gyrA* and *gyrB* genes of levofloxacin resistant *Helicobacter pylori* strains and dual resistance with clarithromycin. *Clin. Lab.* **2021**, *67*, 10. [CrossRef]
14. Gong, M.; Han, Y.; Wang, X.; Tao, H.; Meng, F.; Hou, B.; Sun, B.B.; Wang, G. Effect of temperature on metronidazole resistance in *Helicobacter pylori*. *Front. Microbiol.* **2021**, *1*, 12. [CrossRef] [PubMed]
15. Marais, A.; Bilardi, C.; Cantet, F.; Mendz, G.L.; Mégraud, F. Characterization of the genes rdxA and frxA involved in metronidazole resistance in *Helicobacter pylori*. *Res. Microbiol.* **2003**, *154*, 137–144. [CrossRef]
16. Tran, T.T.; Nguyen, A.T.; Quach, D.T.; Pham, D.T.-H.; Cao, N.M.; Nguyen, U.T.-H.; Dang, A.N.-T.; Tran, M.A.; Quach, L.H.; Tran, K.T. Emergence of amoxicillin resistance and identification of novel mutations of the pbp1A gene in *Helicobacter pylori* in Vietnam. *BMC Microbiol.* **2022**, *2*, 41. [CrossRef]
17. Tseng, Y.-S.; Wu, D.-C.; Chang, C.-Y.; C-H Kuo, C.-H.; Yang, Y.-C.; Jan, C.-M.; Su, Y.-C.; Kuo, F.-C.; Chang, L.-L. Amoxicillin resistance with β-lactamase production in *Helicobacter pylori*. *Eur. J. Clin. Investig.* **2009**, *9*, 807–812. [CrossRef]
18. Qureshi, N.N.; Gallaher, B.; Schiller, N.L. Evolution of amoxicillin resistance of *Helicobacter pylori* In Vitro: Characterization of resistance mechanisms. *Microb Drug Resist.* **2014**, *12*, 509–516. [CrossRef] [PubMed]
19. Kuo, C.-G.; Ke, J.-N.; Kuo, T.; Lin, C.-Y.; Hsieh, S.-Y.; Chiu, Y.-F.; Wu, H.-Y.; Huang, M.-Z.; Bui, N.-N.; Chiu, C.-H. Multiple amino acid substitutions in penicillin-binding protein-1A confer amoxicillin resistance in refractory *Helicobacter pylori* infection. *J. Microbiol. Immunol. Infect.* **2023**, *56*, 40–47. [CrossRef]
20. Contreras, M.; Benejat, L.; Mujica, H.; Peña, L.; García-Amado, M.-A.; Michelangeli, F.; Lehours, P. Real-time PCR detection of 16S rRNA-a single mutation of *Helicobacter pylori* isolates associated with a decrease in susceptibility and resistance to tetracycline in the mucous membrane of gastroesophageal individual hosts. *J. Med. Microbiol.* **2019**, *68*, 1287–1291. [CrossRef]
21. Resina, E.; Gisbert, J.P. Rescue therapy with furazolidone in patients with at least five failures of eradication treatment and multi-resistant *H. pylori* infection. *Antibiotics* **2021**, *10*, 1028. [CrossRef]
22. Srisuphanunt, M.; Wilairatana, P.; Kooltheat, N.; Duangchan, T.; Katzenmeier, G.; Rose, J.B. Molecular Mechanisms of Antibiotic Resistance and Novel Treatment Strategies for *Helicobacter pylori* Infections. *Trop. Med. Infect. Dis.* **2023**, *8*, 163. [CrossRef]
23. Fauzia, K.A.; Miftahussurur, M.; Syam, A.F.; Waskito, L.A.; Doohan, D.; Rezkitha, Y.A.A.; Matsumoto, T.; Tuan, V.P.; Akada, J.; Yonezawa, H. Biofilm formation and antibiotic resistance phenotype of *Helicobacter pylori* clinical isolates. *Toxins* **2020**, *7*, 473. [CrossRef] [PubMed]
24. Miftahussurur, M.; Fauzia, K.A.; Nusi, I.A.; Setiawan, P.B.; Syam, A.F.; Waskito, L.A.; Doohan, D.; Ratnasari, N.; Khomsan, A.; I Ketut Adnyana, I.K.; et al. E-test versus agar dilution for antibiotic susceptibility testing of *Helicobacter pylori*: A comparison study. *BMC Res. Notes* **2020**, *9*, 13–22. [CrossRef] [PubMed]
25. Vilaichone, R.K.; Aumpan, N.; Ratanachu-Ek, T.; Uchida, T.; Tshering, L.; Mahachai, V.; Yamaoka, Y. Population-based study of *Helicobacter pylori* infection and antibiotic resistance in Bhutan. *Int. J. Infect. Dis.* **2022**, *97*, 102–107. [CrossRef] [PubMed]
26. Raro, O.H.F.; Collar, G.S.; Da Silva, R.M.C.; Vezzaro, P.; Mott, M.P.; Da Cunha, G.R.; Riche, C.V.W.; Dias, C.; Caierão, J. Performance of polymyxin B agar-based tests among carbapenem-resistant Enterobacterales. *Lett. Appl. Microbiol.* **2021**, *72*, 767–773. [CrossRef]
27. Patel, J.B. *Performance Standards for Antimicrobial Susceptibility Testing*; Clinical and Laboratory Standards Institute: Wayne, MI, USA, 2017; pp. 1–42.
28. Siavoshi, F.; Saniee, P.; Latifi-Navid, S.; Massarrat, S.; Sheykholeslami, A. Increased resistance of *H. pylori* isolates to metronidazole and tetracycline—Comparison of three 3-year studies. *Arch. Iran. Med.* **2021**, *4*, 1–5.
29. Rebrikov, D.V.; Samatov, G.A.; Trofimov, D.Y.; Semenov, P.A.; Savilova, A.M.; Kofiadi, I.A.; Abramov, I.A. *Real-time PCR-M*; Knowledge Laboratory: Stanford, CA, USA, 2019; 223p.
30. Pichon, M.; Freche, B.; Christophe Burucoa, C. New Strategy for the Detection and Treatment of *Helicobacter pylori* Infections in Primary Care Guided by a Non-Invasive PCR in Stool: Protocol of the French HepyPrim Study. *J. Clin. Med.* **2022**, *3*, 11. [CrossRef]
31. Borodinov, A.G.; Manoilov, V.V.; Zarutsky, I.V.; Petrov, A.I.; Kurochkin, V.E. Generations of DNA sequencing methods. *Sci. Instrum.* **2020**, *4*, 3–20.
32. Ishibashi, F.; Suzuki, S.; Nagai, n.; Mochida, K.; Morishita, T. Optimizing *Helicobacter pylori* Treatment: An Updated Review of Empirical and Susceptibility Test-Based Treatments. *Gut Liver.* **2023**. ahead of print. [CrossRef]
33. Hulten, K.G.; Genta, R.M.; Kalfus, I.N.; Zhou, Y.; Zhang, H.; Graham, D.Y. Comparison of Culture With Antibiogram to Next-Generation Sequencing Using Bacterial Isolates and Formalin-Fixed, Paraffin-Embedded Gastric Biopsies. *Gastroenterology* **2021**, *161*, 1433–1442. [CrossRef]
34. Moss, S.F.; Dang, L.P.; Chua, D.; Sobrado, J.; Zhou, Y.; Graham, D.Y. Comparable Results of *Helicobacter pylori* Antibiotic Resistance Testing of Stools vs Gastric Biopsies Using Next-Generation Sequencing. *Gastroenterology* **2022**, *2*, 27. [CrossRef] [PubMed]
35. Celiberto, F.; Losurdo, G.; Pricci, M.; Girardi, B.; Marotti, A.; Leo, A.D.; Ierardi, E. The State of the Art of Molecular Fecal Investigations for *Helicobacter pylori* (H. pylori) Antibiotic Resistances. *Int. J. Mol. Sci.* **2023**, *24*, 4361. [CrossRef] [PubMed]
36. Megraud, F.; Bruyndonckx, R.; Coenen, S.; Wittkop, L.; Huang, T.-D.; Hoebeke, M.; Bénéjat, L.; Lehours, F.; Goossens, H.; Glupczynski, Y. Helicobacter pylori resistance to antibiotics in Europe in 2018 and its relationship to antibiotic consumption in the community. *Gut* **2021**, *70*, 1815–1822. [CrossRef] [PubMed]
37. Savoldi, A.; Carrara, E.; Graham, D.Y.; Conti, M.; Tacconelli, E. Prevalence of antibiotic resistance in *Helicobacter pylori*: A systematic review and meta-analysis in World Health Organization regions. *Gastroenterology* **2018**, *155*, 1372–1382. [CrossRef]

38. Liu, Y.; Wang, S.; Yang, F.; Chi, W.; Ding, L.; Liu, T.; Zhu, F.; Ji, D.; Zhou, J.; Fang, Y.; et al. Antimicrobial resistance patterns and genetic elements associated with the antibiotic resistance of *Helicobacter pylori* strains from Shanghai. *Gut Pathog.* **2022**, *14*, 14. [CrossRef]
39. Cho, J.H.; Jin, S.Y. Current guidelines for *Helicobacter pylori* treatment in East Asia 2022: Differences am ong China, Japan, and South Korea. *World J. Clin. Cases.* **2022**, *10*, 6349–6359. [CrossRef]
40. Li, J.; Deng, J.; Wang, Z.; Li, H.; Wan, C. Antibiotic resistance of *Helicobacter pylori* strains isolated from pediatric patients in Southwest China. *Front Microbiol.* **2021**, *11*, 621791. [CrossRef]
41. Shu, X.; Ye, D.; Hu, C.; Peng, K.; Zhao, H.; Li, H.; Jiang, M. Alarming antibiotics resistance of *Helicobacter pylori* from children in Southeast China over 6 years. *Sci. Rep.* **2022**, *21*, 66. [CrossRef]
42. Andreev, D.A.; Maev, I.V.; Kucheryavyy, Y.A. *Helicobacter pylori* resistance in the Russian Federation: A meta-analysis of studies over the past 10 years. *Ther. Arch.* **2020**, *92*, 24–30.
43. Nyssen, O.P.; Vaira, D.; Tepes, B.; Kupcinskas, L.; Bordin, D.; Pérez-Aisa, A.; Gasbarrini, A.; Castro-Fernández, M.; Bujanda, L.; Garre, A. Hp-EuReg Investigators. Room for Improvement in the Treatment of *Helicobacter pylori* Infection: Lessons from the European Registry on H. pylori Management (Hp-EuReg). *J. Clin. Gastroenterol.* **2022**, *2*, 98–108. [CrossRef]
44. Bujanda, L.; Nyssen, O.P.; Vaira, D.; Saracino, L.M.; Fiorini, G.; Lerang, F.; Georgopoulos, S.; Tepes, B.; Heluwaert, F.; Antonio Gasbarrini, A. The Hp-EuReg Investigators. Antibiotic Resistance Prevalence and Trends in Patients Infected with *Helicobacter pylori* in the Period 2013-2020: Results of the European Registry on H. pylori Management (Hp-EuReg). *Antibiotics* **2021**, *9*, 1058. [CrossRef] [PubMed]
45. Boyanova, L.; Hadzhiyski, P.; Gergova, R.; Markovska, R. Evolution of *Helicobacter pylori* Resistance to Antibiotics: A Topic of Increasing Concern. *Antibiotics* **2023**, *12*, 332. [CrossRef] [PubMed]
46. Mégraud, F.; Alix, C.; Charron, P.; Bénéjat, L.; Ducournau, A.; Bessède, E.; Lehours, F. Survey of the antimicrobial resistance of *Helicobacter pylori* in France in 2018 and evolution during the previous 5 years. *Helicobacter* **2021**, *26*, e12767. [CrossRef] [PubMed]
47. Mosites, E.; Bruden, D.; Morris, J.; Reasonover, A.; Rudolph, K.; Hurlburt, D.; Hennessy, T.; McMahon, B.; Bruce, M. Antimicrobial resistance among *Helicobacter pylori* isolates in Alaska, 2000–2016. *J. Glob. Antimicrob. Resist.* **2018**, *15*, 148–153. [CrossRef] [PubMed]
48. Mannion, A.; Dzink-Fox, J.; Shen, Z.; Piazuelo, M.B.; Wilson, K.T.; Correa, P.; Peek, R.M., Jr.; Camargo, M.C.; Fox, J.G. Antimicrobial resistance of *Helicobacter pylori* and gene variants in populations with high and low risk of stomach cancer. *J. Clin. Microbiol.* **2021**, *59*, e03203-20. [CrossRef]
49. Alavifard, H.; Mirzaei, N.; Yadegar, A.; Baghaei, K.; Smith, S.M.; Sadeghi, A.; Zali, M.R. Investigation of mutations associated with clarithromycin resistance and *Helicobacter pylori* virulence genotypes isolated from the Iranian population: A cross-sectional study. *Curr. Microbiol.* **2021**, *78*, 244–254. [CrossRef]
50. Subsomwong, P.; Doohan, D.; Fauzia, K.A.; Akada, J.; Matsumoto, T.; Yee, T.T.; Htet, K.; Waskito, L.A.; Tuan, V.; Uchida, T. Next-Generation Sequencing-Based Study of *Helicobacter pylori* Isolates from Myanmar and Their Susceptibility to Antibiotics. *Microorganosms* **2022**, *10*, 196. [CrossRef]
51. Kim, B.J.; Kim, J.G. Substitutions in penicillin-binding protein 1 in amoxicillin-resistant *Helicoobacter pylori* strains isolated from Korean patients. *Gut Liver.* **2013**, *7*, 655–660. [CrossRef]
52. De Palma, G.Z.; Mendiondo, N.; Wonaga, A.; Viola, L.; Ibarra, D.; Campitelli, E.; Salim, N.; Corti, R.; Goldman, C.; Catalano, M. Occurrence of mutations in the antimicrobial target genesrelated to levofloxacin, clarithromycin, and amoxicillin resistance in *Helicobacter pylori* isolates from Buenos Aires city. *Microb. Drug Resist.* **2017**, *23*, 351–358. [CrossRef]
53. Chtourou, L.; Moalla, M.; Mnif, B.; Smaoui, H.; Gdoura, H.; Boudabous, M.; Mnif, L.; Amouri, A.; Hammami, A.; Tahri, N. Prevalence of *Helicobacter pylori* resistance to clarithromycin in Tunisia. *J. Med. Microbiol.* **2022**, *8*, 71. [CrossRef]
54. Albasha, A.M.; Elnosh, M.M.; Osman, E.H.; Zeinalabdin, D.M.; Fadl, A.A.M.; Ali, M.A.; Altayb, H.N. *Helicobacter pylori* 23S rRNA gene A2142G, A2143G, T2182C, and C2195T mutations associated with clarithromycin resistance detected in Sudanese patients. *BMC Microbiol.* **2021**, *2*, 21–38. [CrossRef] [PubMed]
55. Tran, V.H.; Ha, T.M.T.; Le, P.T.Q.; Phan, T.N.; Tran, T.N.H. Characterisation of point mutations in domain V of the 23S rRNA gene of clinical *Helicobacter pylori* strains and clarithromycin-resistant phenotype in central Vietnam. *J. Glob. Antimicrob. Resist.* **2019**, *3*, 87–91. [CrossRef] [PubMed]
56. Tsapkova, L.A.; Polyakova, V.V.; Bodunova, N.A.; Baratova, I.V.; Voynovan, I.N.; Dekhnich, N.N.; Ivanchik, N.V.; Sabelnikova, E.A.; Bordin, D.S. Possibilities of a molecular genetic method for detecting resistance to clarithromycin and levofloxacin in *Helicobacter pylori.* *Eff. Pharmacother.* **2022**, *42*, 16–20.
57. Iannone, A.; Giorgio, F.; Russo, F.; Riezzo, G.; Girardi, B.; Pricci, M.; Palmer, S.C.; Barone, M.; Principi, M.; Strippoli, G.F. New fecal test for non-invasive *Helicobacter pylori* detection: A diagnostic accuracy study. *Clin. Trial* **2018**, *24*, 3021–3029. [CrossRef]
58. Gong, Y.; Zhai, R.; Sun, L.; He, L.; Wang, H.; Guo, Y.; Zhang, J. RdxA Diversity and Mutations Associated with Metronidazole Resistance of *Helicobacter pylori.* *Microbiol. Spectr.* **2023**, *21*, e0390322. [CrossRef]
59. Fauzia, K.A.; Aftab, H.; Tshibangu-Kabamba, E.; Alfaray, R.I.; Saruuljavkhlan, B.; Cimuanga-Mukanya, A.; Matsumoto, T.; Subsomwong, P.; Akada, J.; Miftahussurur, M.; et al. Bangladesh—Mutations Related to Antibiotics Resistance in *Helicobacter pylori* Clinical Isolates from Bangladesh. *Antibiotics* **2023**, *12*, 279. [CrossRef] [PubMed]
60. Domanovich-Asor, T.; Craddock, H.A.; Motro, Y.; Khalfin, B.; Peretz, A.; Moran-Gilad, J. Unraveling antimicrobial resistance in *Helicobacter pylori*: Global resistome meets global phylogeny. *Helicobacter* **2021**, *5*, 25. [CrossRef]

61. Domanovich-Asor, T.; Motro, Y.; Khalfin, B.; Craddock, H.A.; Peretz, A.; Moran-Gilad, J. Genomic Analysis of Antimicrobial Resistance Genotype-to-Phenotype Agreement in *Helicobacter pylori*. *Microorganisms* **2021**, *9*, 2. [CrossRef]
62. Azrad, M.; Vazana, D.; On, A.; Paritski, M.; Rohana, H.; Roshrosh, H.; Agay-Shay, K.; Peretz, A. Antibiotic resistance patterns of *Helicobacter pylori* in North Israel—A six-year study. *Helicobacter* **2022**, *12*, 12932. [CrossRef]
63. Tang, X.; Wang, Z.; Shen, Y.; Song, X.; Benghezal, M.; Marshall, B.J.; Tang, H.; Hong Li, H. Antibiotic resistance patterns of *Helicobacter pylori* strains isolated from the Tibet Autonomous Region, China. *Microbiology* **2022**, *22*, 196. [CrossRef]
64. Lopo, I.; Libânio, D.; Pita, I.; Dinis-Ribeiro, M.; Pimentel-Nunes, P. *Helicobacter pylori* antibiotic resistance in Portugal: Systematic review and meta-analysis. *Helicobacter* **2018**, *8*, 23. [CrossRef]
65. Lee, Y.-C.; Dore, M.P.; Graham, D.Y. Diagnosis and treatment of *Helicobacter pylori* infection. *Annu. Rev. Med.* **2022**, *4*, 183–195. [CrossRef] [PubMed]

Disclaimer/Publisher's Note: The statements, opinions and data contained in all publications are solely those of the individual author(s) and contributor(s) and not of MDPI and/or the editor(s). MDPI and/or the editor(s) disclaim responsibility for any injury to people or property resulting from any ideas, methods, instructions or products referred to in the content.

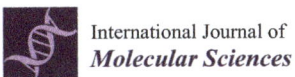

Review

Exploring the Involvement of Gut Microbiota in Cancer Therapy-Induced Cardiotoxicity

Kunika [1,2], Norbert Frey [1,2] and Ashraf Y. Rangrez [1,2,*]

1. Department of Cardiology, Angiology and Pneumology, University Hospital Heidelberg, 69120 Heidelberg, Germany
2. DZHK (German Centre for Cardiovascular Research), Partner Site Heidelberg/Mannheim, 69120 Heidelberg, Germany
* Correspondence: ashrafyusuf.rangrez@med.uni-heidelberg.de

Abstract: Trillions of microbes in the human intestinal tract, including bacteria, viruses, fungi, and protozoa, are collectively referred to as the gut microbiome. Recent technological developments have led to a significant increase in our understanding of the human microbiome. It has been discovered that the microbiome affects both health and the progression of diseases, including cancer and heart disease. Several studies have indicated that the gut microbiota may serve as a potential target in cancer therapy modulation, by enhancing the effectiveness of chemotherapy and/or immunotherapy. Moreover, altered microbiome composition has been linked to the long-term effects of cancer therapy; for example, the deleterious effects of chemotherapy on microbial diversity can, in turn, lead to acute dysbiosis and serious gastrointestinal toxicity. Specifically, the relationship between the microbiome and cardiac diseases in cancer patients following therapy is poorly understood. In this article, we provide a summary of the role of the microbiome in cancer treatment, while also speculating on a potential connection between treatment-related microbial changes and cardiotoxicity. Through a brief review of the literature, we further explore which bacterial families or genera were differentially affected in cancer treatment and cardiac disease. A deeper understanding of the link between the gut microbiome and cardiotoxicity caused by cancer treatment may help lower the risk of this critical and potentially fatal side effect.

Keywords: gut microbiome; dysbiosis; cancer treatment; cardiotoxicity

1. Introduction

Over the past several decades, tremendous efforts have been made to develop a range of treatment options for cancer, including chemotherapy, radiotherapy, immunotherapy, and surgery, all of which have significantly reduced the mortality and morbidity associated with various forms of cancer [1]. Although the benefits of anticancer drugs and therapies are undeniable, safety aspects cannot be overlooked; for example, some treatments have been found to adversely affect the cardiovascular system [2,3]. Cardiotoxicity is a crucial factor to consider for individuals receiving cancer therapy because, even though most patients will recover from cancer, they will then have elevated long-term cardiac risks [4,5]. However, in-depth insights into the underlying molecular mechanisms and causal agents are lacking. Interestingly, a pioneering study including 1526 tumors and their adjacent normal tissues across seven cancer types (breast, lung, ovary, pancreas, melanoma, bone, and brain tumors) reported a distinct microbiome composition specific to cancer types [6]. The authors also correlated bacteria identified in the tumor microenvironment (TME), or their predicted functions, with tumor types and subtypes, smoking status, and response to immunotherapy [6]. Similarly, one of the long-term effects of cancer treatment is a shift in the composition of the gut microbiome, termed gut dysbiosis [7]. Importantly, low-grade chronic inflammation is one of the hallmarks of cardiac diseases and cancers, and is also caused by gut dysbiosis and an altered intestinal permeability barrier. Can the

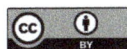

gut microbiome be the missing link? Well-directed and thorough research is required to answer these questions.

The microbiome is defined as a collection of all microbial genomes found in a particular environment. Rapid advances in tools and techniques in recent years have provided new knowledge and insights into the interactions between microorganisms and their hosts [8]. Humans and microbes have evolved together, and microbial communities play a significant role in maintaining human health [9]. The number of gut microbiota, the microbial commensal organisms of the gastrointestinal system, exceeds the number of human cells and constitutes the largest surface area for microbial interactions with the host's immune system. In contrast, alterations in the microbial composition of the gut, or gut dysbiosis, play important physiological roles, primarily promoting the accumulation of proinflammatory substances [9]. Moreover, the gut microbiome plays an important role in regulating the risk of several chronic diseases, including inflammatory bowel disease, obesity, type 2 diabetes, cardiovascular disease, and cancer [9]. Of additional interest, it has been demonstrated that the gut microbiota co-evolves with the host and lies at the intersection of multiple antitumor and oncogenic metabolic, immune, and inflammatory pathways in cancer [10]. Several studies have highlighted that the connection among gut microbiota, genotoxins, and inflammatory responses to microbiota is associated with carcinogenesis [11]. Along these lines, it has been shown that the gut microbiota can vary the host response to chemotherapy through various mechanisms, including immune interactions, xenometabolism, and alterations in community structure [12]. These and similar findings put forth and support the gut microbiome–cancer axis, and a better understanding of these complex interactions may lead to new and better cancer therapy approaches [13,14].

In this review, we provide an overview of the potential relationship between gut microbiota and cancer treatment-induced cardiovascular toxicity (Figure 1). We also briefly discuss microbial signatures that are either unique or distinctly regulated in cancer therapy and heart diseases. Although thorough and targeted research is lacking in this direction, based on the available data on the microbiome in cancer therapy, we postulate a plausible relationship between treatment-induced microbial changes and long-term effects via the microbiota–gut–heart axis.

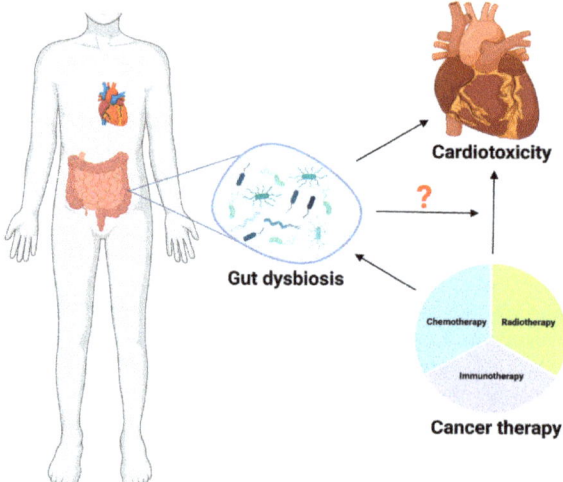

Figure 1. Among the most severe late side effects of cancer treatment in cancer survivors are cardiovascular problems, including heart failure, myocardial ischemia, hypertension, thrombosis, and

arrhythmias. Based on the current literature, we know that cancer therapy could result in gut dysbiosis. On the other hand, it is also recently reported that gut dysbiosis could worsen the cardiac function. However, we still do not know if and how gut dysbiosis play a role in cancer therapy induced cardiotoxicity (as shown with a question mark in the pictorial representation). Large-scale cancer survivor microbiome research may help identify patients at cardiovascular risk who may benefit from a more specialized microbiota-mediated treatment. Additionally, a deeper understanding of the link between the gut microbiome and cardiotoxicity brought on by cancer treatment may make it possible to lower the likelihood of this major and fatal adverse effect. (This Schematic representation was created using Biorender (https://biorender.com/)).

2. Cancer Treatment Efficacy and Toxicity Are Influenced by Gut Microbiota

Over the past century, tremendous progress has been made in cancer treatment, resulting in improved quality of life and survival for cancer patients. However, these advances in cancer treatment are often accompanied by treatment-related complications, including secondary systemic side effects. Recently, there has been increasing evidence that cancer treatments can disrupt the host immune response, leading to gut dysbiosis, disturbed immune system, and reduced effectiveness of the treatment [15,16]. Several studies have shown that the absence of gut microbiota reduces therapeutic efficacy, suggesting that commensal microbes modulate treatment-induced anticancer immune responses through various mechanisms. Ground-breaking results from animal models demonstrated the importance of commensals in regulating the effectiveness of radiation therapy, chemotherapy, and immunotherapy drugs [17–19]. For example, the intestinal microbiota and the myeloid cells that infiltrate tumors while a patient is receiving platinum-based therapy have been linked together [17]. The current understanding of the relationships among gut bacteria, host reactions, and anticancer medication was analyzed by Huang et al. in 2022 [20], with an emphasis on the immunomodulatory function of microbiota, which supports the effectiveness of immune checkpoint inhibitors. Importantly, this work focuses on the intricate and dynamic relationships between the microbiota and anticancer drugs, as well as the possibility for microbiome-based therapies to potentially enhance the effectiveness of cancer treatment. Huang and colleagues discovered that the gut microbiota affects the pharmacokinetics and pharmacodynamics of anticancer drugs. Furthermore, their work emphasizes the possibility of using microbiota-based therapies, such as probiotics or fecal microbiota transplantation, to increase the efficacy and decrease the toxicity of anticancer medications, as well as the response to immunotherapy. Additionally, anticancer medication response and individualized cancer treatment may be predicted using microbiota-based biomarkers. Nevertheless, additional systematic studies are required in order to completely comprehend the complex connections between the microbiota and anticancer therapies and determine the best methods for modifying the microbiota in order to improve cancer treatment outcomes.

Studying the relationship between microbes and cancer will contribute to a better understanding of the role of microbes in the mechanisms underlying tumorigenesis and other types of cancer, and hopefully improve therapeutic efficacy [21]. Sivan et al. [22] showed that the microbiome could be modulated to alter cancer immunotherapy. An important finding of this study was that *Bifidobacterium* alone could enhance tumor control to a level comparable to that of programmed cell death protein 1 ligand 1 (PD-L1) specific antibody therapy (checkpoint blockage) [22]. Antibodies targeting cytotoxic T-lymphocyte-associated antigen 4 (CTLA-4) have been effective in cancer immunotherapy, and specific *Bacteroides* species are required for the anticancer effects of CTLA-4 inhibition [23].

T-cell responses specific to *B. thetaiotaomicron* and *B. fragilis* have been linked to the effectiveness of CTLA-4 inhibition in mice and humans [23]. Nevertheless, thorough research is required in order to fully understand the mechanisms underlying the effects of the gut microbiota on treatment toxicity.

The non-specificity of several chemotherapeutic agents causes damage to healthy, non-cancerous cells [24]. Chemotherapy-related toxicities include cardiovascular and metabolic diseases, secondary cancer, avascular necrosis, cognitive impairment, cancer-related fatigue, poor mental health-related quality of life, nephrotoxicity, hypogonadism, neurotoxicity, pulmonary toxicity, anxiety, and depression. Cardiotoxicity caused by chemotherapy results in severe heart dysfunction, with heart failure (HF) as the most serious outcome. Following radiotherapy or chemotherapy, there is a considerable risk of developing cardiovascular disease (CVD), particularly in individuals with breast cancer and hematological malignancies [25]. Fibrosis, vascular damage, and shrinkage of damaged tissues or organs are examples of chronic toxicities caused by radiotherapy [26]. Although there is a dearth of information about whether and how the microbiota controls the response to radiotherapy, investigations of drug–microbiome interactions have revealed that several chemotherapeutic agents, such as gemcitabine, vidarabine, and etoposide phosphate, have impaired therapeutic efficacy, reduced mouse survival, and increased cytotoxicity [27]. Similarly, according to a previous study [28] pelvic radiation therapy altered the gut microbiota, with a 10% decrease in *Firmicutes* and a 3% increase in *Fusobacterium*. Through several mechanisms, including modulation of immunological responses, the gut microbiota has been shown to influence the efficacy and toxicity of several chemotherapies and immunotherapies [14]. Thus, targeting the microbiota is a potential strategy for increasing the effectiveness of chemotherapy and decreasing its toxicity.

Taken together, these results suggest that the efficacy of cancer therapy and the degree of gastrointestinal toxicity caused by cancer therapy are influenced by gut microbiota. Studies have indicated that gut microbes play an important role in cancer therapy by reversing anticancer effects and modulating the efficacy of drugs that mediate toxicity. These gut microbes may provide new avenues to improve the efficacy, reduce the toxicity of current chemotherapeutic agents, and improve susceptibility to immunotherapy.

2.1. Gut Microbiota and Immunotherapy

Immunotherapy with anti-PD-1/PD-L1 is more successful in tumors with inflamed T cells than in tumors with insufficient T cells because the PD-1/PD-L1 axis is known to play a crucial role in regulating immune system function. Recent research has indicated that gut microbiota may influence the PD-1/PD-L1 axis and the development of innate and adaptive immune systems [22,29]. According to a univariate study, gut microbiota diversity, *Faecalibacterium* abundance, and *Bacteroidetes* diversity were the best indicators of immunotherapy effectiveness. The effect of *Faecalibacterium* on the treatment response was proven by the FMT of responders and non-responders to anti-PD-1 in mice. One study also discovered that the biggest predictor of response to anti-PD-1 medication was the ratio of advantageous to non-beneficial operational taxonomic units (OTUs) [30]. Patients with a baseline majority of *Faecalibacterium* and other *Firmicutes* had longer Progression Free Survival (PFS) than those with a baseline predominance of Bacteroidetes, according to a study by Chaput et al. that analyzed the feces of 26 melanoma patients receiving ipilimumab [31]. Zheng et al. demonstrated a connection between certain gut flora and the effectiveness of immunotherapy in the treatment of liver cancer. The study discovered that *Akkermansia* and *Ruminococcus* were more prevalent in the gut microbiota of responders in hepatocellular carcinoma patients following PD-1 inhibitor therapy [32].

2.2. Gut Microbiota and Chemotherapy

Galloway-Pea et al. found a steady decline in the overall microbial diversity over time in the microbiota of AML patients after chemotherapy [33]. They observed an increase in Lactobacillus and a decrease in the anaerobic species *Blautia* [33]. Remarkably, chemotherapy increased the incidence of intestinal domination, a condition in which more than 30% of intestinal bacteria originate from a single taxon. The majority of the dominant incidents were caused by opportunistic pathogenic bacteria, such as *Staphylococcus, Enterobacter*, and *Escherichia* [33]. Deng et al. also compared the fecal microbiota composition of 33 healthy controls and 14 colorectal cancer (CRC) patients receiving tegafur and oxaliplatin [34]. Only CRC patients had *Veillonella dispar* in their systems, as opposed to healthy controls. *Prevotella copri* and *Bacteroides plebeius* were also enriched in chemotherapy patients compared with controls [34]. Another study (n = 43) of CRC patients with stages II–IV reported increased ratios of *Bacteroidetes* to *Firmicutes*, *Bacteroidetes*, *Bilophila Comamonas*, *Collinsella*, *Butyricimonas*, *Eggerthella*, and *Anaerostipes*, and decreased ratios of *Morganella*, *Pyramidobacter*, *Proteus*, and *Escherichia-Shigella* following CTX [35]. Diversity and composition of the gut microbiome were compared using feces from patients (n = 28) before and after CTX [36]. At the genus level, *Ruminococcus*, *Oscillospira*, *Blautia*, *Lachnospira*, *Roseburia*, *Dorea*, *Coprococcus*, *Anaerostipes*, *Clostridium*, *Collin-sella*, *Adlercreutzia*, and *Bifidobacterium* are significantly less common [36]. To date, there is a paucity of literature elucidating the specific mechanisms by which the gut microbiota may contribute to the development of cardiovascular disease in patients who have undergone chemotherapy, and it is an important limitation of this review. Although some studies have indicated a potential link between changes in the gut microbiome and cardiovascular risk factors, such as inflammation and insulin resistance [37], the exact pathways underlying these changes remain poorly understood. Chemotherapy can cause negative effects on the heart, commonly known as chemotherapy-induced cardiotoxicity, which may lead to various clinical symptoms, such as reduced ejection fraction, cardiac arrhythmias, hypertension, and ischemia/myocardial infarction [38]. These cardiotoxic effects can have a significant negative impact on the quality of life and outcomes of cancer patients. Although several categories of chemotherapy agents have been associated with an increased risk of cardiotoxicity, the underlying mechanisms are not yet fully elucidated. Identifying patients at high risk of cardiotoxicity before treatment and monitoring them closely during and after therapy are critical measures in minimizing the effects of chemotherapy-induced cardiotoxicity on patient outcomes. On the other hand, recent studies suggest that the gut microbiota can indirectly influence the development of chemotherapy-induced cardiotoxicity, through the production of metabolites and other signaling molecules [39]. For instance, specific bacteria in the gut can produce compounds (such as butyrate) that interact with the immune system and modify the expression of genes involved in cardiac function and repair [40]. A growing body of evidence indicates that the gut microbiome plays a significant role in protecting against chemotherapy-induced bloodstream infections. Montassier et al. proposed a microbiota-based predictive risk index model that could potentially be utilized to stratify patients at risk of complications before treatment [41]. This model is based on the observation that microbiome diversity decreases before the commencement of therapy. Moreover, the gut microbiota can influence the metabolism of chemotherapy drugs, which could result in increased toxicity or altered efficacy. For example, Wallace et al. showed that gastrointestinal biota can metabolize the chemotherapy drug irinotecan into a toxic by-product, which, in turn, can cause severe diarrhea in some patients [42]. The researchers identified a bacterial enzyme, beta-glucuronidase, responsible for this process, and demonstrated that inhibiting the enzyme reduced the toxicity of irinotecan in mice [42]. These findings indicate that the microbiota can influence the metabolism of chemotherapy drugs, which may result in increased toxicity or altered efficacy.

Trimethylamine N-oxide (TMAO) is a metabolite that is produced by certain gut bacteria from dietary nutrients, such as choline and carnitine [43]. Chemotherapy-induced changes in the gut microbiota can increase the production of TMAO, which has been linked to an increased risk of atherosclerosis and cardiovascular disease. In addition, TMAO can also be implicated in chemotherapy-induced cardiotoxicity by exacerbating the negative effects of chemotherapy on the cardiovascular system. Research has shown that the composition of gut microbiota can affect the production of TMAO, and that certain gut bacteria are more efficient at producing TMAO than others [44]. Chemotherapy can cause changes in the gut microbiota, leading to an increase in the abundance of bacteria that produce TMAO. This increase in TMAO production can contribute to the development of cardiovascular disease, and may also exacerbate chemotherapy-induced cardiotoxicity [45]. Thus, gut metabolites such as TMAO might serve as a link between gut microbiota-induced cardiotoxicity and chemotherapy-induced cardiotoxicity. In addition, an imbalance in gut microbiota composition and function can lead to chronic inflammation, oxidative stress, and other factors that can contribute to the development of cardiovascular disease, including cardiotoxicity induced by chemotherapy [43,46]. While the exact mechanisms underlying the relationship between gut microbiota and chemotherapy-induced cardiotoxicity are not yet fully understood, these findings suggest that targeting the microbiome may be a promising strategy for mitigating the cardiovascular side effects of cancer treatment. However, more research is required in order to gain a better understanding of the complex interactions among the gut microbiota, cancer therapies, and cardiovascular health.

2.3. Gut Microbiota and Radiotherapy

Radiotherapy results in dysregulation of the gut microbiota, which negatively affects the diversity and richness of gut bacterial diversity, potentially causing an enrichment of harmful microbiota (*Proteobacteria* and *Fusobacteria*) and a decrease in beneficial microbiota (*Faecalibacterium* and *Bifidobacterium*) [47,48]. El Alam et al. discovered a significant alteration in the gut microbiome composition during pelvic chemotherapy and radiotherapy (CRT), with increases in *Proteobacteria* and decreases in *Clostridiales*, whereas after CRT, the gut microbiome composition changed, with increases in *Bacteroides* species [49]. Intestinal radiation injury is a disorder that can be influenced by radiotherapy, by altering bacteria that produce short-chain fatty acids (SCFAs) [48]. Uncertainty persists regarding the effect of SCFAs on the prevalence of various disorders.

2.4. Gut Microbiota and TME

The gut microbiota shapes the immune system in the early years of life, and alterations in the gut microbiota later in life have a significant impact on numerous immune system functions [50]. The relationship between the gut microbiota and the host immune system increases the likelihood that the TME will interact with larger systemic microbial–immune networks, which serves as a reminder that the gut microbiota is increasingly acting as a crucial TME regulator [51–55]. The intestinal bacterium *B. pseudolongum* produces the metabolite inosine, which, by acting on the adenosine A2A receptor on T cells, significantly promotes Th1 cell differentiation in the presence of exogenous IFN-γ and improves the therapeutic response to immune checkpoint inhibitor (ICI) therapy, including anti-CTLA-4 and anti-PD-L1 [56]. A study showed that some gut bacteria, including *Bacteroides* and *Ruminococcaceae*, can contribute to the development of hepatocellular carcinoma by escalating hepatocyte inflammation, building up toxic substances, and causing liver steatosis [57]. According to the "holobiont" idea, it was recently proposed that the gut microbiome influences the "TME", which in turn affects tumor growth [52,58]. Ohtani et al. reported that the intestinal microbiota of obese individuals increases the amount of deoxycholic acid in the blood, which in turn promotes liver carcinogenesis by causing hepatic stellate cells to exhibit a senescence-associated secretory phenotype [59,60]. Altogether, these findings strongly suggest the crucial role that gut dysbiosis plays in the influence on TME microbiota and the efficacy of cancer therapeutic drugs/modes.

3. Cancer Treatment-Induced Cardiovascular Toxicity

The two major causes of death worldwide, accounting for approximately 50% of all deaths, are cancer and cardiovascular disease [61]. Recent cancer treatment strategies have improved patient survival rates. Nonetheless, many cancer therapies have undesired deleterious side effects on the cardiovascular system [62,63]. For example, breast cancer survivors have been shown to be at a significantly higher risk of death due to cardiovascular disease, outweighing the mortality risk of the original cancer or its recurrence [64]. Through an interdisciplinary approach involving cardiologists and oncologists, the cardio-oncology field is working to develop optimal strategies for patients with cardiovascular disease or risk factors from cancer diagnosis throughout the rest of their lives, even after treatment ends. Heart failure, myocardial ischemia, and myocardial infarction are just a few of the conditions that fall under the umbrella term "cardiotoxicity", which also covers a wide range of other conditions. Increasing therapeutic effectiveness has increased cancer patient survival; however, the long-term cardiovascular effects of these therapies have gained clinical significance. With more than 3.5 million breast cancer survivors in the US, both conventional chemotherapy (such as anthracyclines and radiotherapy) and targeted medicines (such as HER2 inhibitors and CDK4/6 inhibitors) have significantly improved patient care. Since then, cardiovascular disease has overtaken other conditions as the main killer and morbidity factor in this group [65,66]. Owing to their well-known cardiovascular side effects and comparatively high incidence of heart failure, anthracyclines have been the most extensively researched medication for decades [67]. Hoffmann et al. [68] reported that doxorubicin and trastuzumab treatment of nude mice in an orthotopic mouse model of human breast cancer led to a cardiovascular defect. In order to effectively treat cancer, new strategies are urgently needed to prevent potential cardiovascular diseases. Changes may occur years after therapy is over, and may be abrupt or persistent [69].

4. Gut Microbiota and Cardiovascular Toxicity

Heart failure has long been associated with impaired intestinal barrier function, which leads to gut dysbiosis and bacterial translocation [70–72]. Interestingly, the gut microbiome is increasingly reported to influence cancer development and progression in different ways [73]; for example, on one hand, several types of cancers result in altered gut microbiota, whereas the efficacy of cancer therapies, chemo- and immunotherapy, for example, is found to be strongly influenced by microbiome composition [74,75]. The chemo–gut study, a cross-sectional survey exploring physical, mental, and gastrointestinal health outcomes in cancer survivors, has recently provided novel insights into the strong association between chemotherapy and chronic, moderate-to-severe gastrointestinal symptoms lasting for years after cancer treatment, which are associated with worse mental and physical health [76,77]. Thus, is the gut microbiome a common link between cancer therapy and cardiotoxicity? The answer to this question is still not clear, due to the lack of concrete data on the relationship among microbiota, vascular damage, and heart failure in cancer patients after therapy; however, a few recent studies have suggested that the postulated link is not far-fetched. For example, Huang et al. [78] and Liu et al. [79] have recently shown that an imbalance in the gut microbiome composition and its functional alterations are likely to be among the major etiological mechanisms underlying doxorubicin-induced cardiotoxicity. Importantly, Huang et al. [78] showed that the gut dysbiosis due to doxorubicin contributes to the development of cardiotoxicity, by altering doxorubicin metabolism and increasing inflammation. Furthermore, they observed improved cardiac function and reduced doxorubicin-induced cardiotoxicity upon microbial depletion with the use of antibiotics. Overall, these results strongly suggests that the gut microbiota may potentially serve as new therapeutic target for cardiotoxicity and cardiovascular diseases. Similarly, Zhao et al. [80] observed that cisplatin, one of the chemotherapy drugs that is known to cause cardiotoxicity, led to a dramatic reduction in *Firmicutes* and elevated levels of pathogenic bacteria. On the other hand, *Lactobacillus* supplementation in cisplatin-treated mice increased body weight, improved cardiac function, and attenuated inflammation. The study thus showed that probiotics may help avoid cardiotoxicity brought on by chemotherapy, but additional validation studies are required in order to establish the best probiotic strain, dosage, and duration for this usage.

Similarly, Lin et al. demonstrated that yellow wine polyphenolic compounds protect against doxorubicin-induced cardiotoxicity by modulating the composition and metabolic function of gut microbiota [81]. Thus, it will not be surprising if researchers in the near future consider the gut microbiota as a new target for the treatment of cardiotoxicity and cardiovascular diseases. Large-scale cancer survivor microbiome investigations may help identify individuals at cardiovascular risk who could benefit from more specialized microbiome-mediated treatment. Furthermore, a deeper understanding of the connection between gut microbiota and cardiotoxicity caused by cancer therapies may pave the way for lowering the risk of these grave and potentially deadly side effects.

4.1. Gut Microbiota and Heart Failure

Heart failure (HF) is a serious health problem that negatively affects mortality and morbidity worldwide [82]. The levels of several proinflammatory cytokines in plasma are correlated with the severity and prognosis of the disease in patients with heart failure, who are thought to experience a persistent systemic inflammatory response [83,84]. The gut is a blood-demanding organ, and because of its restricted blood supply, the villi (and microvilli) are vulnerable to functional ischemia. A drop in the pH of the intestinal mucosa can result in intestinal ischemia in patients with HF [85]. A decline in intestinal mucosal pH is an indicator of intestinal ischemia in patients with HF [86]. Gut microbiota composition and metabolic parameters of patients with chronic heart failure (CHF) were significantly different from those of the control group, according to a fecal metagenomic study of 53 patients with chronic heart failure and 41 control participants [87]. Patients with HF are almost invariably found to have impaired intestinal barriers [88]. *Yersinia enterocolitica*, *Candida*, *Campylobacter*, *Salmonella*, *Shigella*, and other pathogenic bacteria are more prevalent in patients with CHF than in healthy controls [89]. According to the NYHA scale, these changes are strongly associated with HF severity [89].

4.2. Gut Microbiota and Atherosclerosis

Atherosclerosis is a chronic inflammatory condition characterized by a lipid core and an outer fibrous cap that mostly affects the middle and major arteries. A substantial cause of mortality, atherosclerosis is an immunoinflammatory condition that results in blockages in the large and medium arteries and acute CVD [90]. The presence of bacteria in the atherosclerotic plaques of patients with coronary artery disease was confirmed by fluorescence in situ hybridization and conserved polymerase chain reaction [91]. Macrogenomic sequencing of the feces of the subjects was performed in a case-control study of 218 patients with atherosclerotic cardiovascular disease (ACVD) and 187 healthy controls. This study found increased copy numbers of bacterial genes encoding TMA lytic enzymes (enzymes associated with TMAO production), increased TMAO production, and increased abundance of the atherosclerotic cardiovascular disease (ACVD) gut microbiome comprising *Enterobacteriaceae* and *Streptococcus*, among other significant metabolic alterations functionally associated with ASCVD [92]. New approaches for the identification and management of atherosclerosis may emerge from the study of gut microbiota and its metabolites. Dietary factors and gut flora are strongly linked to the development of atherosclerosis, with inflammation also playing a role. For instance, an increase in *Bacteroides fragilis* resulted in a decrease in *Lactobacilli* and an increase in *Desulfovibrionaceae*, which caused dysfunctional lipid or glucose metabolism and worsened the inflammatory response [93]. Peanut skin extract reduced the serum total and low-density lipoprotein cholesterol content, and increased the high-density lipoprotein cholesterol content in atherosclerotic mice, thereby decreasing the development of atheromatous plaques [94].

Dysbiotic intestinal flora can worsen cardiovascular diseases. Through altered gut microbiota composition, immune cell activation, and metabolic dysfunction, an imbalance in the gut microbiota caused by poor diet, aging, and antibiotic usage might exacerbate cardiovascular diseases. Disruption of the gut microbiota may, in turn, be further promoted by cardiovascular disorders (Figure 2). A balanced gut microbiota may prevent the progression of CVD.

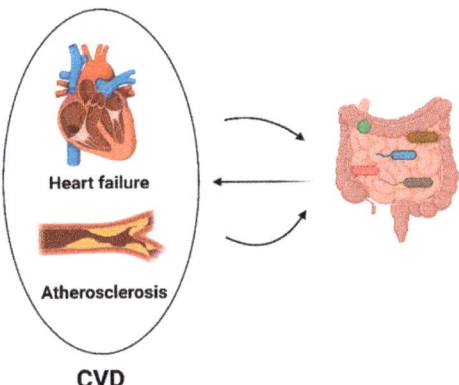

Figure 2. Crosstalk between cardiovascular disease and gut microbiota. Various microbes in the gut are represented with different colors. (This Schematic representation was created using Biorender (https://biorender.com/)).

5. Microbial Signatures Associated with Cancer Treatment and Cardiac Diseases

The most prevalent bacterial phyla in a healthy gut microbiome are *Firmicutes* and *Bacteroidetes*, followed by *Proteobacteria*, *Actinobacteria*, *Fusobacteria*, and *Verrucomicrobia* [95]. *Prevotella* spp. and *Bacteroides* spp. are the most prominent *Bacteroidetes* members, whereas *Bifidobacterium* is the most significant *Actinobacteria* representative [96]. However, gut microbial composition is dramatically altered in several cardiovascular diseases and distinct forms of cancer (Table 1). Interestingly, gut microbial alterations associated with the progression or pathogenicity of many of the cardiovascular diseases have similarly been reported in many cancer therapies, suggesting a potential link between cancer therapy-induced cardiotoxicity and gut dysbiosis. Thus, it is important to understand whether and what kind of correlations exist among cancer therapies, gut dysbiosis, and cardiovascular diseases.

Table 1. Some of the gut bacteria associated with cardiac diseases and cancer treatment.

Cancer Treatment	Cardiac Diseases
Bacteroides fragilis, Helicobacter pylori, Salmonella tyhimunum, Burkholderia cepacian, Akkerman-sia muciniphila, Faecalibacterium prausnitzii and Bifidobacterium longum, Brevundii monas and Staphylococci, Firmicutes and Actinobacteria, Lactobacillus, and Escherichia coli, Clostridium difficile, Faecalisbacterium, and Burkholderia cepacian, Aristipes shahi, Burkholderia cepacian, Akkermansia, and Alistipes	Bacteroidetes Lactobacillales Candida Faecalibacterium prausnitzii Roseburia intestinalis and Faecalibacterium cf. prausnitzii

Types of bacteria in cancer treatment:

Some cancer chemotherapies, radiotherapy, and immunotherapies have been reported to be affected by the gut microbiota, in terms of both their effectiveness and toxicity. Chemotherapeutic treatments used to treat cancer cause gut dysbiosis, which is followed by a decline in commensal microorganisms, such as *Bifidobacterium* and *Lactobacillus*, and an increase in opportunistic pathogens, such as *Clostridium difficile* [96]. By controlling the immune system, the intestinal microbiota can affect the therapeutic efficacy of medications for tumors. In contrast to non-responders (NR), PD-1 responders (R) with lung cancer in both Europe and the US had a higher relative abundance of *Akkermansia muciniphila* [97]. Studies also revealed a tendency toward a higher frequency of *Corynebacterium aurimucosum* and *Staphylococcus haemolyticus* in NR patients and a higher frequency of *Enterococcus hirae* in R patients [98]. According to some reports, Fluorouracil (5-FU) therapy results in dysbiosis in mice. After 5-FU administration, the abundance of *Bacteroides* and *Lactobacillus* species decreased, whereas that of *Staphylococcus* and *Clostridium* species increased [99].

Compared to controls, fecal samples from 36 juvenile leukemia patients receiving high-dose methotrexate chemotherapy and 36 healthy children showed a substantial decrease in *Bifidobacterium*, *Lactobacillus*, and *Escherichia coli* [100]. The intestinal barrier is broken and intestinal crypts undergo apoptosis as a result of radiotherapy [101]. In a small pilot study, radiotherapy plus antibiotics reduced *Firmicute* abundance and increased *Proteobacteria* abundance in three pediatric cancer patients with pelvic rhabdomyosarcoma [102].

Types of bacteria in cardiac diseases:

Recent studies have highlighted a possible contribution of the gut microbiome to CVD. CVDs is linked to a higher *Firmicutes/Bacteroidetes* (F/B) proportion. The phylum *Bacteroidetes* was found to be negatively associated with ischemic heart disease (IHD), and the order *Lactobacillales* was positively associated with IHD in a small case-control study (n = 128) [98]. Type 2 diabetes mellitus, a key CVD risk factor, has been sparsely linked to *Acidaminococcus*, *Aggregatibacter*, *Anaerostipes*, *Blautia*, *Desulfovibrio*, *Dorea*, and *Faecalibacterium* [103]. The reduced abundance of bacteria that produce short-chain fatty acids (SCFAs), such as *Roseburia*, *Faecalibacterium*, and *Eubacterium rectale*, and an increased abundance of host opportunistic pathogens, such as *Escherichia coli*, *Clostridium ramosum*, *Bacteroides caccae*, and *Eggerthella lenta* have been linked to a higher risk of CVDs [104,105]. Researchers have found that, compared to healthy controls, patients with atherosclerosis have reduced relative abundances of *Roseburia* and *Eubacterium* and greater relative abundances of *Collinsella* [106]. Intestinal mucosal barrier degradation and dysbacteriosis caused by lower cardiac output in HF are accompanied by elevated levels of pathogenic bacteria, such as *Candida*, and decreased levels of anti-inflammatory bacteria, such as *Faecalibacterium prausnitzii*. Additionally, elevated levels of some gut bacterial species, such as *Escherichia coli*, *Klebsiella pneumonia*, and *Streptococcus viridans* have been linked to heart failure [107].

Altogether, gut bacteria, unique or common to cancer treatment and cardiac diseases, offer a new avenue for research to learn more about clinical outcomes, potential treatments, and diagnosis, as well as a better understanding of the role of microbes in the development of cancer treatment-induced cardiotoxicity. Gut microbiota can be used as a biomarker to predict the effects of cancer therapy. Populations at high risk may receive more specialized treatment, depending on their microbiota compared to a generic one.

6. Gut Microbiota-Derived Metabolites in Cancer Treatment

Numerous metabolic illnesses, such as obesity, type 2 diabetes, nonalcoholic fatty liver disease, and cardiovascular disease, are influenced by the gut microbiome and its metabolites. The maintenance of host physiology depends on communication between microbes and their hosts, which is mediated by metabolites generated by the microbiota [108]. These metabolites have been found to affect both the toxicity and effectiveness of cancer treatment, through modulation of immune processes and protective epithelial functions, respectively (Figure 3). Metabolites such as SCFAs, secondary bile acids, polyamines, lipids, and vitamins are produced by gut microbiota [109]. The colon produces SCFAs, primarily acetate, butyrate, and propionate, from dietary fiber and polysaccharides. The most common bacterial species that produce SCFAs include *Faecalibacterium prausnitzii*, *Clostridium leptum*, *Eubacterium rectale*, and *Roseburia* species, as well as lactate-utilizing species such as *Anaerostipes* and *Eubacterium hallii*, which synthesize SCFAs from lactate and acetate [110]. The regulation of T cell homeostasis has been associated with SCFAs that can control the differentiation of T cells into effector or regulatory (Treg) cells in response to immunological conditions, such as the presence or absence of important cytokines [72] Gut microbial metabolites, including bacteriocins, short-chain fatty acids, and phenylpropanoid-derived metabolites, display direct and indirect anticancer activities via different molecular mechanisms [111]. Recent studies have confirmed the differential expression of SCFA in immunotherapy responders compared to non-responders. SCFAs are well known for their anti-inflammatory and antioxidant effects on the host, which help stop the proliferation of cancer cells. Bile acid profiles may change as a result of bacterial bile acid transformation, which may then affect systemic inflammatory and fibrotic processes [72]. In terms of cancer development and anticancer activity, the mechanisms of the action of gut microbial metabolites are not fully understood.

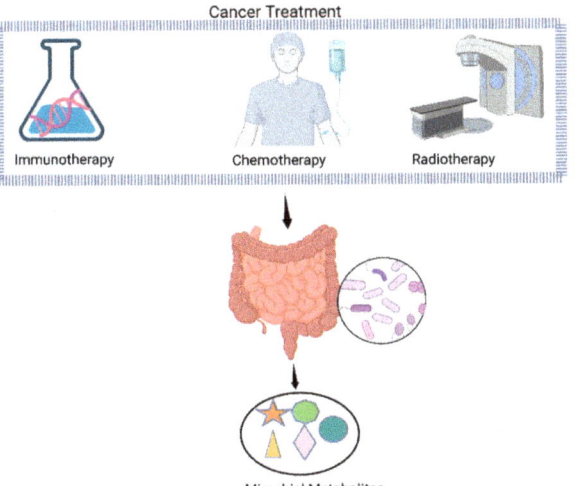

Figure 3. Metabolites produced by the gut microbiota have a key role in controlling the activity of intestinal cells, as well as local and systemic immunological and inflammatory responses. The most effective method for dealing with gut microbiota-derived metabolites and their widespread impacts in order to enhance cancer therapy outcomes will need to be determined. Different colors in circle represent different gut microbes, whereas, different shapes in oval form represent individual metabolite, e.g., star shape for metabolite A, triangle for metabolite B, etc. (This Schematic representation was created using Biorender (https://biorender.com/)).

7. Conclusions

Patients with cancer endure a variety of immediate and long-term side effects throughout the body, including gastrointestinal- and cardiotoxicity. Preclinical and clinical research, in addition to reports on the link between microbiota and cancer, has revealed that this subject may be a key mediator of how the body reacts to cancer treatment. Clinical trials on a substantial cohort of cancer survivors are urgently needed and may open up novel possibilities for microbiota-mediated therapies to stop or lessen the long-term side effects of cancer therapy. Future therapies may employ techniques that can help achieve more precise manipulation of microbiota composition, such as the relative proportion of a particular bacterial genus in the microbiota. In order to discover dysbiotic conditions linked to negative or poor cancer treatment outcomes and to identify microbial targets that can be modified, personalized biomarkers are urgently needed. Improving the physical well-being of cancer survivors requires a thorough understanding of the microbiota–gut–heart axis and the effects of the changed intestinal microbiome on immunological and metabolic pathways. We can only maximize the regulation of the intestinal microbiota and enhance the potential of cancer treatment by fully comprehending which intestinal bacteria and their metabolic product(s) could be altered. Overall, our review aimed to shed light on the potential complex interplay among the microbiome, cancer treatment, and cardiovascular health, and to identify potential avenues for future research into this important area of study. However, direct evidence supporting proposed postulations and hypotheses is still missing. This lack of significant direct evidence suggests that further research is needed in order to explore the potential effects of gut microbiota and its metabolites in cardiotoxicity, which may lead to new therapeutic opportunities and the identification of predictive biomarkers.

Author Contributions: Conceptualization, K. and A.Y.R.; Resources, N.F. and A.Y.R.; Writing—original draft preparation, K.; Writing—review and editing, N.F. and A.Y.R.; Supervision, N.F. and A.Y.R.; Funding acquisition, N.F. and A.Y.R. All authors have read and agreed to the published version of the manuscript.

Funding: This research was funded by the German Research Foundation (Deutsche Forschungsgemeinschaft) (grant numbers RA 2717/4-1 and FR 1289/17-1).

Institutional Review Board Statement: Not applicable.

Informed Consent Statement: Not applicable.

Data Availability Statement: Not applicable.

Conflicts of Interest: The authors declare no conflict of interest.

References

1. Santucci, C.; Carioli, G.; Bertuccio, P.; Malvezzi, M.; Pastorino, U.; Boffetta, P.; Negri, E.; Bosetti, C.; La Vecchia, C. Progress in cancer mortality, incidence, and survival: A global overview. *Eur. J. Cancer Prev.* **2020**, *29*, 367–381. [CrossRef] [PubMed]
2. Yeh, E.T.H.; Bickford, C.L. Cardiovascular complications of cancer therapy: Incidence, pathogenesis, diagnosis, and management. *J. Am. Coll. Cardiol.* **2009**, *53*, 2231–2247. [CrossRef] [PubMed]
3. Raschi, E.; Vasina, V.; Ursino, M.G.; Boriani, G.; Martoni, A.; De Ponti, F. Anticancer drugs and cardiotoxicity: Insights and perspectives in the era of targeted therapy. *Pharmacol. Ther.* **2010**, *125*, 196–218. [CrossRef] [PubMed]
4. Oeffinger, K.C.; Mertens, A.C.; Sklar, C.A.; Kawashima, T.; Hudson, M.M.; Meadows, A.T.; Friedman, D.L.; Marina, N.; Hobbie, W.; Kadan-Lottick, N.S.; et al. Chronic health conditions in adult survivors of childhood cancer. *N. Engl. J. Med.* **2006**, *355*, 1572–1582. [CrossRef] [PubMed]
5. Lipshultz, S.E.; Adams, M.J.; Colan, S.D.; Constine, L.S.; Herman, E.H.; Hsu, D.T.; Hudson, M.M.; Kremer, L.C.; Landy, D.C.; Miller, T.L.; et al. Long-term cardiovascular toxicity in children, adolescents, and young adults who receive cancer therapy: Pathophysiology, course, monitoring, management, prevention, and research directions: A scientific statement from the American Heart Association. *Circulation* **2013**, *128*, 1927–1995. [CrossRef]
6. Nejman, D.; Livyatan, I.; Fuks, G.; Gavert, N.; Zwang, Y.; Geller, L.T.; Rotter-Maskowitz, A.; Weiser, R.; Mallel, G.; Gigi, E.; et al. The human tumor microbiome is composed of tumor type–specific intracellular bacteria. *Science* **2020**, *368*, 973–980. [CrossRef]
7. Deleemans, J.M.; Chleilat, F.; Reimer, R.A.; Henning, J.-W.; Baydoun, M.; Piedalue, K.-A.; McLennan, A.; Carlson, L.E. The chemo-gut study: Investigating the long-term effects of chemotherapy on gut microbiota, metabolic, immune, psychological and cognitive parameters in young adult Cancer survivors; study protocol. *BMC Cancer* **2019**, *19*, 1243. [CrossRef] [PubMed]
8. Laudadio, I.; Fulci, V.; Palone, F.; Stronati, L.; Cucchiara, S.; Carissimi, C. Quantitative Assessment of Shotgun Metagenomics and 16S rDNA Amplicon Sequencing in the Study of Human Gut Microbiome. *OMICS* **2018**, *22*, 248–254. [CrossRef]
9. Groussin, M.; Mazel, F.; Alm, E.J. Co-evolution and Co-speciation of Host-Gut Bacteria Systems. *Cell Host Microbe* **2020**, *28*, 12–22. [CrossRef]
10. Nicholson, J.K.; Holmes, E.; Kinross, J.; Burcelin, R.; Gibson, G.; Jia, W.; Pettersson, S. Host-gut microbiota metabolic interactions. *Science* **2012**, *336*, 1262–1267. [CrossRef]
11. Rajagopala, S.V.; Vashee, S.; Oldfield, L.M.; Suzuki, Y.; Venter, J.C.; Telenti, A.; Nelson, K.E. The Human Microbiome and CancerThe Human Microbiome and Cancer. *Cancer Prev. Res.* **2017**, *10*, 226–234. [CrossRef] [PubMed]
12. Perez-Chanona, E.; Trinchieri, G. The role of microbiota in cancer therapy. *Curr. Opin. Immunol.* **2016**, *39*, 75–81. [CrossRef]
13. Sepich-Poore, G.D.; Zitvogel, L.; Straussman, R.; Hasty, J.; Wargo, J.A.; Knight, R. The microbiome and human cancer. *Science*, **2021**, *371*, eabc4552. [CrossRef] [PubMed]
14. Alexander, J.L.; Wilson, I.D.; Teare, J.; Marchesi, J.R.; Nicholson, J.K.; Kinross, J.M. Gut microbiota modulation of chemotherapy efficacy and toxicity. *Nat. Rev. Gastroenterol. Hepatol.* **2017**, *14*, 356–365. [CrossRef] [PubMed]
15. Liu, Z.; Cao, C.; Ren, Y.; Weng, S.; Liu, L.; Guo, C.; Wang, L.; Han, X.; Ren, J.; Liu, Z. Antitumor effects of fecal microbiota transplantation: Implications for microbiome modulation in cancer treatment. *Front. Immunol.* **2022**, *13*, 4788.
16. Yin, B.; Wang, X.; Yuan, F.; Li, Y.; Lu, P. Research progress on the effect of gut and tumor microbiota on antitumor efficacy and adverse effects of chemotherapy drugs. *Front. Microbiol.* **2022**, *13*, 899111. [CrossRef]
17. Iida, N.; Dzutsev, A.; Stewart, C.A.; Smith, L.; Bouladoux, N.; Weingarten, R.A.; Molina, D.A.; Salcedo, R.; Back, T.; Cramer, S.; et al. Commensal bacteria control cancer response to therapy by modulating the tumor microenvironment. *Science* **2013**, *342*, 967–970. [CrossRef]
18. Shiao, S.L.; Kershaw, K.M.; Limon, J.J.; You, S.; Yoon, J.; Ko, E.Y.; Guarnerio, J.; Potdar, A.A.; McGovern, D.P.; Bose, S.; et al. Commensal bacteria and fungi differentially regulate tumor responses to radiation therapy. *Cancer Cell* **2021**, *39*, 1202–1213.e6. [CrossRef]
19. Pernigoni, N.; Zagato, E.; Calcinotto, A.; Troiani, M.; Mestre, R.P.; Calì, B.; Attanasio, G.; Troisi, J.; Minini, M.; Mosole, S.; et al. Commensal bacteria promote endocrine resistance in prostate cancer through androgen biosynthesis. *Science* **2021**, *374*, 216–224. [CrossRef]

20. Huang, J.; Liu, W.; Kang, W.; He, Y.; Yang, R.; Mou, X.; Zhao, W. Effects of microbiota on anticancer drugs: Current knowledge and potential applications. *EBioMedicine* **2022**, *83*, 104197. [CrossRef]
21. Goubet, A.-G.; Daillère, R.; Routy, B.; Derosa, L.; Roberti, P.M.; Zitvogel, L. The impact of the intestinal microbiota in therapeutic responses against cancer. *Comptes Rendus Biol.* **2018**, *341*, 284–289. [CrossRef] [PubMed]
22. Sivan, A.; Corrales, L.; Hubert, N.; Williams, J.B.; Aquino-Michaels, K.; Earley, Z.M.; Benyamin, F.W.; Lei, Y.M.; Jabri, B.; Alegre, M.-L.; et al. Commensal Bifidobacterium promotes antitumor immunity and facilitates anti–PD-L1 efficacy. *Science* **2015**, *350*, 1084–1089. [CrossRef]
23. Vétizou, M.; Pitt, J.M.; Daillère, R.; Lepage, P.; Waldschmitt, N.; Flament, C.; Rusakiewicz, S.; Routy, B.; Roberti, M.P.; Duong, C.P.M.; et al. Anticancer immunotherapy by CTLA-4 blockade relies on the gut microbiota. *Science* **2015**, *350*, 1079–1084. [CrossRef] [PubMed]
24. Galluzzi, L.; Humeau, J.; Buqué, A.; Zitvogel, L.; Kroemer, G. Immunostimulation with chemotherapy in the era of immune checkpoint inhibitors. *Nat. Rev. Clin. Oncol.* **2020**, *17*, 725–741. [CrossRef]
25. Finet, J.E.; Tang, W.H.W. Protecting the heart in cancer therapy. *F1000Research* **2018**, *7*, 1566. [CrossRef]
26. Nam, Y.-D.; Kim, H.J.; Seo, J.-G.; Kang, S.W.; Bae, J.-W. Impact of pelvic radiotherapy on gut microbiota of gynecological cancer patients revealed by massive pyrosequencing. *PLoS ONE* **2013**, *8*, e82659. [CrossRef]
27. Lehouritis, P.; Cummins, J.; Stanton, M.; Murphy, C.T.; McCarthy, F.O.; Reid, G.; Urbaniak, C.; Byrne, W.L.; Tangney, M. Local bacteria affect the efficacy of chemotherapeutic drugs. *Sci. Rep.* **2015**, *5*, 14554. [CrossRef] [PubMed]
28. Barnett, G.C.; West, C.; Dunning, A.M.; Elliott, R.M.; Coles, C.E.; Pharoah, P.D.P.; Burnet, N.G. Normal tissue reactions to radiotherapy: Towards tailoring treatment dose by genotype. *Nat. Rev. Cancer* **2009**, *9*, 134–142. [CrossRef] [PubMed]
29. Alsaab, H.O.; Sau, S.; Alzhrani, R.; Tatiparti, K.; Bhise, K.; Kashaw, S.K.; Iyer, A.K. PD-1 and PD-L1 Checkpoint Signaling Inhibition for Cancer Immunotherapy: Mechanism, Combinations, and Clinical Outcome. *Front. Pharmacol.* **2017**, *8*, 561. [CrossRef]
30. Matson, V.; Fessler, J.; Bao, R.; Chongsuwat, T.; Zha, Y.; Alegre, M.-L.; Luke, J.J.; Gajewski, T.F. The commensal microbiome is associated with anti-PD-1 efficacy in metastatic melanoma patients. *Science* **2018**, *359*, 104–108. [CrossRef]
31. Chaput, N.; Lepage, P.; Coutzac, C.; Soularue, E.; Le Roux, K.; Monot, C.; Boselli, L.; Routier, E.; Cassard, L.; Collins, M.; et al. Baseline gut microbiota predicts clinical response and colitis in metastatic melanoma patients treated with ipilimumab. *Ann. Oncol.* **2017**, *28*, 1368–1379. [CrossRef]
32. Zheng, Y.; Wang, T.; Tu, X.; Huang, Y.; Zhang, H.; Tan, D.; Jiang, W.; Cai, S.; Zhao, P.; Song, R.; et al. Gut microbiome affects the response to anti-PD-1 immunotherapy in patients with hepatocellular carcinoma. *J. Immunother. Cancer* **2019**, *7*, 193. [CrossRef]
33. Galloway-Pena, J.R.; Smith, D.P.; Sahasrabhojane, P.; Ajami, N.J.; Wadsworth, W.D.; Daver, N.G.; Chemaly, R.F.; Marsh, L.; Ghantoji, S.S.; Pemmaraju, N.; et al. The role of the gastrointestinal microbiome in infectious complications during induction chemotherapy for acute myeloid leukemia. *Cancer* **2016**, *122*, 2186–2196. [CrossRef] [PubMed]
34. Deng, X.; Li, Z.; Li, G.; Li, B.; Jin, X.; Lyu, G. Comparison of Microbiota in Patients Treated by Surgery or Chemotherapy by 16S rRNA Sequencing Reveals Potential Biomarkers for Colorectal Cancer Therapy. *Front. Microbiol.* **2018**, *9*, 1607. [CrossRef] [PubMed]
35. Kong, C.; Gao, R.; Yan, X.; Huang, L.; He, J.; Li, H.; You, J.; Qin, H. Alterations in intestinal microbiota of colorectal cancer patients receiving radical surgery combined with adjuvant CapeOx therapy. *Sci. China Life Sci.* **2019**, *62*, 1178–1193. [CrossRef] [PubMed]
36. Montassier, E.; Gastinne, T.; Vangay, P.; Al-Ghalith, G.A.; Bruley des Varannes, S.; Massart, S.; Moreau, P.; Potel, G.; De La Cochetière, M.F.; Batard, E.; et al. Chemotherapy-driven dysbiosis in the intestinal microbiome. *Aliment. Pharmacol. Ther.* **2015**, *42*, 515–528. [CrossRef]
37. Astudillo, A.A.; Mayrovitz, H.N. The Gut Microbiome and Cardiovascular Disease. *Cureus* **2021**, *13*, e14519. [CrossRef]
38. Abdul-Rahman, T.; Dunham, A.; Huang, H.; Bukhari, S.M.A.; Mehta, A.; Awuah, W.A.; Ede-Imafidon, D.; Cantu-Herrera, E.; Talukder, S.; Joshi, A.; et al. Chemotherapy Induced Cardiotoxicity: A State of the Art Review on General Mechanisms, Prevention, Treatment and Recent Advances in Novel Therapeutics. *Curr. Probl. Cardiol.* **2023**, *48*, 101591. [CrossRef] [PubMed]
39. Ciernikova, S.; Mego, M.; Chovanec, M. Exploring the Potential Role of the Gut Microbiome in Chemotherapy-Induced Neurocognitive Disorders and Cardiovascular Toxicity. *Cancers* **2021**, *13*, 782. [CrossRef] [PubMed]
40. Belkaid, Y.; Hand, T.W. Role of the microbiota in immunity and inflammation. *Cell* **2014**, *157*, 121–141. [CrossRef]
41. Montassier, E.; Al-Ghalith, G.A.; Ward, T.; Corvec, S.; Gastinne, T.; Potel, G.; Moreau, P.; de la Cochetiere, M.F.; Batard, E.; Knights, D. Pretreatment gut microbiome predicts chemotherapy-related bloodstream infection. *Genome Med.* **2016**, *8*, 49. [CrossRef] [PubMed]
42. Wallace, B.D.; Wang, H.; Lane, K.T.; Scott, J.E.; Orans, J.; Koo, J.S.; Venkatesh, M.; Jobin, C.; Yeh, L.-A.; Mani, S.; et al. Alleviating cancer drug toxicity by inhibiting a bacterial enzyme. *Science* **2010**, *330*, 831–835. [CrossRef] [PubMed]
43. Zhen, J.; Zhou, Z.; He, M.; Han, H.-X.; Lv, E.-H.; Wen, P.-B.; Liu, X.; Wang, Y.-T.; Cai, X.-C.; Tian, J.-Q.; et al. The gut microbial metabolite trimethylamine N-oxide and cardiovascular diseases. *Front. Endocrinol.* **2023**, *14*, 1085041. [CrossRef] [PubMed]
44. Liu, Y.; Dai, M. Trimethylamine N-Oxide Generated by the Gut Microbiota Is Associated with Vascular Inflammation: New Insights into Atherosclerosis. *Mediat. Inflamm.* **2020**, *2020*, 4634172. [CrossRef]
45. Wang, Z.; Roberts, A.B.; Buffa, J.A.; Levison, B.S.; Zhu, W.; Org, E.; Gu, X.; Huang, Y.; Zamanian-Daryoush, M.; Culley, M.K.; et al. Non-lethal Inhibition of Gut Microbial Trimethylamine Production for the Treatment of Atherosclerosis. *Cell* **2015**, *163*, 1585–1595. [CrossRef]

46. Chou, R.H.; Chen, C.-Y.; Chen, I.-C.; Huang, H.-L.; Lu, Y.-W.; Kuo, C.-S.; Chang, C.-C.; Huang, P.-H.; Chen, J.-W.; Lin, S.-J. Trimethylamine N-Oxide, Circulating Endothelial Progenitor Cells, and Endothelial Function in Patients with Stable Angina. *Sci. Rep.* **2019**, *9*, 4249. [CrossRef]
47. Fernandes, A.; Oliveira, A.; Guedes, C.; Fernandes, R.; Soares, R.; Barata, P. Effect of Radium-223 on the Gut Microbiota of Prostate Cancer Patients: A Pilot Case Series Study. *Curr. Issues Mol. Biol.* **2022**, *44*, 4950–4959. [CrossRef]
48. Li, Y.; Zhang, Y.; Wei, K.; He, J.; Ding, N.; Hua, J.; Zhou, T.; Niu, F.; Zhou, G.; Shi, T.; et al. Review: Effect of Gut Microbiota and Its Metabolite SCFAs on Radiation-Induced Intestinal Injury. *Front. Cell. Infect. Microbiol.* **2021**, *11*, 577236. [CrossRef]
49. El Alam, M.B.; Sims, T.T.; Kouzy, R.; Biegert, G.W.G.; Jaoude, J.A.B.I.; Karpinets, T.V.; Yoshida-Court, K.; Wu, X.; Delgado-Medrano, A.Y.; Mezzari, M.P.; et al. A prospective study of the adaptive changes in the gut microbiome during standard-of-care chemoradiotherapy for gynecologic cancers. *PLoS ONE* **2021**, *16*, e0247905. [CrossRef]
50. Maynard, C.L.; Elson, C.O.; Hatton, R.D.; Weaver, C.T. Reciprocal interactions of the intestinal microbiota and immune system. *Nature* **2012**, *489*, 231–241. [CrossRef]
51. Erdman, S.E.; Poutahidis, T. Cancer inflammation and regulatory T cells. *Int. J. Cancer* **2010**, *127*, 768–779. [CrossRef]
52. Erdman, S.E.; Poutahidis, T. Gut bacteria and cancer. *Biochim. Biophys. Acta* **2015**, *1856*, 86–90. [CrossRef]
53. Erdman, S.E.; Rao, V.P.; Olipitz, W.; Taylor, C.L.; Jackson, E.A.; Levkovich, T.; Lee, C.-W.; Horwitz, B.H.; Fox, J.G.; Ge, Z.; et al. Unifying roles for regulatory T cells and inflammation in cancer. *Int. J. Cancer* **2010**, *126*, 1651–1665. [CrossRef] [PubMed]
54. Lakritz, J.R.; Poutahidis, T.; Levkovich, T.; Varian, B.J.; Ibrahim, Y.M.; Chatziagiagkos, A.; Mirabal, S.; Alm, E.J.; Erdman, S.E. Beneficial bacteria stimulate host immune cells to counteract dietary and genetic predisposition to mammary cancer in mice. *Int. J. Cancer* **2013**, *135*, 529–540. [CrossRef] [PubMed]
55. Rao, V.P.; Poutahidis, T.; Fox, J.G.; Erdman, S.E. Breast cancer: Should gastrointestinal bacteria be on our radar screen? *Cancer Res.* **2007**, *67*, 847–850. [CrossRef] [PubMed]
56. Mager, L.F.; Burkhard, R.; Pett, N.; Cooke, N.C.A.; Brown, K.; Ramay, H.; Paik, S.; Stagg, J.; Groves, R.A.; Gallo, M.; et al. Microbiome-derived inosine modulates response to checkpoint inhibitor immunotherapy. *Science* **2020**, *369*, 1481–1489. [CrossRef]
57. Ponziani, F.R.; Nicoletti, A.; Gasbarrini, A.; Pompili, M. Diagnostic and therapeutic potential of the gut microbiota in patients with early hepatocellular carcinoma. *Ther. Adv. Med. Oncol.* **2019**, *11*, 1758835919848184. [CrossRef]
58. Erdman, S.E.; Poutahidis, T. The microbiome modulates the tumor macroenvironment. *Oncoimmunology* **2014**, *3*, e28271. [CrossRef]
59. Ohtani, N. Microbiome and cancer. *Semin. Immunopathol.* **2015**, *37*, 65–72. [CrossRef]
60. Yoshimoto, S.; Loo, T.M.; Atarashi, K.; Kanda, H.; Sato, S.; Oyadomari, S.; Iwakura, Y.; Oshima, K.; Morita, H.; Hattori, M.; et al. Obesity-induced gut microbial metabolite promotes liver cancer through senescence secretome. *Nature* **2013**, *499*, 97–101. [CrossRef]
61. Murphy, S.L.; Kochanek, K.D.; Xu, J.Q.; Arias, E. *Mortality in the United States, 2014*; NCHS Data Brief, No. 229; National Center for Health Statistics: Hyattsville, MD, USA, 2015.
62. Herrmann, J. Adverse cardiac effects of cancer therapies: Cardiotoxicity and arrhythmia. *Nat. Rev. Cardiol.* **2020**, *17*, 474–502. [CrossRef] [PubMed]
63. Lenneman, C.G.; Sawyer, D.B. Cardio-Oncology: An Update on Cardiotoxicity of Cancer-Related Treatment. *Circ. Res.* **2016**, *118*, 1008–1020. [CrossRef] [PubMed]
64. Bodai, B.I.; Tuso, P. Breast cancer survivorship: A comprehensive review of long-term medical issues and lifestyle recommendations. *Perm. J.* **2015**, *19*, 48. [CrossRef]
65. Gulati, M.; Mulvagh, S.L. The connection between the breast and heart in a woman: Breast cancer and cardiovascular disease. *Clin. Cardiol.* **2018**, *41*, 253–257. [CrossRef] [PubMed]
66. Mehta, L.S.; Beckie, T.M.; DeVon, H.A.; Grines, C.L.; Krumholz, H.M.; Johnson, M.N.; Lindley, K.J.; Vaccarino, V.; Wang, T.Y.; Watson, K.E.; et al. Acute myocardial infarction in women: A scientific statement from the American Heart Association. *Circulation* **2016**, *133*, 916–947. [CrossRef]
67. Cardinale, D.; Colombo, A.; Bacchiani, G.; Tedeschi, I.; Meroni, C.A.; Veglia, F.; Civelli, M.; Lamantia, G.; Colombo, N.; Curigliano, G.; et al. Early detection of anthracycline cardiotoxicity and improvement with heart failure therapy. *Circulation* **2015**, *131*, 1981–1988. [CrossRef]
68. Hoffman, R.K.; Kim, B.-J.; Shah, P.D.; Carver, J.; Ky, B.; Ryeom, S. Damage to cardiac vasculature may be associated with breast cancer treatment-induced cardiotoxicity. *Cardio-Oncology* **2021**, *7*, 15. [CrossRef]
69. Chanan-Khan, A.; Srinivasan, S.; Czuczman, M.S. Prevention and management of cardiotoxicity from antineoplastic therapy. *J. Support. Oncol.* **2004**, *2*, 251–256.
70. Anker, S.D.; Egerer, K.R.; Volk, H.-D.; Kox, W.J.; Poole-Wilson, P.A.; Coats, A.J. Elevated soluble CD14 receptors and altered cytokines in chronic heart failure. *Am. J. Cardiol.* **1997**, *79*, 1426–1430. [CrossRef]
71. Krack, A.; Sharma, R.; Figulla, H.R.; Anker, S.D. The importance of the gastrointestinal system in the pathogenesis of heart failure. *Eur. Heart J.* **2005**, *26*, 2368–2374. [CrossRef]
72. Tang, W.H.W.; Li, D.Y.; Hazen, S.L. Dietary metabolism, the gut microbiome, and heart failure. *Nat. Rev. Cardiol.* **2019**, *16*, 137–154. [CrossRef] [PubMed]
73. Zitvogel, L.; Daillère, R.; Roberti, M.P.; Routy, B.; Kroemer, G. Anticancer effects of the microbiome and its products. *Nat. Rev. Genet.* **2017**, *15*, 465–478. [CrossRef] [PubMed]

74. Karin, M.; Jobin, C.; Balkwill, F. Chemotherapy, immunity and microbiota—A new triumvirate? *Nat. Med.* **2014**, *20*, 126–127. [PubMed]
75. Roy, S.; Trinchieri, G. Microbiota: A key orchestrator of cancer therapy. *Nat. Rev. Cancer* **2017**, *17*, 271–285. [CrossRef] [PubMed]
76. Deleemans, J.M.; Toivonen, K.; Reimer, R.A.; Carlson, L.E. The Chemo-Gut Study: A Cross-Sectional Survey Exploring Physical, Mental, and Gastrointestinal Health Outcomes in Cancer Survivors. *Glob. Adv. Health Med.* **2022**, *11*, 2164957X221145940. [CrossRef]
77. Deleemans, J.M.; Chleilat, F.; Reimer, R.A.; Baydoun, M.; Piedalue, K.-A.; Lowry, D.E.; Henning, J.-W.; Carlson, L.E. The Chemo-Gut Pilot Study: Associations between Gut Microbiota, Gastrointestinal Symptoms, and Psychosocial Health Outcomes in a Cross-Sectional Sample of Young Adult Cancer Survivors. *Curr. Oncol.* **2022**, *29*, 2973–2994. [CrossRef]
78. Huang, J.; Wei, S.; Jiang, C.; Xiao, Z.; Liu, J.; Peng, W.; Zhang, B.; Li, W. Involvement of Abnormal Gut Microbiota Composition and Function in Doxorubicin-Induced Cardiotoxicity. *Front. Cell. Infect. Microbiol.* **2022**, *12*, 808837. [CrossRef]
79. Liu, X.; Liu, Y.; Chen, X.; Wang, C.; Chen, X.; Liu, W.; Huang, K.; Chen, H.; Yang, J. Multi-walled carbon nanotubes exacerbate doxorubicin-induced cardiotoxicity by altering gut microbiota and pulmonary and colonic macrophage phenotype in mice. *Toxicology* **2020**, *435*, 152410. [CrossRef]
80. Zhao, L.; Xing, C.; Sun, W.; Hou, G.; Yang, G.; Yuan, L. Lactobacillus supplementation prevents cisplatin-induced cardiotoxicity possibly by inflammation inhibition. *Cancer Chemother. Pharmacol.* **2018**, *82*, 999–1008. [CrossRef]
81. Lin, H.; Meng, L.; Sun, Z.; Sun, S.; Huang, X.; Lin, N.; Zhang, J.; Lu, W.; Yang, Q.; Chi, J.; et al. Yellow Wine Polyphenolic Compound Protects Against Doxorubicin-Induced Cardiotoxicity by Modulating the Composition and Metabolic Function of the Gut Microbiota. *Circ. Heart Fail.* **2021**, *14*, e008220. [CrossRef]
82. Ni, H.; Xu, J.Q. *Recent Trends in Heart Failure Related Mortality: United States, 2000–2014*; NCHS Data Brief, No. 231; National Center for Health Statistics: Hyattsville, MD, USA, 2015.
83. Pullen, A.B.; Jadapalli, J.K.; Rhourri-Frih, B.; Halade, G.V. Re-evaluating the causes and consequences of non-resolving inflammation in chronic cardiovascular disease. *Heart Fail. Rev.* **2019**, *25*, 381–391. [CrossRef] [PubMed]
84. Sarhene, M.; Wang, Y.; Wei, J.; Huang, Y.; Li, M.; Li, L.; Acheampong, E.; Zhengcan, Z.; Xiaoyan, Q.; Yunsheng, X.; et al. Biomarkers in heart failure: The past, current and future. *Heart Fail. Rev.* **2019**, *24*, 867–903. [CrossRef] [PubMed]
85. Takala, J. Determinants of splanchnic blood flow. *Br. J. Anaesth.* **1996**, *77*, 50–58. [CrossRef]
86. Krack, A.; Richartz, B.M.; Gastmann, A.; Greim, K.; Lotze, U.; Anker, S.D.; Figulla, H.R. Studies on intragastric PCO2 at rest and during exercise as a marker of intestinal perfusion in patients with chronic heart failure. *Eur. J. Heart Fail.* **2004**, *6*, 403–407. [CrossRef] [PubMed]
87. Cui, X.; Ye, L.; Li, J.; Jin, L.; Wang, W.; Li, S.; Bao, M.; Wu, S.; Li, L.; Geng, B.; et al. Metagenomic and metabolomic analyses unveil dysbiosis of gut microbiota in chronic heart failure patients. *Sci. Rep.* **2018**, *8*, 635. [CrossRef]
88. Witkowski, M.; Weeks, T.L.; Hazen, S.L. Gut Microbiota and Cardiovascular Disease. *Circ. Res.* **2020**, *127*, 553–570. [CrossRef]
89. Pasini, E.; Aquilani, R.; Testa, C.; Baiardi, P.; Angioletti, S.; Boschi, F.; Verri, M.; Dioguardi, F.S. Pathogenic Gut Flora in Patients With Chronic Heart Failure. *JACC Heart Fail.* **2016**, *4*, 220–227. [CrossRef]
90. Kobiyama, K.; Ley, K. Atherosclerosis. *Circ. Res.* **2018**, *123*, 1118–1120. [CrossRef]
91. Ott, S.J.; El Mokhtari, N.E.; Musfeldt, M.; Hellmig, S.; Freitag, S.; Rehman, A.; Kühbacher, T.; Nikolaus, S.; Namsolleck, P.; Blaut, M.; et al. Detection of diverse bacterial signatures in atherosclerotic lesions of patients with coronary heart disease. *Circulation* **2006**, *113*, 929–937. [CrossRef]
92. Jie, Z.; Xia, H.; Zhong, S.-L.; Feng, Q.; Li, S.; Liang, S.; Zhong, H.; Liu, Z.; Gao, Y.; Zhao, H.; et al. The gut microbiome in atherosclerotic cardiovascular disease. *Nat. Commun.* **2017**, *8*, 845. [CrossRef]
93. Shi, G.; Lin, Y.; Wu, Y.; Zhou, J.; Cao, L.; Chen, J.; Li, Y.; Tan, N.; Zhong, S. *Bacteroides fragilis* Supplementation Deteriorated Metabolic Dysfunction, Inflammation, and Aorta Atherosclerosis by Inducing Gut Microbiota Dysbiosis in Animal Model. *Nutrients* **2022**, *14*, 2199. [CrossRef]
94. Xu, Y.; Lv, C.; Wang, H.; Lu, Q.; Ye, M.; Zhu, X.; Liu, R. Peanut skin extract ameliorates high-fat diet-induced atherosclerosis by regulating lipid metabolism, inflammation reaction and gut microbiota in ApoE$^{-/-}$ mice. *Food Res. Int.* **2022**, *154*, 111014. [CrossRef] [PubMed]
95. Arumugam, M.; Raes, J.; Pelletier, E.; Le Paslier, D.; Yamada, T.; Mende, D.R.; Fernandes, G.R.; Tap, J.; Bruls, T.; Batto, J.M.; et al. Enterotypes of the human gut microbiome. *Nature* **2011**, *473*, 174–180. [CrossRef] [PubMed]
96. Emoto, T.; Yamashita, T.; Sasaki, N.; Hirota, Y.; Hayashi, T.; So, A.; Kasahara, K.; Yodoi, K.; Matsumoto, T.; Mizoguchi, T.; et al. Analysis of gut microbiota in coronary artery disease patients: A possible link between gut microbiota and coronary artery disease. *J. Atheroscler. Thromb.* **2016**, *23*, 908–921. [CrossRef]
97. Yang, Q.; Lin, S.L.; Kwok, M.K.; Leung, G.M.; Schooling, C.M. The roles of 27 genera of human gut microbiota in ischemic heart disease, type 2 diabetes mellitus, and their risk factors: A Mendelian randomization study. *Am. J. Epidemiol.* **2018**, *187*, 1916–1922. [CrossRef]
98. Routy, B.; le Chatelier, E.; DeRosa, L.; Duong, C.P.M.; Alou, M.T.; Daillère, R.; Fluckiger, A.; Messaoudene, M.; Rauber, C.; Roberti, M.P.; et al. Gut microbiome influences efficacy of PD-1–based immunotherapy against epithelial tumors. *Science* **2018**, *359*, 91–97. [CrossRef]
99. Yan, Q.; Gu, Y.; Li, X.; Yang, W.; Jia, L.; Chen, C.; Han, X.; Huang, Y.; Zhao, L.; Li, P.; et al. Alterations of the gut microbiome in hypertension. *Front. Cell. Infect. Microbiol.* **2017**, *7*, 381. [CrossRef]

100. Karlsson, F.H.; Fåk, F.; Nookaew, I.; Tremaroli, V.; Fagerberg, B.; Petranovic, D.; Bäckhed, F.; Nielsen, J. Symptomatic atherosclerosis is associated with an altered gut metagenome. *Nat. Commun.* **2012**, *3*, 1245. [CrossRef]
101. Tang, W.W.; Kitai, T.; Hazen, S.L. Gut microbiota in cardiovascular health and disease. *Circ. Res.* **2017**, *120*, 1183–1196. [CrossRef]
102. Zwielehner, J.; Lassl, C.; Hippe, B.; Pointner, A.; Switzeny, O.J.; Remely, M.; Kitzweger, E.; Ruckser, R.; Haslberger, A.G. Changes in human fecal microbiota due to chemotherapy analyzed by TaqMan-PCR, 454 sequencing and PCR-DGGE fingerprinting. *PLoS ONE* **2011**, *6*, e28654. [CrossRef]
103. Stringer, A.M.; Gibson, R.J.; Logan, R.M.; Bowen, J.M.; Yeoh, A.S.J.; Hamilton, J.; Keefe, D.M.K. Gastrointestinal microflora and mucins may play a critical role in the development of 5-fluorouracil-induced gastrointestinal mucositis. *Exp. Biol. Med.* **2009**, *234*, 430–441. [CrossRef]
104. Huang, Y.; Yang, W.; Liu, H.; Duan, J.; Zhang, Y.; Liu, M.; Li, H.; Hou, Z.; Wu, K.K. Effect of high-dose methotrexate chemotherapy on intestinal Bifidobacteria, Lactobacillus and Escherichia coli in children with acute lymphoblastic leukemia. *Exp. Biol. Med.* **2012**, *237*, 305–311. [CrossRef]
105. Barker, H.E.; Paget, J.T.E.; Khan, A.A.; Harrington, K.J. The tumour microenvironment after radiotherapy: Mechanisms of resistance and recurrence. *Nat. Rev. Cancer* **2015**, *15*, 409–425. [CrossRef]
106. Sahly, N.; Moustafa, A.; Zaghloul, M.; Salem, T.Z. Effect of radiotherapy on the gut microbiome in pediatric cancer patients: A pilot study. *PeerJ* **2019**, *7*, e7683. [CrossRef] [PubMed]
107. Schroeder, B.O.; Bäckhed, F. Signals from the gut microbiota to distant organs in physiology and disease. *Nat. Med.* **2016**, *22*, 1079–1089. [CrossRef]
108. O'keefe, S.J.D. Diet, microorganisms and their metabolites, and colon cancer. *Nat. Rev. Gastroenterol. Hepatol.* **2016**, *13*, 691–706. [CrossRef] [PubMed]
109. Parada Venegas, D.; De la Fuente, M.K.; Landskron, G.; González, M.J.; Quera, R.; Dijkstra, G.; Harmsen, H.J.M.; Faber, K.N.; Hermoso., M.A. Short chain fatty acids (SCFAs)-mediated gut epithelial and immune regulation and its relevance for inflammatory bowel diseases. *Front. Immunol.* **2019**, *10*, 277. [CrossRef] [PubMed]
110. Park, J.; Kim, M.; Kang, S.; Jannasch, A.; Cooper, B.; Patterson, J.; Kim, C. Short-chain fatty acids induce both effector and regulatory T cells by suppression of histone deacetylases and regulation of the mTOR–S6K pathway. *Mucosal Immunol.* **2014**, *8*, 80–93. [CrossRef] [PubMed]
111. Jaye, K.; Li, C.G.; Chang, D.; Bhuyan, D.J. The role of key gut microbial metabolites in the development and treatment of cancer. *Gut Microbes* **2022**, *14*, 2038865. [CrossRef]

Disclaimer/Publisher's Note: The statements, opinions and data contained in all publications are solely those of the individual author(s) and contributor(s) and not of MDPI and/or the editor(s). MDPI and/or the editor(s) disclaim responsibility for any injury to people or property resulting from any ideas, methods, instructions or products referred to in the content.

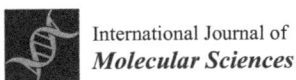

Article

Colon Cancer Microbiome Landscaping: Differences in Right- and Left-Sided Colon Cancer and a Tumor Microbiome-Ileal Microbiome Association

Barbara Kneis [1,2], Stefan Wirtz [3], Klaus Weber [2], Axel Denz [2], Matthias Gittler [2], Carol Geppert [4], Maximilian Brunner [2], Christian Krautz [2], Alexander Reinhard Siebenhüner [5], Robert Schierwagen [6], Olaf Tyc [7], Abbas Agaimy [4], Robert Grützmann [2], Jonel Trebicka [6], Stephan Kersting [8,†] and Melanie Langheinrich [8,*,†]

1. Department of Nephrology, University Hospital Erlangen, 91054 Erlangen, Germany
2. Department of Surgery, University Hospital Erlangen, 91054 Erlangen, Germany
3. Department of Internal Medicine I, University Hospital Erlangen, 91054 Erlangen, Germany
4. Institute of Pathology, University Hospital Erlangen, 91054 Erlangen, Germany
5. Department of Gastroenterology and Hepatology, University Hospital Zurich and University Zurich, 8091 Zürich, Switzerland
6. Department of Internal Medicine B, University Hospital Münster, 48149 Münster, Germany
7. Department of Internal Medicine I, University Clinic Frankfurt, 60590 Frankfurt, Germany
8. Department of Surgery, University Hospital Greifswald, 17475 Greifswald, Germany
* Correspondence: melanie.langheinrich@med.uni-greifswald.de
† These authors contributed equally to this work.

Abstract: In the current era of precision oncology, it is widely acknowledged that CRC is a heterogeneous disease entity. Tumor location (right- or left-sided colon cancer or rectal cancer) is a crucial factor in determining disease progression as well as prognosis and influences disease management. In the last decade, numerous works have reported that the microbiome is an important element of CRC carcinogenesis, progression and therapy response. Owing to the heterogeneous nature of microbiomes, the findings of these studies were inconsistent. The majority of the studies combined colon cancer (CC) and rectal cancer (RC) samples as CRC for analysis. Furthermore, the small intestine, as the major site for immune surveillance in the gut, is understudied compared to the colon. Thus, the CRC heterogeneity puzzle is far from being solved, and more research is necessary for prospective trials that separately investigate CC and RC. Our prospective study aimed to map the colon cancer landscape using 16S rRNA amplicon sequencing in biopsy samples from the terminal ileum, healthy colon tissue, healthy rectal tissue and tumor tissue as well as in preoperative and postoperative stool samples of 41 patients. While fecal samples provide a good approximation of the average gut microbiome composition, mucosal biopsies allow for detecting subtle variations in local microbial communities. In particular, the small bowel microbiome has remained poorly characterized, mainly because of sampling difficulties. Our analysis revealed the following: (i) right- and left-sided colon cancers harbor distinct and diverse microbiomes, (ii) the tumor microbiome leads to a more consistent cancer-defined microbiome between locations and reveals a tumor microbiome–ileal microbiome association, (iii) the stool only partly reflects the microbiome landscape in patients with CC, and (iv) mechanical bowel preparation and perioperative antibiotics together with surgery result in major changes in the stool microbiome, characterized by a significant increase in the abundance of potentially pathogenic bacteria, such as *Enterococcus*. Collectively, our results provide new and valuable insights into the complex microbiome landscape in patients with colon cancer.

Keywords: microbiome; colon cancer; right-sided colon cancer; left-sided colon cancer; tumor microbiome; gut microbiome

Citation: Kneis, B.; Wirtz, S.; Weber, K.; Denz, A.; Gittler, M.; Geppert, C.; Brunner, M.; Krautz, C.; Siebenhüner, A.R.; Schierwagen, R.; et al. Colon Cancer Microbiome Landscaping: Differences in Right- and Left-Sided Colon Cancer and a Tumor Microbiome-Ileal Microbiome Association. *Int. J. Mol. Sci.* 2023, 24, 3265. https://doi.org/10.3390/ijms24043265

Academic Editor: Maria Teresa Mascellino

Received: 30 November 2022
Revised: 1 February 2023
Accepted: 3 February 2023
Published: 7 February 2023

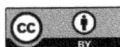

Copyright: © 2023 by the authors. Licensee MDPI, Basel, Switzerland. This article is an open access article distributed under the terms and conditions of the Creative Commons Attribution (CC BY) license (https://creativecommons.org/licenses/by/4.0/).

1. Introduction

Colorectal cancer (CRC) is the third leading cause of cancer death worldwide and the second leading cause of cancer mortality in Europe [1,2]. Although CRC incidence and mortality rates have decreased over the past decades, global trends have shown that the incidence among young adults aged 20–49 has increased [3]. While the prognosis of patients with early-stage disease is excellent, 40% of patients across all disease stages ultimately die from their disease within five years [4]. In the last decade, it became clear that differences in oncological outcome can be partly explained by differences in tumor biology. CRC is a highly heterogeneous group of tumors, and the pathogenesis of CRC is a complex and multifactorial process involving the accumulation of various genetic and epigenetic alterations [5]. Beyond these alterations, it is widely accepted that tumor location (right- and left-sided colon cancer, rectal cancer) is a crucial factor involved in disease progression as well as prognosis and influences disease management [6–8]. Right-sided colon cancer (RSCC) occurs within the cecum, ascending colon, hepatic flexure and transverse colon, while left-sided colon cancer (LSCC) arises in the splenic flexure, descending colon and sigmoid colon. The right- and left-sided colon have distinct embryological origins, developing from the mid- and hindgut [6]. Moreover, differences in clinical and molecular characteristics have been observed. In particular, RSCC presents with microsatellite instability, BRAF mutations, high immunogenicity and a worse prognosis [9,10]. To date, colon cancer (CC) and rectal cancer (RC) are synonymously termed CRC. However, based on experimental, translational and clinical research, there is more and more evidence to divide CC and RC as self-standing tumor entities [11].

Epidemiologic studies have identified a number of environmental factors that affect the risk of CRC carcinogenesis, including lifestyle, nutritional factors and the microbiome [12,13]. Microbes have been linked to cancer in 10–20% of cases [14–16]. Novel data have demonstrated that locations previously considered sterile, such as the liver, pancreas and even tumor tissue, harbor their own site-specific microbiome [17–19]. The human intestinal microbiome primarily comprises *Firmicutes*, *Bacteroidetes*, *Actinobacteria*, and *Proteobacteria* [16]. After rapid changes in the first years of life, the gut microbiome remains relatively stable for decades and displays gradual changes with advancing age. High diversity might be a key feature of a healthy microbiome [20–24]. Dysbiosis refers to an abnormality in the composition and/or function of the host's symbiotic microbial ecosystem that exceeds its constitutive capacity and, as a result, has adverse effects on the host [25]. The microbiome can impact cancer initiation, progression and response to therapy [26–28]. In 2022, the microbiome is mentioned as a distinctive enabling characteristic for the acquisition of hallmarks of cancer capabilities [16,29]. The hallmarks of cancer, first published in 2000 by Hanahan and Weinberg and updated in 2011, are defined as a core set of functional capabilities acquired by human cells through their way to form malignant tumors [29,30]. Nevertheless, uncertainty remains regarding the direct and indirect effects of the microbiome in cancer [31–33]. Sequencing and association studies have demonstrated changes in microbial composition and ecology in patients with CRC, specifically, a decrease in commensal bacterial species (e.g., butyrate-producing bacteria) and the enrichment of opportunistic pathogens (e.g., proinflammatory). Moreover, there is strong evidence that the gut microbiome influences the efficacy of immune checkpoint inhibitors (ICIs) in CRC and other types of cancers [34–39]. However, recent studies have revealed that the ileal microbiota also determines the prognostic and predictive features and therapeutic responses of CC [40,41].

Altogether, most microbiome studies in CRC have focused on the analysis of fecal rather than tumor or mucosal samples. Furthermore, most studies have considered colon and rectal cancers as one disease entity, CRC. As mentioned before, obvious differences exist in tumor biology, molecular carcinogenesis, treatment and response to therapy. In surgical oncology, for decades researchers have been becoming aware that CC and RC are different diseases, based on multimodal treatments, surgical techniques, complication rates and relapse patterns. To overcome the heterogeneous nature of the microbiome, research should concentrate on separately describing results for CC and RC.

To address these aspects, we focused our attention on mapping associations between the microbiota and clinicopathologic features of tumor tissue and healthy tissue of the ileum, colon or rectum as well as fecal samples collected before and after surgery from patients with primarily untreated CC. The results provide a deeper understanding of the complex microbiome landscape in patients with colon cancer.

2. Results

2.1. Patient Characteristics

The study cohort consisted of 41 newly diagnosed, treatment-naive CC patients scheduled for elective surgery and included 23 male (56.1%) and 18 female (43.9%) patients, of whom 24 patients were with RSCC and 17 patients were with LSCC (only CC, no rectal cancer patients), aged from 39 to 90 years. The baseline clinical and pathological characteristics are shown in Table 1; no significant differences were observed between patients with RSCC and LSCC.

Table 1. Clinicopathological characteristics of the study participants.

Patient Characteristics	Right-Sided Colon Cancer n (%)	Left-Sided Colon Cancer n (%)	p Value
Age			
○ overall, years	40–90	39–88	
○ mean, years	70.9	67.4	
○ group 1: ≤60 years	3 (12.5)	5 (29.4)	
○ group 2: 61–79 years	16 (66.7)	10 (58.8)	
○ group 3: ≥80 years	5 (20.8)	2 (11.8)	0.36
Sex			
○ Male	12 (50)	11 (64.7)	
○ Female	12 (50)	6 (35.3)	0.35
BMI			
○ <18.5 Underweight	0	0	
○ 18.5–24.9 Normal weight	11 (45.8)	4 (23.5)	
○ 25.0–29.9 Preobesity	9 (57.5)	8 (47.1)	
○ 30.0–34.9 Obesity class 1	3 (12.5)	4 (23.5)	
○ 35.0–39.9 Obesity class 2	1 (4.2)	1 (5.9)	
○ ≥40 Obesity class 3	0	0	0.50
Dietary patterns			
○ omnivorous	23 (95.8)	16 (94.1)	
○ vegan/vegetarian	1 (4.2)	1 (5.9)	0.80
Smoking			
○ yes	2 (8.3)	3 (17.6)	
○ no	22 (91.6)	14 (82.4)	0.37
Medication			
○ no	3 (12.5)	4 (23.5)	
○ yes (1–3)	12 (50)	6 (35.3)	
○ yes (3–5)	4 (16.7)	4 (23.5)	
○ yes (>5)	5 (20.8)	3 (17.6)	0.68

Table 1. Cont.

Patient Characteristics	Right-Sided Colon Cancer n (%)	Left-Sided Colon Cancer n (%)	p Value
T-stage			
○ 1	3 (12.5)	2 (11.8)	
○ 2	6 (25)	0	
○ 3	11 (45.8)	14 (82.4)	0.06
○ 4	4 (16.7)	1 (5.9)	
N-stage			
○ 0	19 (79.2)	13 (76.5)	
○ 1	4 (16.7)	4 (23.5)	0.62
○ 2	1 (4.2)	0	
Differentiation (G)			
○ 1 (well differentiated)	0	0	
○ 2 (moderately differentiated)	11 (45.8)	9 (52.9)	0.65
○ 3 (poorly differentiated)	13 (54.2)	8 (47.1)	
R-status			
○ local R0	24	17	n/a
M-status			
○ 0	21 (87.5)	15 (88.2)	0.94
○ 1	3 (12.5)	2 (11.8)	
MSS status			
○ MSS	16 (66.7)	15 (88.2)	0.11
○ MSI	8 (33.3)	2 (11.8)	

2.2. Microbiome Profile of the Study Cohort

2.2.1. The Microbiome Landscape across the Locations

First, we analyzed all sample types (ileal tissue, healthy colon tissue, healthy rectal tissue, tumor tissue, preoperative stool and postoperative stool). The most abundant phyla in all samples were *Firmicutes* and *Bacteroidetes*, followed by *Actinobacteria*, *Proteobacteria*, *Verrucomicrobia* and *Fusobacteria*, to different degrees (Figure 1a). The microbiota profile at the genus level in all samples is shown in Figure 1b. The profile of the microbiota in the different analyzed samples differed from those found in the quality controls (mock community, water).

To estimate the richness and diversity of the different habitats, the alpha diversity indices were analyzed. We compared the Observed, Chao, ACE, Shannon, Simpson and Fisher indices of the different sample types at the genus level. The overall structure of the microbiota in the microhabitats was significantly different based on all indices: the Observed index (p value: 0.000002; (ANOVA) F value: 7.4813) (Figure 2a), the Chao1 index (p value: 0.00001; (ANOVA) F value: 6.4832), the ACE index (p value: 0.00004; (ANOVA) F value: 5.9738), the Shannon index (p value: 0.000000006; (ANOVA) F value: 10.664), the Simpson index (p value: 0.00000004; (ANOVA) F value: 9.6125) and the Fisher index (p value: 0.000002; (ANOVA) F value: 7.5182). The diversity was lowest in postoperative stool samples, which could be explained by the bowel preparation (mechanical and antibiotics) and surgical stress.

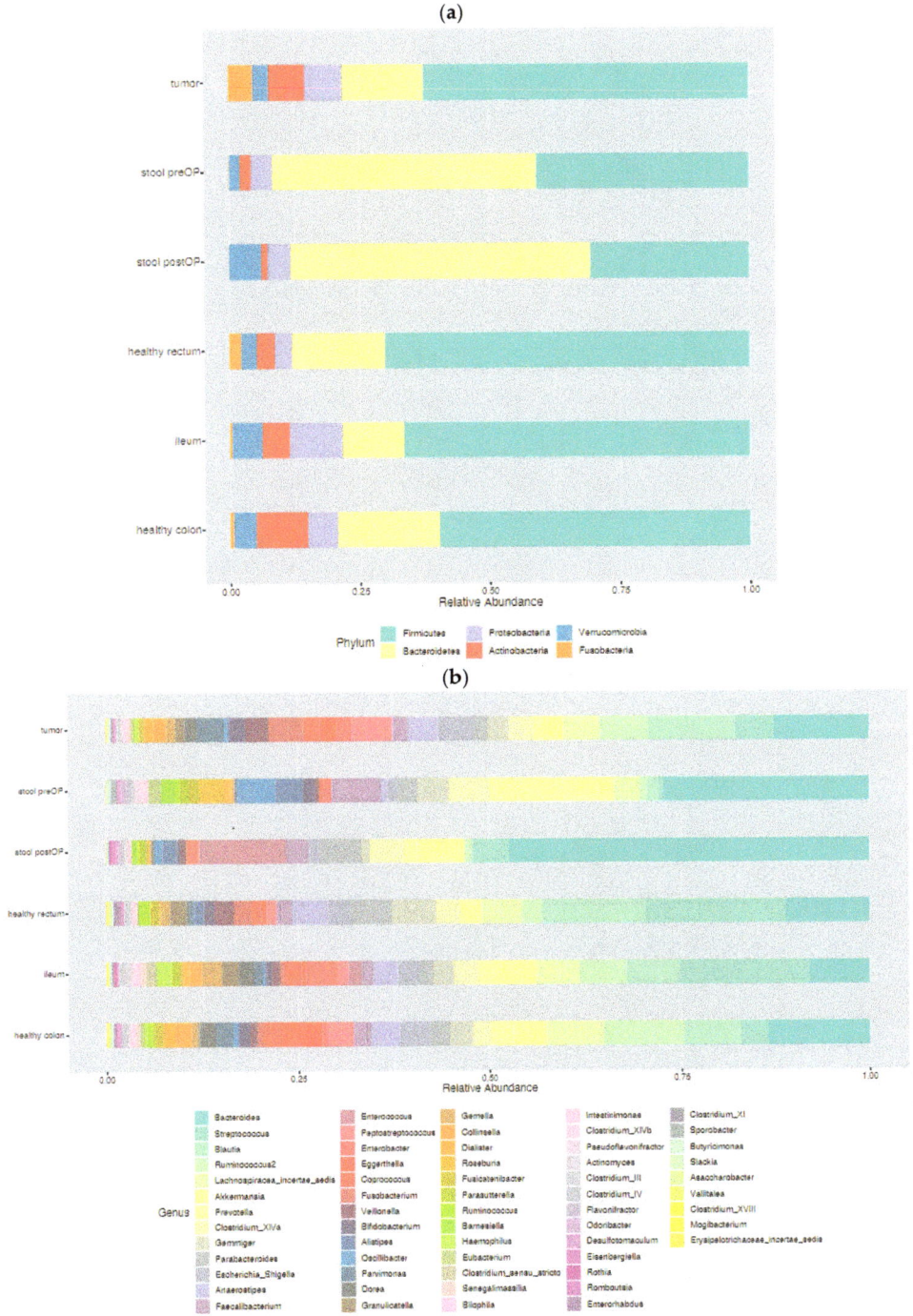

Figure 1. Taxonomic analysis of the microbiome in the different habitats of CC patients: represented at the phylum level (**a**) and genus level (**b**).

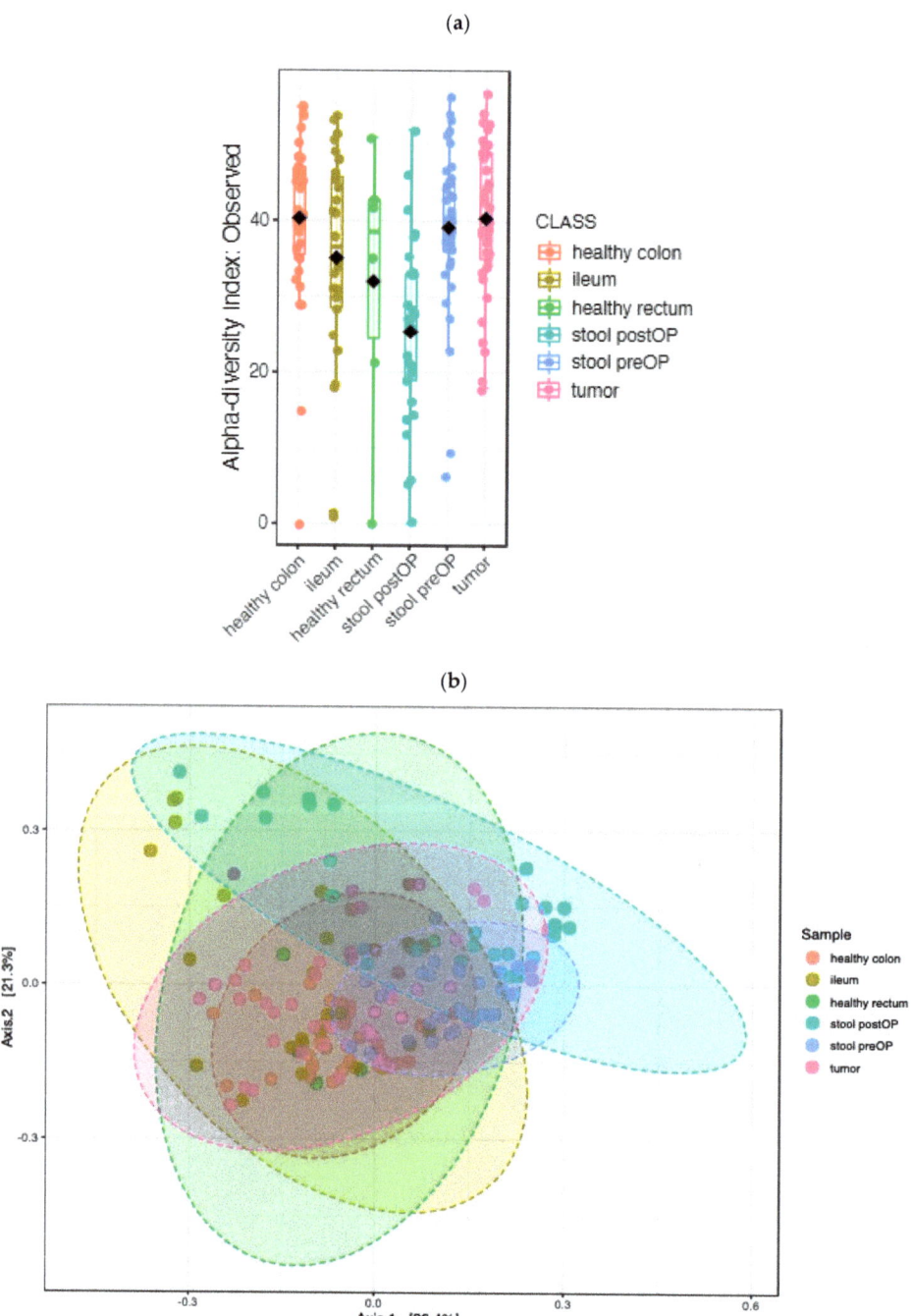

Figure 2. Microbiome diversity comparison between the locations of CC patients: alpha diversity box plot (Observed, *p* value < 0.001) (**a**) and principal coordinate analysis (PCoA) using Jensen–Shannon metric distances of beta diversity (**b**) at the genus level, *p* value < 0.001.

Moreover, a beta diversity analysis was performed. At the genus level, the analysis revealed that the overall structure of the microbiota in the analyzed habitats was significantly different (PCoA Jensen–Shannon (PERMANOVA) F value: 9.5743, R-squared: 0.22074, p value < 0.001; Figure 2b).

A linear discriminant analysis (LDA) coupled with effect size measurements (LEfSe) was applied to identify key taxa that were differentially abundant between the analyzed samples. A total of 46 key taxa were identified at the genus level (Figure 3, LDA score > 3, p value < 0.05, FDR-adjusted p value < 0.1; Supplementary Figure S1).

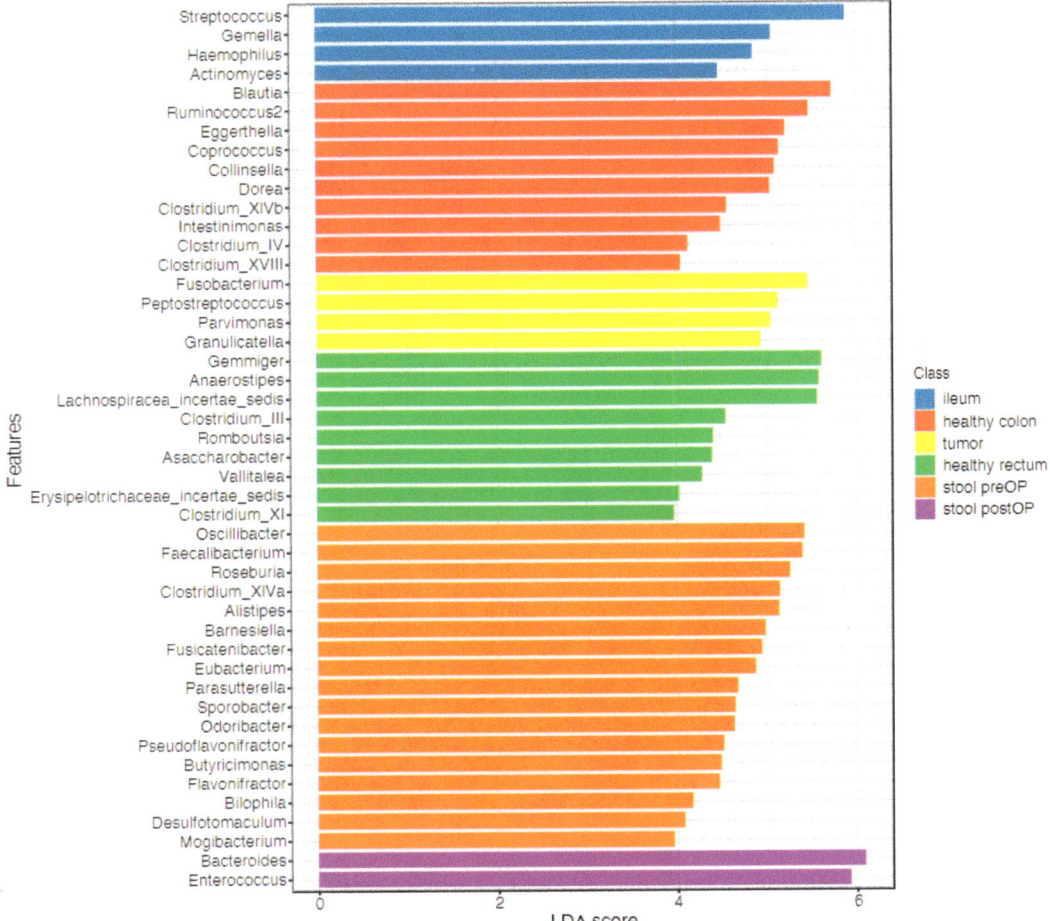

Figure 3. Microbiome communities are significantly different between the locations: LEfSe analysis computed from genera differentially abundant in the analyzed microhabitats, p value < 0.05.

2.2.2. The Microbiome Communities Are Significantly Different between Tumor and Stool Samples

The early detection of CC is of great prognostic importance, and stool samples are a potential source of microbial biomarkers. We compared tumor tissue and preoperative stool samples and analyzed differences in the microbiota composition. The beta diversity comparisons showed significantly different bacterial community clusters between the tumor and stool samples (PCoA Jensen–Shannon divergence (PERMANOVA) F value: 18.721, R-squared: 0.19558, p value < 0.001, Figure 4a). The LEfSe analysis identified

35 genera whose abundances significantly differed between the tumor and stool samples (LDA score > 3, *p* value < 0.05, FDR-adjusted *p* value < 0.05; Figure 4b). No significant differences in the alpha diversity were observed between the tumor and stool samples (Figure 5a). The random forest classification machine learning algorithm was used to confirm the data. Using 120 trees, the algorithm achieved the best prediction with a classification error of 0.0253 (Supplementary Figure S1). The top five ranked genera to discriminate between stools and tumors were Flavonifractor, Oscillibacter, Odoribacter, Roseburia and Eggerthella (Supplementary Figure S2).

To determine whether the composition of the microbiome differs according to clinical factors, additional analyses were performed based on location (RSCC, LSCC) and pathologic parameters (T stage, differentiation, nodal stage, MSS status). The alpha diversity of the whole microbiome of the stool and tumor tissue was significantly different between the RSCC and LSCC groups (Observed index *p* value: 0.014561; (*t* test) statistics: 2.4996; Chao1 index *p* value: 0.017411; (*t* test) statistics: 2.4305). The MSS and MSI tumor groups were slightly but not significantly different (Chao1 index *p* value: 0.0508; (*t* test) statistics: −2.0505) (Figure 5b,c).

The tumor tissue of grade 3 tumors was significantly enriched in *Fusobacterium* and *Parvimonas*, while *Fusicatenibacter*, *Blautia*, *Intestimonas* and *Romboutsia* were significantly increased in grade 2 tumors (*p* value < 0.01, FDR-adjusted *p* value < 0.1). There was no significant difference among the T or N stages; we think that this was due to the stage-specific distribution: early T1/2 stages (*n* = 11) compared to T3/4 (*n* = 29) and more N-negative (*n* = 32) than N-positive patients (*n* = 9). In tumor tissue, no significant differences according to MSS status were observed.

In contrast, the preoperative stool of grade 2 patients was associated with *Dialister* and *Intestimonas*, while grade 3 tumors were significantly enriched in E. shigella (*p* value < 0.01, FDR-adjusted *p* value < 0.1). Furthermore, the stool of MSI patients was significantly enriched with *Clostridium_XIVb* (*p* value < 0.01, FDR-adjusted *p* value < 0.1). Taken together, these findings suggest that the stool microbiome (preoperative) only partly reflects the tumor microbiome.

(a)

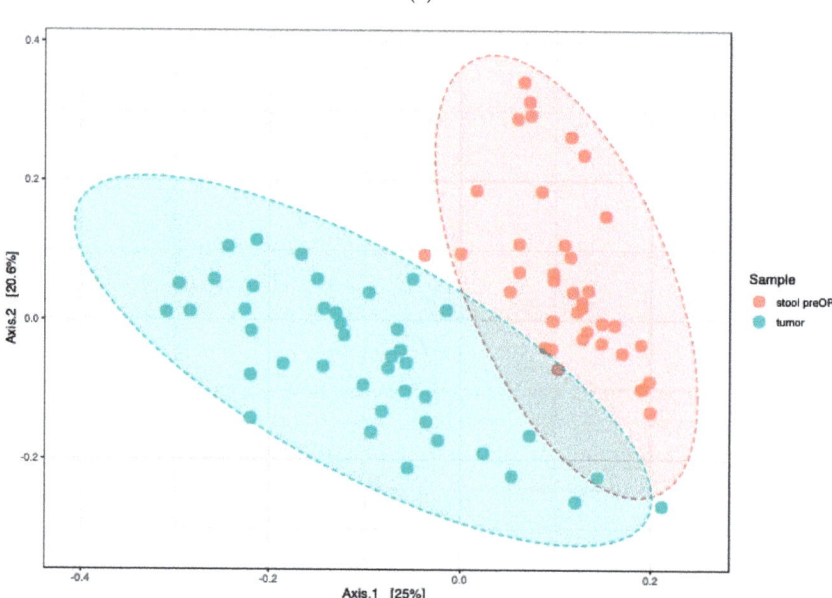

Figure 4. *Cont.*

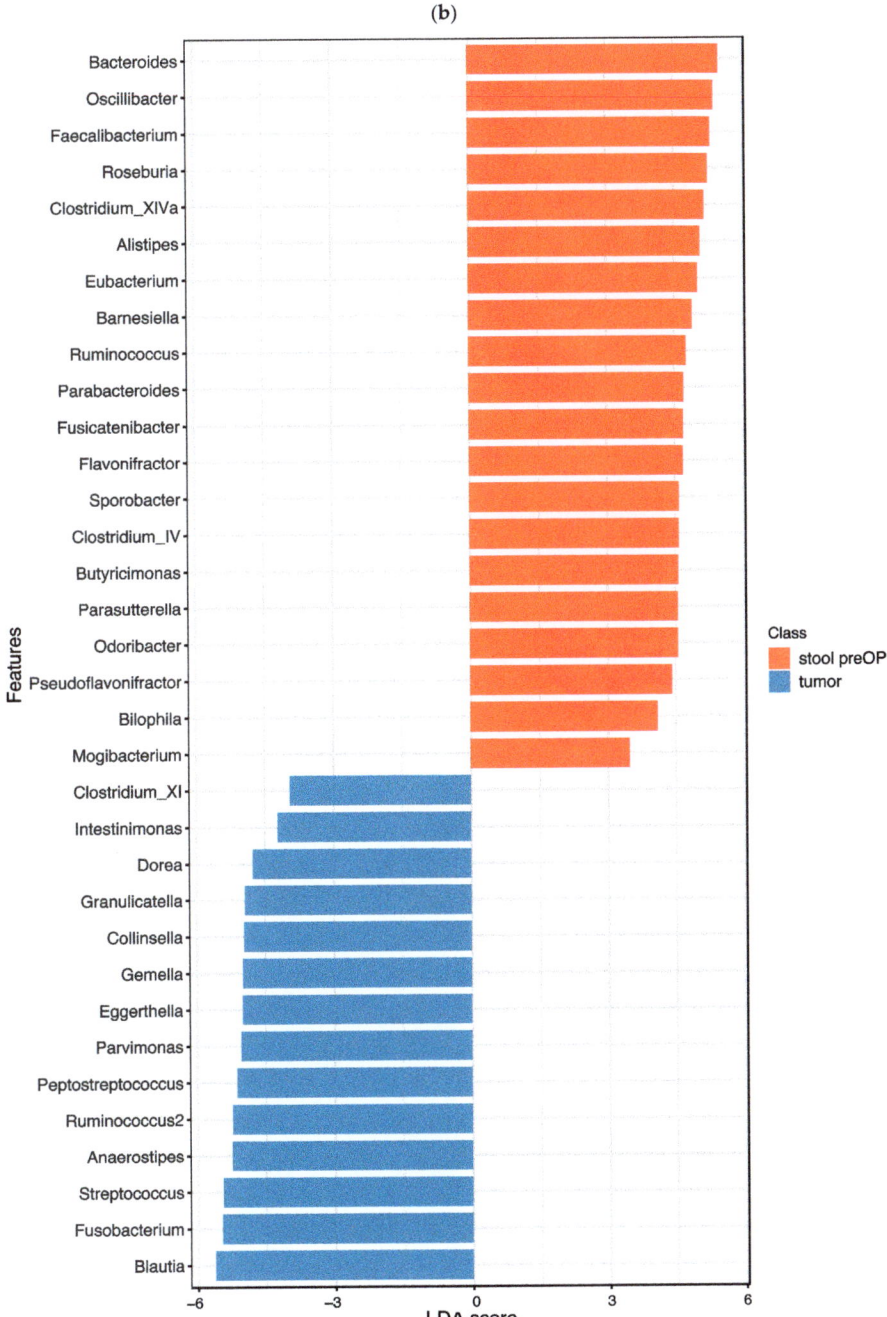

Figure 4. Stool microbiome only partly reflects the microbiome landscape in CC patients: PCoA using Jensen–Shannon divergence of beta diversity between tumor and preoperative stool, p value < 0.001 (**a**), LEfSe detected marked differences in the predominance of bacterial communities between tumor and preoperative stool, p value < 0.05 (**b**).

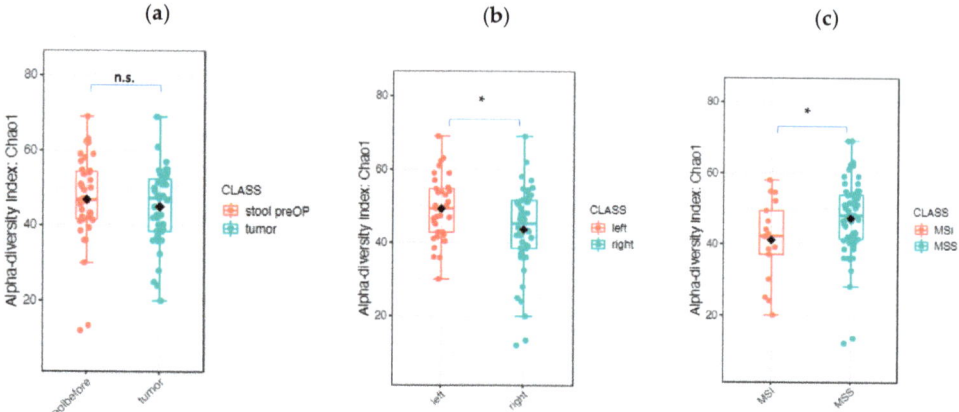

Figure 5. Microbiome composition according to tumor sidedness and MSS status: (**a**) diversity analysis using the Chao1 alpha diversity index between tumor and preoperative stool; (**b**) overall microbiome of the tumor and preoperative stool according to sidedness RSCC and LSCC; and (**c**) overall microbiome of the tumor and preoperative stool according to MSS status (* $p < 0.05$, n.s, not significant).

The core microbiome, based on sample prevalence (>50%) and relative abundance (0.01%), is displayed in Figure 6. The core analysis revealed six genera as the core taxa across all samples. Among them, *Parabacteroides* was prevalent in more than half of the samples from the RSCC patients, while *Bifidobacterium* and *Roseburia* were prevalent in more than half of the LSCC patients. Taken together, these findings indicate that RSCC and LSCC harbored a diverse core microbiome, with *Bacteroides* as the predominant genus (Figure 6) in both.

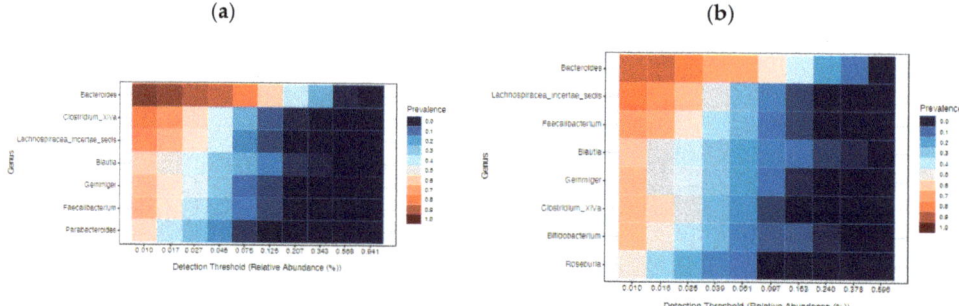

Figure 6. Heatmap of the core microbiome: the overall core microbiome of stool and tumor between RSCC (**a**) and LSCC patients clustered differentially (**b**).

2.2.3. The Tumor Microbiome Profile: Significant Differences between RSCC and LSCC

For a deeper understanding of the intratumoral microbiome, we further analyzed the tumor tissue and sidedness (Figure 7). We first assessed the general tumor landscape. The top taxa in RSCC patients (Figure 7b) at the genus level were *Bacteroides* (15%), *Ruminococcus2* (10%), *Blautia* (8%), *Peptostreptococcus* (7%) and *Veillonella* (5%), and the top taxa in LSCC patients (Figure 7c) were *Blautia* (15%), *Bacteroides* (11%), *Streptococcus* (7%), *Parvimonas* (7%) and *Fusobacterium* (6%). The MSI patients (Figure 7d) harbored *Bacteroides* (18%), *Clostridium_XIVa* (11%), *Coprococcus* (9%) and *Blautia* (8%), while in the MSS patients (Figure 7e), the top taxa were *Bacteroides* (12%), *Blautia* (12%), *Ruminococcus2* (6%) and *Peptostreptococcus* (6%).

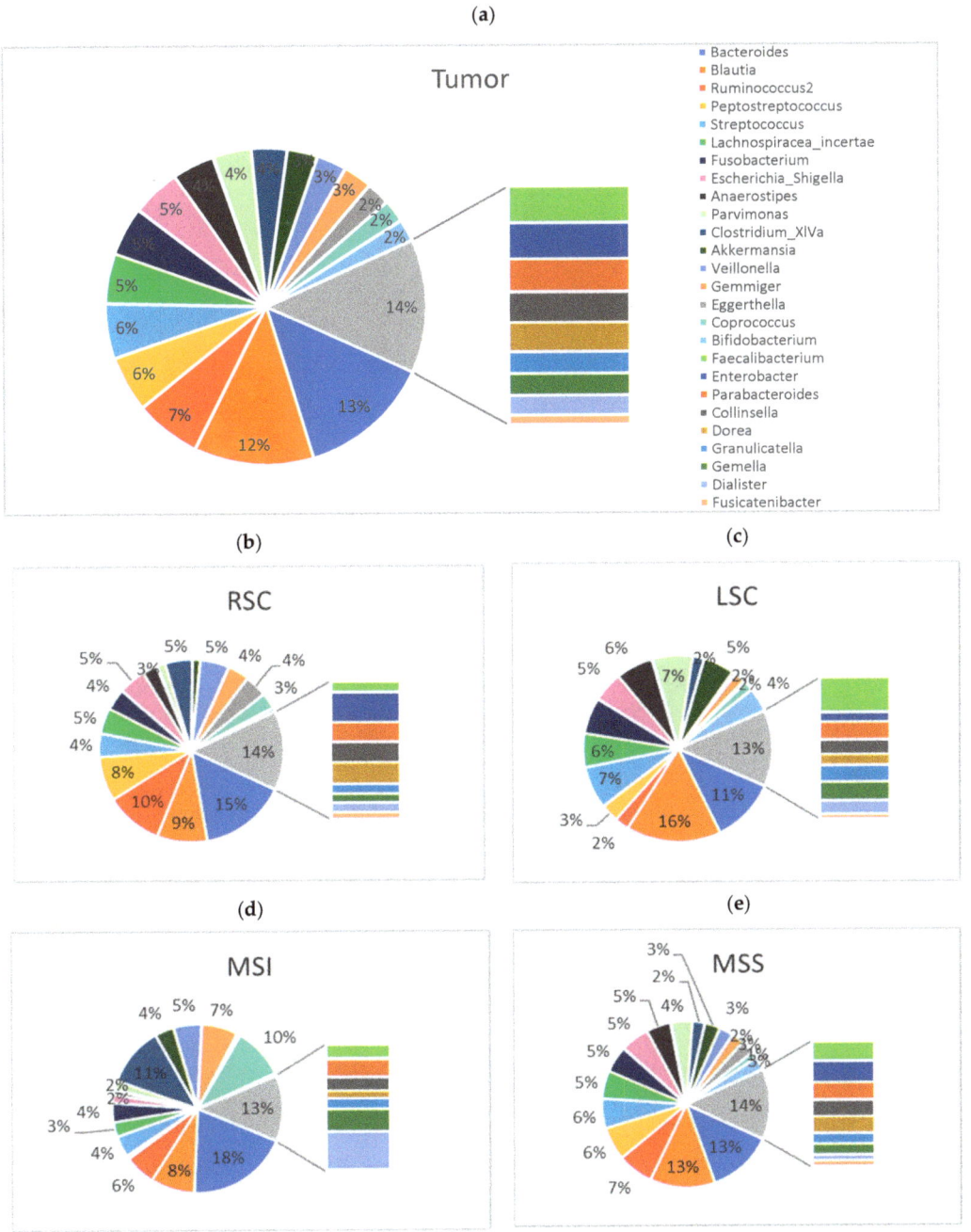

Figure 7. Taxonomic analysis of the tumor microbiome composition: Pie chart showing the abundance profile of the tumor samples (**a**), RSCC subgroup (**b**), LSCC subgroup (**c**), MSI subgroup (**d**) and MSS subgroup (**e**) at the genus level.

A comparison of alpha diversity revealed significant differences between RSCC and LSCC at the genus level. Based on the Chao1 (p value: 0.018981; (t test) statistics: 2.4735;

Figure 8) and Observed (*p* value < 0.05) indices, the alpha diversity was significantly higher in LSCC than in RSCC (Figure 8a). There were no significant differences in alpha diversity based on sex, age, T stage, N stage or differentiation, while for the MSS status, these indices were significantly different (Chao1 index *p* value: 0.014618; (*t* test) statistics: −2.8349, Figure 8b).

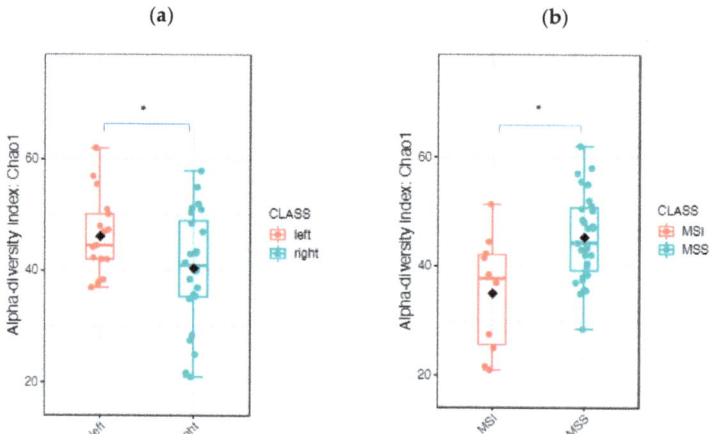

Figure 8. Tumor microbiome diversity comparison: the alpha diversity analysis revealed significant differences between RSCC and LSCC (**a**) and between MSS and MSI patients (**b**) at the genus level (* *p* < 0.05).

The differential abundance analysis, which shows the highest power to compare groups, especially for less than 20 samples per group, revealed a significant increase in the abundance of *Haemophilus* and *Veilonella* in the tumor tissue of RSCC patients, while increased *Bifidobacterium*, *Akkermansia*, *Roseburia* and *Ruminococcus* were associated with LSCC (genus level, *p* value < 0.001, FDR-adjusted *p* value < 0.05). The FDR-adjusted LEfSe analysis revealed two significantly different genera, *Bifidobacterium* and *Romboutsia*, in LSCC patients (genus level, *p* value < 0.05, LDA > 3.0, FDR-adjusted *p* value < 0.05). The original LEfSe analysis revealed 10 significantly different genera: *Bifidobacterium, Romboutsia, Clostridium_III, Ruminococcus, Anaerostipes, Akkermansia, Clostridium_sensu_stricto* and *Asaccharobacter* in LSC patients and *Haemophilus* and *Veillonella* in RSCC patients (genus level, *p* value < 0.05, LDA > 3.0). In regard to MSS status, the original LEfSe analysis revealed seven significantly different genera: *Asaccharobacter, Actinomyces, Eubacterium, Pseudoflavonifractor, Fusicatenibacter* and *Anaerostipes* in tumor specimens from the MSS patients and *Clostridium_III* in tumor tissue from the MSI patients (genus level, *p* value < 0.05, LDA > 3.0). The FDR-adjusted LEfSe revealed no significant differences. The abundances of *Fusobacterium, Peptostreptococcus* and *Desulfotomaculum* were significantly different in grade 3 tumor specimens (original LEfSe, genus level, *p* value < 0.05, LDA > 3.0), but no significant differences were identified based on the FDR-adjusted *p* value (<0.05).

2.2.4. The Microbiome of the Terminal Ileum: Tumor-Associated Alterations

We next assessed the general ileum landscape (Figure 9). The most abundant phylum was Firmicutes, followed by Bacteroidetes and Proteobacteria. The top 5 taxa at the family level were *Lachnospiraceae* (32%), *Streptococcaceae* (18%), *Bacteroidaceae* (8%), *Enterobacteriaceae* (8%) and *Verrucomicrobiaceae* (6%) (Figure 9a). The terminal ileum core microbiota, defined as genera with a threshold over 50%, are displayed in Figure 10. The typical ileal microbiota is dominated by the facultative anaerobic genus *Streptococcus* and the strict anaerobic genera *Bacteroides, Lachnospiraceae_incertae_sedis* and *Clostridium cluster XIV*.

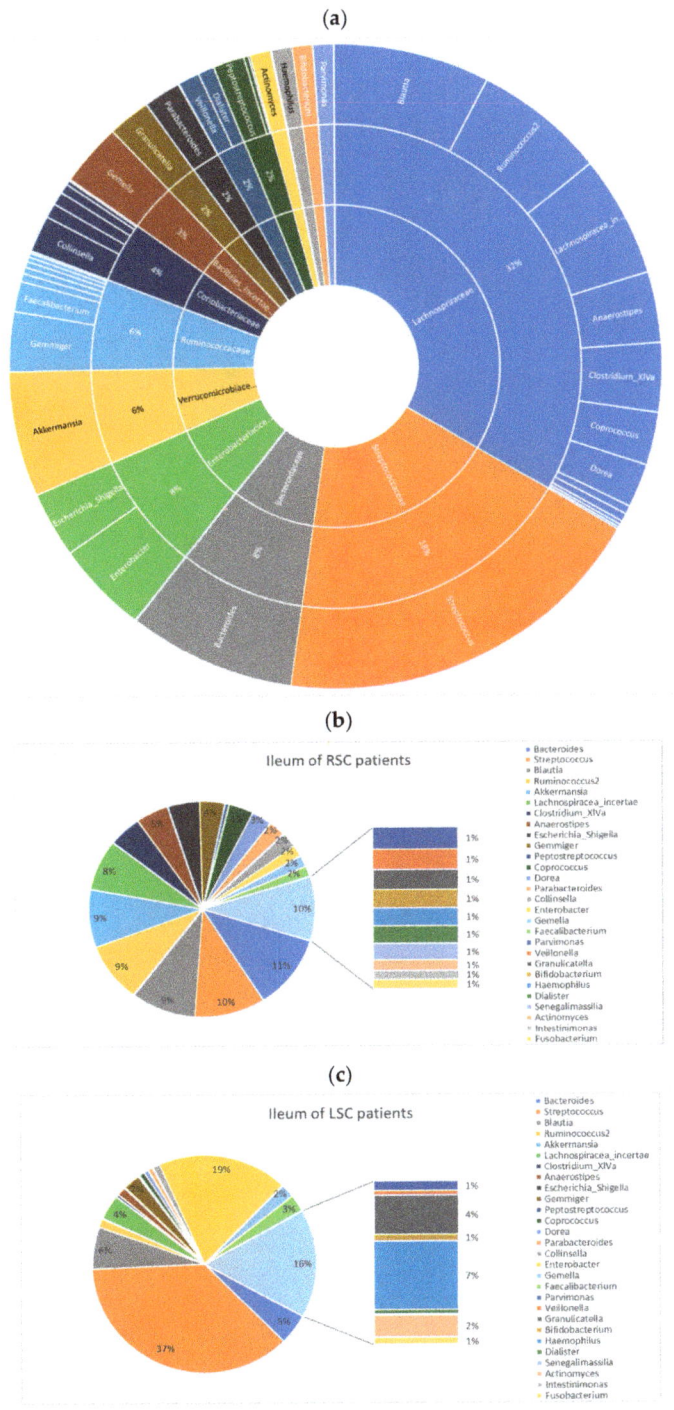

Figure 9. Cont.

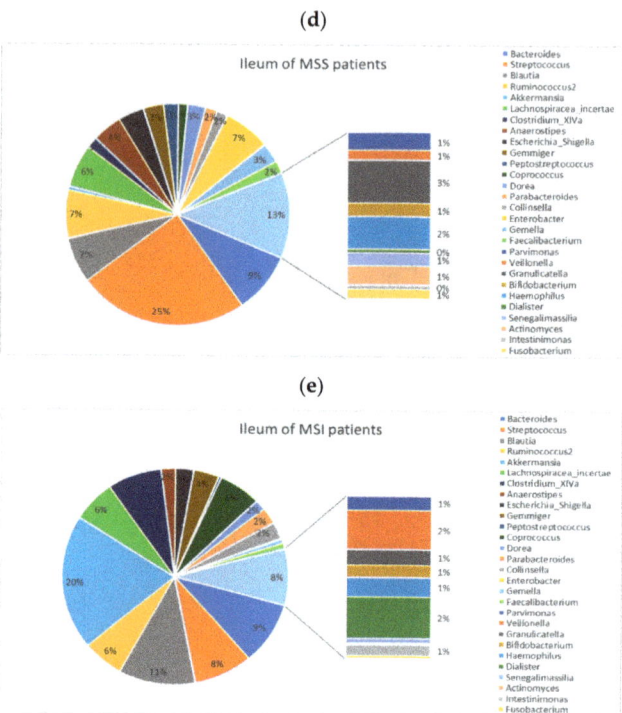

Figure 9. The ileal microbiome profile, taxonomic analysis: (**a**) Pie chart of the microbiome abundance profile of the terminal ileum. The inner circle represents the family level, and the outer circle represents the genus level. Microbiome profiles classified according to tumor location and MSS status: RSCC (**b**), LSCC (**c**), MSS (**d**) and MSI (**e**).

From five LSCC patients, we also had specimens of the terminal ileum. In these patients, the top taxa at the genus level were *Streptococcus* (37% versus 10% in patients with RSC) and *Enterobacter* (19% versus 2% in patients with RSC). Due to the small sample size, no significant differences were observed in regard to sidedness. The core microbiome analysis further revealed that the ileal microbiome of the RSCC and LSCC patients as well as of the MSS and MSI patients harbored a diverse core microbiome (Figure 10c,d). The differential abundance analysis with the highest power to compare groups, especially for less than 20 samples per group, revealed five significantly different features for MSS status: *Enterobacter*, *Actinomyces* and *Streptococcus* for the MSS patients and *Eisenbergiella* and *Parasutterella* for the MSI patients. The original LEfSe analysis revealed three significantly different features, *Actinomyces*, *Abiotrophia* and *Atopobium*, in the MSS patients (p value < 0.05, LDA > 3.0), but the FDR-adjusted p values revealed no differences.

Between the ileal samples and preoperative stool samples, the alpha (Observed index p value < 0.01, [t test] statistics: -2.61) and beta diversity (PCoA Jensen–Shannon (PERMANOVA) F value: 18.525, R-squared: 0.23592, p value < 0.001) clustered significantly differently (Supplementary Figure S3). The LEfSe analysis revealed 23 genera with a significantly different abundance (p value < 0.05, LDA > 3.0, FDR-adjusted p value < 0.05, Supplementary Figure S4).

Next, we compared ileal samples and tumor tissue and interestingly did not reveal a significant difference in the alpha and beta diversity (Figure 11b). The original LEfSe analysis revealed only one significantly different abundant genus, *Atopobium* (p value < 0.05, LDA > 3.0), in specimens of the terminal ileum, and the FRD-adjusted analysis (<0.05) revealed no significant differences.

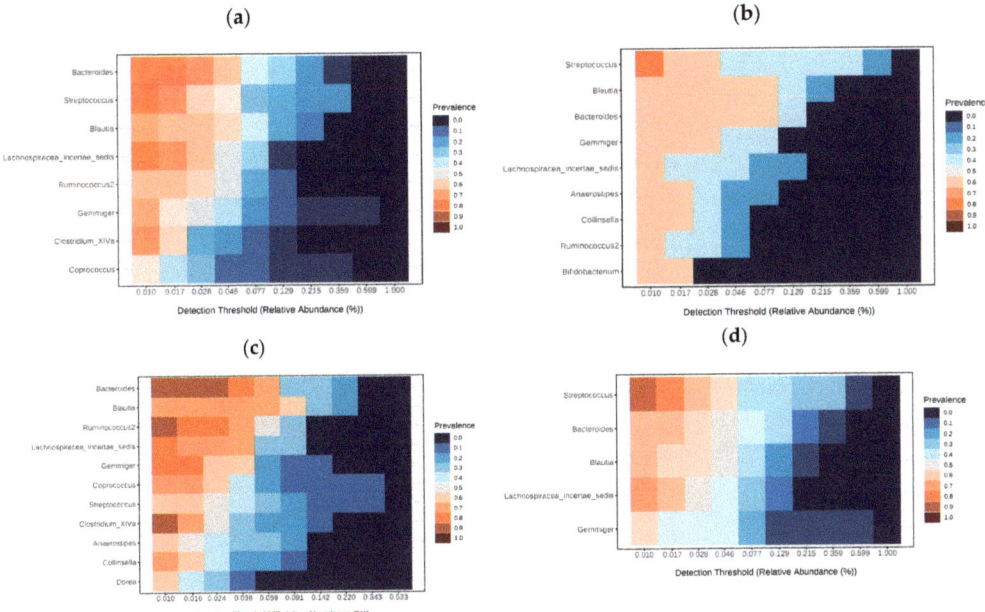

Figure 10. Heatmap of the core microbiome of the terminal ileum (defined as genera present in >50% of samples), based on tumor location: RSCC (**a**) and LSCC (**b**), and on MSS status: MSI (**c**) and MSS (**d**).

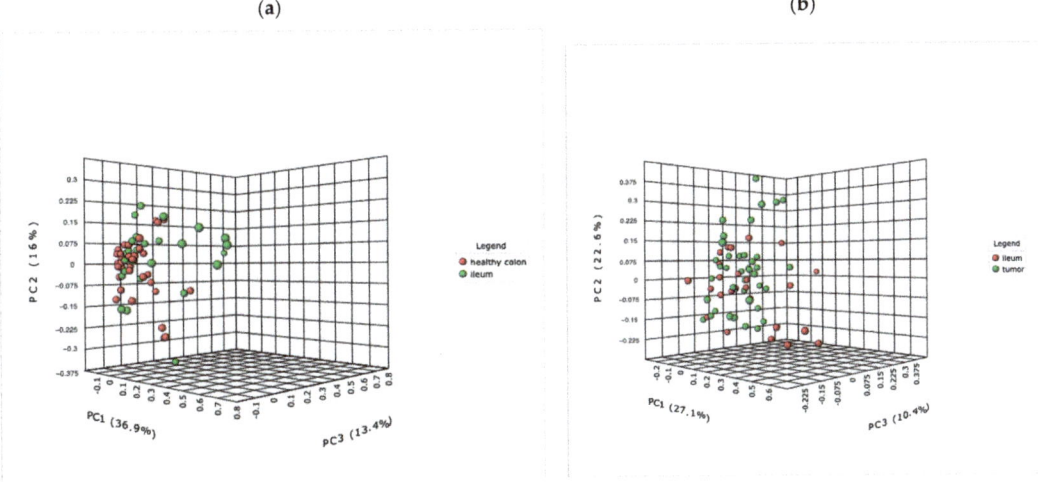

Figure 11. The tumor microbiome–ileal microbiome association: PCoA using Jensen–Shannon divergence of beta diversity between ileal and healthy colon tissue was significantly different, p value < 0.05 (**a**), while no significant differences were observed between ileal samples and tumor samples (**b**).

Additionally, between the ileal samples and healthy colon tissue samples, no significant differences in alpha diversity were observed, while the beta diversity was significantly different (PCoA Jensen–Shannon (PERMANOVA) F value: 3.8652, R-squared: 0.063505,

p value < 0.03; [PERMDISP] F value 4.7804, p value < 0.03; Figure 11a). The LEfSe analysis revealed three genera with significantly different abundances in specimens of the terminal ileum: *Streptococcus, Gemella* and *Granulicatella* (p value < 0.05, LDA > 3.0).

2.2.5. The Stool Microbiome Structure: Sequential Analysis before and after Surgery Revealed Major Changes

Due to bowel preparation, perioperative antibiotic prophylaxis and surgery, the stool microbiome underwent major changes before and after surgery. The ratio between *Firmicutes* and *Bacteroidetes* (regarded as dysbiosis) was decreased: the preoperative stool samples harbored 41% *Firmicutes* and 51% *Bacteroides*, while the postoperative samples consisted of 29% *Firmicutes* and 60% *Bacteroides* (Figure 12a). The microbiome composition differed strikingly at the genus level between the timepoints (beta diversity analysis (PERMANOVA) F value: 14.506; R-squared: 0.18019; p value < 0.001) (Figure 12c). Bacterial richness and evenness were significantly lower in the postoperative stool samples, and the postoperative stool samples were characterized by a significant increase in the abundance of *Enterococcus* (p value < 2.20×10^9), LDA −5.84), a lactic-acid-producing bacterial genus that includes potentially pathogenic strains.

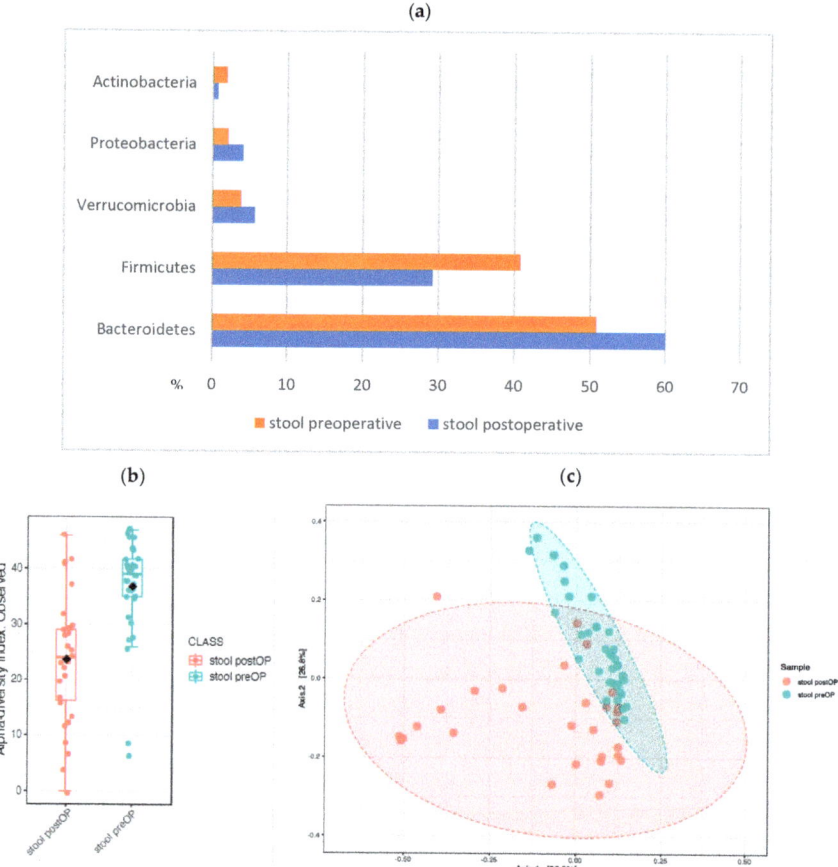

Figure 12. The stool microbiome preoperative and postoperative showed major differences: (**a**) Phylum level abundance profile of preoperative and postoperative samples. Comparison of pre- and postoperative stool revealed significant differences at the genus level: (**b**) alpha diversity and (**c**) beta diversity, (p < 0.001).

3. Discussion

To date, CC and RC are regarded as a single disease entity, termed CRC. Biologically, CRC is a heterogeneous group of tumors, characterized by high interpatient and intratumor heterogeneity with variable clinical features and outcomes. Tumor sidedness (CC versus RC) is one aspect of heterogeneity, and it correlates with distinct biological and molecular characteristics, as well as with different disease management strategies. In surgical clinical oncology, for decades researchers have been becoming aware of the fact that CC and RC are different diseases, based on their surgical procedures and challenges, as well as complication rates and local recurrence patterns.

We believe that understanding CRC heterogeneity and regarding CC and RC as two different tumor entities is fundamental to overcoming the inconsistent study results and the heterogeneous nature of microbiomes. Thus, our prospective, observational study aimed to characterize the microbiome landscape of different body sites in patients with treatment-naive CC. Moreover, we correlated the microbiome with sidedness (RSCC versus LSCC) and other clinicopathologic features of tumor progression (such as stage, lymph node involvement and tumor grade). Right or extended right hemicolectomy with complete mesocolic excision involves the resection of the tumor along with nonmalignant tissues, including the terminal ileum. These procedures provide surgical access to the ileal lumen. Studies investigating the bacterial composition of CC via a comparison of matched samples from multiple locations in the body, such as feces, tumor tissue and normal-healthy mucosa tissue, are rare and have reported inconsistent results. As mentioned before, one reason might be that the majority of these studies combined CC and RC samples as CRC for their analyses. Furthermore, analyzing the gut microbiome using stools does not capture all the microbes in the gut, in particular mucosally adherent microbes and microbes in the small intestine (ileal microbiota). Most of our knowledge has been derived from studies of ileal biopsies during colonoscopies or naso-ileal catheters. However, data must be interpreted cautiously because accessing the ileal microbiome via retrograde examinations is prone to contamination [34,35,40,42–45]. The ileal microbiota is oral-like and more variable than its colonic counterpart, and across several studies, the ileal core microbiome is constituted by *Firmicutes*, *Proteobacteria* and *Actinobacteria*. Villmones et al. reported the ileal microbiome of 27 patients based on samples collected during radical cystectomies with urinary diversion. They demonstrated that the distal part of the ileum harbors a distinct niche that differs from the colonic flora. The REIMAGINE study revealed that the stool microbiome was a good proxy for that of the large intestine but differed substantially from that of the small intestine [19]. The Zitvogel and Roberti group recently reported that the ileal immune tonus was affected by colonic carcinogenesis in RSCC, indicated by the fact that the growth of heterotopic or orthotopic CCs induced this upregulation of ileal immune gene products [34,35]. They also demonstrated that the ileal microbiome governed the efficacy of chemotherapy and PD-1 blockade in CC independent of microsatellite instability. Our study further reveals that the presence of a colonic tumor leads to a more consistent cancer-defined microbiome and shapes the normal spatial heterogeneity existing along the intestinal tract. No significant differences in alpha or beta diversity were identified between the ileal samples and tumor samples. In our cohort, due to operational reasons, in several cases of LSCC, an extended operation was needed, and from those patients, we also collected terminal ileum specimens. Interestingly, also in this subgroup, we did not observe a significant difference in beta diversity between the tumor and ileum. *Bifidobacterium* was significantly associated with LSCC and was found in the core microbiome of more than half of the ileal samples of the LSCC patients. In contrast, *Bifidobacterium* was not found to be a core microbiota in the ileal samples of the RSCC patients. Furthermore, the abundance profile of the terminal ileum revealed that samples from the patients with LSCC harbored 37% *Streptococcus* and 19% *Enterobacter*, while samples from the patients with RSCC harbored 10% *Streptococcus* and only 2% *Enterobacter*. The subgroup of the MSI patients harbored 20% *Akkermansia* and 25% *Streptococcus*, while in the MSS patients, the percentage of *Akkermansia* was less than 1%, and the amount of *Streptococcus* was 8%.

A limitation of the study is that the microbiome shifts might have been induced by the preoperative bowel preparation, but colonoscopy sampling also requires bowel preparation.

However, we know that the fecal microbiota differs from the microbiota of mucosal tissue in regards to oxygen and nutrition needs [46]. Analyzing the bacterial composition, especially the similarity or dissimilarity, between tumors, healthy mucosa and stool from the same individual provides information regarding changes in the microenvironment that have occurred that favor growth in the right- or left-sided colon. Most microbiota identified from human feces belong to the phyla *Firmicutes, Bacteroidetes, Proteobacteria, Actinobacteria* and *Verrucomicrobia*, with 90% belonging to *Firmicutes* or *Bacteroidetes*. Although a disease-specific microbiota signature has yet to be identified, patients with CRC have reduced bacterial diversity and richness compared to healthy individuals. Specific bacteria, such as Fusobacterium nucleatum, as well as certain *Bacteroides fragilis* and *E. coli* species, are known CRC-associated pathobionts. We confirm previous observations that CC tumors harbor orally derived opportunistic pathogens [47,48]. Furthermore, we observed that the stool microbiome only partially reflects the tumor microbiome. We identified 35 genera whose abundance significantly differed between tumor and stool samples. Interestingly, between paired tumor and nontumor healthy colon tissue, no significant differences were observed. We think the presence of a colonic tumor leads to a more consistent microbiota profile. This finding supports previous studies by Murphy et al. and Liu et al., which demonstrated that the microbiotas in tumor tissue and normal mucosa tissue of patients with CRC were similar [49,50]. We further observed that RSCC and LSCC patients harbor distinct microbiomes, characterized by differences in microbial diversity and bacterial taxa. The alpha diversity in the LSCC patients was significantly higher than that in the RSCC patients. Consistent with our results, Phipps et al. showed that patients with RSCC showed fewer taxonomic differences than those with left-sided carcinomas [51]. However, unlike our study, the study of Phipps et al. included rectal cancer patients. Furthermore, we were able to show that the tumor tissue of RSCC patients was characterized by a significant increase in the abundances of *Haemophilus* and *Veilonella*, while increased abundances of *Bifidobacterium* and *Ruminococcus* were associated with LSCC. Overall, grade 3 tumors were significantly enriched in *Fusobacterium* and *Parvimonas*. Little is known about *Parvimonas*, but interestingly, *Parvimonas micra* and *Fusobacterium* have been shown to aggregate and form biofilms in vitro [52,53]. Biofilm formation is linked to inflammatory bowel disease and CC. Due to dysbiosis, biofilm formation occurs within the inner mucus layer, normally free from microorganisms, which could result in direct contact between bacteria and epithelial cells [54]. As mentioned in the introduction, CRC numbers are rising in younger people worldwide. The increased incidence of early-onset CRC can be the consequence of environmental influences (e.g., having a Western diet, food quality and additive-laden food). Early onset is more frequent in left-sided colon. We consider the microbiome of someone developing colorectal cancer at an age over 80 years to be different from someone with early-onset colorectal cancer. Unfortunately, we have too few patients in the "younger age" group for a detailed analysis. In line with the group of P. O'Toole, we recommend adjusting for age to improve the identification of gut microbiome alterations in multiple diseases.

Accumulating evidence suggests a critical role of intestinal dysbiosis in surgical site infections and anastomotic leakage after CRC surgeries. Despite improvements in surgical techniques, new energy devices and intensive care management, anastomotic leakage is still a significant problem in daily clinical practice. We recently linked the microbiome to surgical complications in pancreatic surgeries [18]. In CRC surgeries, the microbiome has also been linked to postoperative complications [55–57]. Many factors beyond geography, diet and lifestyle affect tumors, independent of the microbiome composition, prior gastrointestinal surgery, antibiotic treatment or preoperative bowel preparation regimen. To prevent this type of possible bias, we designed a study in which all patients received the same preoperative bowel preparation regimen on the day prior to their surgery and perioperative antibiotic prophylaxis (most of the studies did not even report this treatment). Furthermore, we excluded upfront confounding variables, such as antibiotic usage, four weeks prior to surgery and systemic conditions related to bowel dysfunction, and only patients who lived in Franconia (Germany) for at least six months were included. We observed that the pre- and postoperative stool microbiomes differed strikingly. Bacterial richness and evenness were significantly lower in the postoperative stool samples. Furthermore, postoperative stool samples were highly dysbiotic and characterized by a significant increase in the abundance of *Enterococcus*, a potentially pathogenic bacterium. These findings suggest that bowel preparation, perioperative antibiotic treatment and surgery had a major effect on the stool microbiome. We aim to begin a new study analyzing the impact of mechanical bowel preparation on the intestinal microbiome in the context of surgery and outcomes.

4. Materials and Methods

4.1. Study Design

This study population consisted of 41 patients from the prospective Erlanger microbiome study, an observational trial approved by the local ethics committee (Protocol Number: 420_18 B). Treatment-naive patients undergoing elective surgery for histologically proven or suspected CC were screened for eligibility for study participation. Patients with antibiotic therapy within 4 weeks prior to surgery, diseases significantly affecting gastrointestinal function (Crohn's, Ileus) and patients who needed emergency surgery were excluded. Each patient received the same mechanical oral bowel preparation and a standardized single shot of a 3rd generation cephalosporine and metronidazole approximately 30 min before the surgical procedure. The participants were prospectively recruited between 2018 and 2019. CC tumor samples and paired healthy mucosal tissue samples of the proximal resection margin (terminal ileum or healthy colon) and distal resection margin (healthy colon or healthy rectal tissue) of the resected specimen were obtained intraoperatively. Preoperative and postoperative stool samples were self-collected by the patients according to a well-explained protocol.

4.2. Sample Processing and DNA Purification

Stool samples were collected and stabilized before surgery and bowel preparation (stool preOp) and after surgery (stool postOp) on days 5–7 using the Omnigene Gut system (DNA Genotek, Ottawa, ON, Canada) and stored at −80 °C until DNA extraction. DNA was extracted from stool using the PSP Stool DNA stool kit according to the specifications of the manufacturer (Invitek Molecular, Berlin, Germany). Specimens of tumor tissue and mucosal tissue were collected immediately after resection, suspended in Qiagen RNA later buffer and stored at −80 °C. DNA from tumor tissue and mucosal tissue of the proximal and distal resection margins was extracted using Dulbecco's phosphate buffered saline (Sigma Aldrich Chemistry GmbH, St. Louis, MO, USA) and the Qiamp Microbiome Kit (Qiagen, Hilden Germany) according to the manufacturer's recommendations. DNA from stool samples was extracted using a PSP® Spin Stool DNA Kit (Invitek Molecular) and LookOut® DNA Erase (Sigma Life Science, St. Louis, MO, USA). DNA was subsequently quantified using a Qubit device (Thermo Fisher Scientific, Waltham, MA, USA).

4.3. 16S rDNA Amplification

The V3+4 region of the 16S rRNA gene was amplified using 10 ng of bacterial template DNA with degenerate region-specific primers (341F: 5′-ACTCCTACGGGAGGCAGCAG-3′ and 806R: 5′-123 GGACTACHVGGGTWTCTAAT-3′), containing barcodes and Illumina flow cell adaptor sequences [58], in a reaction consisting of 25 (stool) or 35 (tissue) PCR cycles (98 °C 15 s, 58 °C 20 s, and 72 °C 40 s) using the NEBNext Ultra II Q5 Master Mix (New England Biolabs, Ipswich, MA, USA). Amplicons were purified with Agencourt AMPure XP Beads (Beckmann Coulter, Brea, CA, USA), normalized and pooled before sequencing on an Illumina MiSeq device using a 600-cycle paired-end kit and the standard Illumina HP10 and HP11 sequencing primers.

4.4. Bioinformatic Processing of the Sequencing Data

For bioinformatic processing, the terminal 15 bases of both forward and reverse reads were removed before merging and quality filtering using fastq_mergepairs and fastq_filter_options from Usearch 10 [58]. Subsequently, merged fastq files were demultiplexed and trimmed using Cutadapt [59]. For 16S sequence determination, the Uparse and Sintax algorithms within Usearch using the Silva 16S rRNA database (v123) were applied. All reads were mapped to OTUs, and an OTU table was created using a Qubit device (Thermo Fisher Scientific). The V3+4 region of the 16S rRNA gene was amplified using 10 ng of bacterial template DNA with degenerate region-specific primers (341F: 5′-ACTCCTACGGGAGGCAGCAG-3′; 806R: 5′-123 GGACTACHVGGGTWTCTAAT-3′) containing barcodes and Illumina flow cell adaptor sequences in a reaction consisting of 25 (stool) or 35 (tissue) PCR cycles (98 °C 15 s, 58 °C 20 s, 72 °C 40 s) using the NEBNext Ultra II Q5 Master Mix (New England Biolabs, Ipswich, MA, USA). Amplicons were purified with Agencourt AMPure XP Beads (Beckmann Coulter, Brea, CA, USA), normalized and pooled before sequencing on an Illumina MiSeq device using a 600-cycle paired-end kit and the standard Illumina HP10 and HP11 sequencing primers. For bioinformatic processing, the terminal 15 bases of both forward and reverse reads were removed before merging and quality filtering using fastq_mergepairs and fastq_filter_options from Usearch 10 [58]. Subsequently, merged fastq files were demultiplexed and trimmed using Cutadapt [59]. The 16S Uparse and Sintax [60] algorithms were performed within Usearch using the silva 16S rRNA database (v123) [61,62].

4.5. Microbiome Analyses

The Microbiome Analyst platform [63,64] was used to calculate alpha and beta diversities and to compare the relative abundance of bacterial taxa. For richness measurements, we used Observed (amount of unique OTUs found in each sample) and Chao1 (also accounting for unobserved species based on low-abundance OTUs). For evenness measurement, Shannon diversity was used, which accounts for both richness and abundance. A p value of <0.05 was considered significant. Beta diversity represents the diversity between microbial communities. Bray–Curtis dissimilarity or the Jensen–Shannon distance was calculated to measure beta diversity, and then, principal coordinates analysis (PCoA) was applied for visualization. For differential analysis, DESeq2 was used for samples less than 20 samples per sample; it is computationally intensive but more robust with low false positive rates, and a p value of <0.05 was considered significant.

Linear discriminant analysis effect size (LEfSe) was used to identify the key microbial taxa associated with the different locations. This analysis integrates statistical significance with biological consistency (effect size) estimation. It uses a nonparametric factorial Kruskal–Wallis (KW) rank sum test to detect features with significant differential abundance with respect to the class of interest, followed by linear discriminant analysis to estimate the effect size of each differentially abundant feature. The original LEfSe implementation uses original p values when determining significant taxa, and an LDA score > 3 (effect size) and a p value of <0.05 were considered statistically significant. Meanwhile, the Microbiome Analyst implementation provides the option to use either original or FDR-adjusted p value cutoffs to identify significant features.

5. Conclusions

In summary, our findings provide the following new insights. RSCC and LSCC harbor distinct niches and have different microbiome compositions. The presence of a colonic tumor leads to a more consistent cancer-defined microbiome and shapes the normal spatial heterogeneity existing along the intestinal tract. The tumor microbiome may contribute towards shaping a favorable microbiome across the large intestine border into the ileum and also in LSCC. The stool microbiome only partly reflects the microbiome landscape of patients with CC. Mechanical bowel preparation and perioperative antibiotics together with surgery resulted in major changes in the stool microbiome, characterized by a significant increase in the abundance of potentially pathogenic bacteria, such as *Enterococcus*.

We believe that regarding CC and RC as two different tumor entities is fundamental to overcoming the inconsistent study results and the heterogeneous nature of microbiomes. Overall, our results have implications for understanding the role and impact of the microbiome in right- and left-sided CC.

Supplementary Materials: The following supporting information can be downloaded at: https://www.mdpi.com/article/10.3390/ijms24043265/s1.

Author Contributions: M.L. and S.K. initiated the study and were responsible for the study design. The authors responsible for data collection were B.K., M.G. and M.L. B.K. performed the experiments as part of her doctoral thesis and was assisted by S.W. The original draft was written by B.K., S.K. and M.L. S.W., K.W., A.D., M.B., C.K., C.G., A.A., O.T., R.S., R.G., A.R.S. and J.T. critically revised the manuscript. S.K. and M.L. are primarily responsible for the final manuscript. All authors have read and agreed to the published version of the manuscript.

Funding: This work was financially supported by the Tumorzentrum Erlangen (ID 3007971).

Institutional Review Board Statement: The study was conducted in accordance with the Declaration of Helsinki and approved by the Ethics Committee of the University of Erlangen (Protocol Number: 420_18 B).

Informed Consent Statement: Informed consent was obtained from all subjects involved in the study.

Data Availability Statement: The data are available on reasonable request from the corresponding author.

Conflicts of Interest: The authors declare no conflict of interest.

References

1. Bray, F.; Ferlay, J.; Soerjomataram, I.; Siegel, R.L.; Torre, L.A.; Jemal, A. Global cancer statistics 2018: GLOBOCAN estimates of incidence and mortality worldwide for 36 cancers in 185 countries. *CA A Cancer J. Clin.* **2018**, *68*, 394–424. [CrossRef] [PubMed]
2. Ferlay, J.; Colombet, M.; Soerjomataram, I.; Dyba, T.; Randi, G.; Bettio, M.; Gavin, A.; Visser, O.; Bray, F. Cancer incidence and mortality patterns in Europe: Estimates for 40 countries and 25 major cancers in 2018. *Eur. J. Cancer* **2018**, *103*, 356–387. [CrossRef] [PubMed]
3. Vuik, F.E.; Nieuwenburg, S.A.; Bardou, M.; Lansdorp-Vogelaar, I.; Dinis-Ribeiro, M.; Bento, M.J.; Zadnik, V.; Pellise, M.; Esteban, L.; Kaminski, M.F.; et al. Increasing incidence of colorectal cancer in young adults in Europe over the last 25 years. *Gut* **2019**, *68*, 1820–1826. [CrossRef] [PubMed]
4. Brenner, H.; Kloor, M.; Pox, C.P. Colorectal cancer. *Lancet* **2014**, *383*, 1490–1502. [CrossRef]
5. Lee, M.S.; Menter, D.G.; Kopetz, S. Right Versus Left Colon Cancer Biology: Integrating the Consensus Molecular Subtypes. *J. Natl. Compr. Cancer Netw.* **2017**, *15*, 411–419. [CrossRef]
6. Stintzing, S.; Tejpar, S.; Gibbs, P.; Thiebach, L.; Lenz, H.J. Understanding the role of primary tumour localisation in colorectal cancer treatment and outcomes. *Eur. J. Cancer* **2017**, *84*, 69–80. [CrossRef]
7. Nagai, Y.; Kiyomatsu, T.; Gohda, Y.; Otani, K.; Deguchi, K.; Yamada, K. The primary tumor location in colorectal cancer: A focused review on its impact on surgical management. *Glob. Health Med.* **2021**, *3*, 386–393. [CrossRef]
8. Kerr, D.J.; Domingo, E.; Kerr, R. Is sidedness prognostically important across all stages of colorectal cancer? *Lancet Oncol.* **2016**, *17*, 1480–1482. [CrossRef]
9. Baran, B.; Mert Ozupek, N.; Yerli Tetik, N.; Acar, E.; Bekcioglu, O.; Baskin, Y. Difference Between Left-Sided and Right-Sided Colorectal Cancer: A Focused Review of Literature. *Gastroenterol. Res.* **2018**, *11*, 264–273. [CrossRef]
10. Xie, M.Z.; Li, J.L.; Cai, Z.M.; Li, K.Z.; Hu, B.L. Impact of primary colorectal Cancer location on the KRAS status and its prognostic value. *BMC Gastroenterol.* **2019**, *19*, 46. [CrossRef]
11. Paschke, S.; Jafarov, S.; Staib, L.; Kreuser, E.D.; Maulbecker-Armstrong, C.; Roitman, M.; Holm, T.; Harris, C.C.; Link, K.H.; Kornmann, M. Are Colon and Rectal Cancer Two Different Tumor Entities? A Proposal to Abandon the Term Colorectal Cancer. *Int. J. Mol. Sci.* **2018**, *19*, 2577. [CrossRef] [PubMed]
12. Song, M.; Chan, A.T.; Sun, J. Influence of the Gut Microbiome, Diet, and Environment on Risk of Colorectal Cancer. *Gastroenterology* **2020**, *158*, 322–340. [CrossRef]
13. Jeon, J.; Du, M.; Schoen, R.E.; Hoffmeister, M.; Newcomb, P.A.; Berndt, S.I.; Caan, B.; Campbell, P.T.; Chan, A.T.; Chang-Claude, J.; et al. Determining Risk of Colorectal Cancer and Starting Age of Screening Based on Lifestyle, Environmental, and Genetic Factors. *Gastroenterology* **2018**, *154*, 2152–2164. [CrossRef] [PubMed]
14. de Martel, C.; Ferlay, J.; Franceschi, S.; Vignat, J.; Bray, F.; Forman, D.; Plummer, M. Global burden of cancers attributable to infections in 2008: A review and synthetic analysis. *Lancet Oncol.* **2012**, *13*, 607–615. [CrossRef]

15. Goodman, B.; Gardner, H. The microbiome and cancer. *J. Pathol.* **2018**, *244*, 667–676. [CrossRef]
16. Hanahan, D. Hallmarks of Cancer: New Dimensions. *Cancer Discov.* **2022**, *12*, 31–46. [CrossRef]
17. Group, N.H.W.; Peterson, J.; Garges, S.; Giovanni, M.; McInnes, P.; Wang, L.; Schloss, J.A.; Bonazzi, V.; McEwen, J.E.; Wetterstrand, K.A.; et al. The NIH Human Microbiome Project. *Genome Res.* **2009**, *19*, 2317–2323. [CrossRef] [PubMed]
18. Langheinrich, M.; Wirtz, S.; Kneis, B.; Gittler, M.M.; Tyc, O.; Schierwagen, R.; Brunner, M.; Krautz, C.; Weber, G.F.; Pilarsky, C.; et al. Microbiome Patterns in Matched Bile, Duodenal, Pancreatic Tumor Tissue, Drainage, and Stool Samples: Association with Preoperative Stenting and Postoperative Pancreatic Fistula Development. *J. Clin. Med.* **2020**, *9*, 2785. [CrossRef]
19. Kartal, E.; Schmidt, T.S.B.; Molina-Montes, E.; Rodriguez-Perales, S.; Wirbel, J.; Maistrenko, O.M.; Akanni, W.A.; Alashkar Alhamwe, B.; Alves, R.J.; Carrato, A.; et al. A faecal microbiota signature with high specificity for pancreatic cancer. *Gut* **2022**, *71*, 1359–1372. [CrossRef]
20. Lynch, S.V.; Pedersen, O. The Human Intestinal Microbiome in Health and Disease. *N. Engl. J. Med.* **2016**, *375*, 2369–2379. [CrossRef]
21. Kim, S.; Jazwinski, S.M. The Gut Microbiota and Healthy Aging: A Mini-Review. *Gerontology* **2018**, *64*, 513–520. [CrossRef] [PubMed]
22. Maffei, V.J.; Kim, S.; Blanchard, E.t.; Luo, M.; Jazwinski, S.M.; Taylor, C.M.; Welsh, D.A. Biological Aging and the Human Gut Microbiota. *J. Gerontol. A Biol. Sci. Med. Sci.* **2017**, *72*, 1474–1482. [CrossRef]
23. O'Toole, P.W.; Jeffery, I.B. Gut microbiota and aging. *Science* **2015**, *350*, 1214–1215. [CrossRef] [PubMed]
24. Rinninella, E.; Raoul, P.; Cintoni, M.; Franceschi, F.; Miggiano, G.A.D.; Gasbarrini, A.; Mele, M.C. What is the Healthy Gut Microbiota Composition? A Changing Ecosystem across Age, Environment, Diet, and Diseases. *Microorganisms* **2019**, *7*, 14. [CrossRef] [PubMed]
25. Scott, A.J.; Alexander, J.L.; Merrifield, C.A.; Cunningham, D.; Jobin, C.; Brown, R.; Alverdy, J.; O'Keefe, S.J.; Gaskins, H.R.; Teare, J.; et al. International Cancer Microbiome Consortium consensus statement on the role of the human microbiome in carcinogenesis. *Gut* **2019**, *68*, 1624–1632. [CrossRef]
26. Elinav, E.; Garrett, W.S.; Trinchieri, G.; Wargo, J. The cancer microbiome. *Nat. Rev. Cancer* **2019**, *19*, 371–376. [CrossRef]
27. Newsome, R.C.; Yang, Y.; Jobin, C. The microbiome, gastrointestinal cancer, and immunotherapy. *J. Gastroenterol. Hepatol.* **2021**, *37*, 263–272. [CrossRef]
28. Vogtmann, E.; Hua, X.; Zeller, G.; Sunagawa, S.; Voigt, A.Y.; Hercog, R.; Goedert, J.J.; Shi, J.; Bork, P.; Sinha, R. Colorectal Cancer and the Human Gut Microbiome: Reproducibility with Whole-Genome Shotgun Sequencing. *PLoS ONE* **2016**, *11*, e0155362. [CrossRef]
29. Hanahan, D.; Weinberg, R.A. Hallmarks of cancer: The next generation. *Cell* **2011**, *144*, 646–674. [CrossRef]
30. Hanahan, D.; Weinberg, R.A. The hallmarks of cancer. *Cell* **2000**, *100*, 57–70. [CrossRef]
31. Zhang, Q.; Zhao, H.; Wu, D.; Cao, D.; Ma, W. A comprehensive analysis of the microbiota composition and gene expression in colorectal cancer. *BMC Microbiol.* **2020**, *20*, 308. [CrossRef] [PubMed]
32. Purcell, R.V.; Visnovska, M.; Biggs, P.J.; Schmeier, S.; Frizelle, F.A. Distinct gut microbiome patterns associate with consensus molecular subtypes of colorectal cancer. *Sci. Rep.* **2017**, *7*, 11590. [CrossRef] [PubMed]
33. Eisele, Y.; Mallea, P.M.; Gigic, B.; Stephens, W.Z.; Warby, C.A.; Buhrke, K.; Lin, T.; Boehm, J.; Schrotz-King, P.; Hardikar, S.; et al. Fusobacterium nucleatum and Clinicopathologic Features of Colorectal Cancer: Results from the ColoCare Study. *Clin. Colorectal. Cancer* **2021**, *20*, e165–e172. [CrossRef] [PubMed]
34. Picard, M.; Yonekura, S.; Slowicka, K.; Petta, I.; Rauber, C.; Routy, B.; Richard, C.; Iebba, V.; Tidjani Alou, M.; Becharef, S.; et al. Ileal immune tonus is a prognosis marker of proximal colon cancer in mice and patients. *Cell Death Differ.* **2021**, *28*, 1532–1547. [CrossRef]
35. Roberti, M.P.; Yonekura, S.; Duong, C.P.M.; Picard, M.; Ferrere, G.; Tidjani Alou, M.; Rauber, C.; Iebba, V.; Lehmann, C.H.K.; Amon, L.; et al. Chemotherapy-induced ileal crypt apoptosis and the ileal microbiome shape immunosurveillance and prognosis of proximal colon cancer. *Nat. Med.* **2020**, *26*, 919–931. [CrossRef]
36. Routy, B.; Le Chatelier, E.; Derosa, L.; Duong, C.P.M.; Alou, M.T.; Daillere, R.; Fluckiger, A.; Messaoudene, M.; Rauber, C.; Roberti, M.P.; et al. Gut microbiome influences efficacy of PD-1-based immunotherapy against epithelial tumors. *Science* **2018**, *359*, 91–97. [CrossRef]
37. Seesaha, P.K.; Chen, X.; Wu, X.; Xu, H.; Li, C.; Jheengut, Y.; Zhao, F.; Liu, L.; Zhang, D. The interplay between dietary factors, gut microbiome and colorectal cancer: A new era of colorectal cancer prevention. *Future Oncol.* **2020**, *16*, 293–306. [CrossRef]
38. DeDecker, L.; Coppedge, B.; Avelar-Barragan, J.; Karnes, W.; Whiteson, K. Microbiome distinctions between the CRC carcinogenic pathways. *Gut Microbes* **2021**, *13*, 1854641. [CrossRef]
39. Kostic, A.D.; Gevers, D.; Pedamallu, C.S.; Michaud, M.; Duke, F.; Earl, A.M.; Ojesina, A.I.; Jung, J.; Bass, A.J.; Tabernero, J.; et al. Genomic analysis identifies association of Fusobacterium with colorectal carcinoma. *Genome Res.* **2012**, *22*, 292–298. [CrossRef]
40. Roberti, M.P.; Rauber, C.; Kroemer, G.; Zitvogel, L. Impact of the ileal microbiota on colon cancer. *Semin. Cancer Biol.* **2021**, *86*, 955–966. [CrossRef]
41. Fidelle, M.; Yonekura, S.; Picard, M.; Cogdill, A.; Hollebecque, A.; Roberti, M.P.; Zitvogel, L. Resolving the Paradox of Colon Cancer Through the Integration of Genetics, Immunology, and the Microbiota. *Front. Immunol.* **2020**, *11*, 600886. [CrossRef] [PubMed]

42. Villmones, H.C.; Haug, E.S.; Ulvestad, E.; Grude, N.; Stenstad, T.; Halland, A.; Kommedal, O. Species Level Description of the Human Ileal Bacterial Microbiota. *Sci. Rep.* **2018**, *8*, 4736. [CrossRef] [PubMed]
43. Booijink, C.C.; El-Aidy, S.; Rajilic-Stojanovic, M.; Heilig, H.G.; Troost, F.J.; Smidt, H.; Kleerebezem, M.; De Vos, W.M.; Zoetendal, E.G. High temporal and inter-individual variation detected in the human ileal microbiota. *Environ. Microbiol.* **2010**, *12*, 3213–3227. [CrossRef] [PubMed]
44. Hayashi, H.; Takahashi, R.; Nishi, T.; Sakamoto, M.; Benno, Y. Molecular analysis of jejunal, ileal, caecal and recto-sigmoidal human colonic microbiota using 16S rRNA gene libraries and terminal restriction fragment length polymorphism. *J. Med. Microbiol.* **2005**, *54*, 1093–1101. [CrossRef]
45. Donaldson, G.P.; Lee, S.M.; Mazmanian, S.K. Gut biogeography of the bacterial microbiota. *Nat. Rev. Microbiol.* **2016**, *14*, 20–32. [CrossRef] [PubMed]
46. Albenberg, L.; Esipova, T.V.; Judge, C.P.; Bittinger, K.; Chen, J.; Laughlin, A.; Grunberg, S.; Baldassano, R.N.; Lewis, J.D.; Li, H.; et al. Correlation between intraluminal oxygen gradient and radial partitioning of intestinal microbiota. *Gastroenterology* **2014**, *147*, 1055–1063.e1058. [CrossRef]
47. Flemer, B.; Lynch, D.B.; Brown, J.M.; Jeffery, I.B.; Ryan, F.J.; Claesson, M.J.; O'Riordain, M.; Shanahan, F.; O'Toole, P.W. Tumour-associated and non-tumour-associated microbiota in colorectal cancer. *Gut* **2017**, *66*, 633–643. [CrossRef]
48. Zwinsova, B.; Petrov, V.A.; Hrivnakova, M.; Smatana, S.; Micenkova, L.; Kazdova, N.; Popovici, V.; Hrstka, R.; Sefr, R.; Bencsikova, B.; et al. Colorectal Tumour Mucosa Microbiome Is Enriched in Oral Pathogens and Defines Three Subtypes That Correlate with Markers of Tumour Progression. *Cancers* **2021**, *13*, 4799. [CrossRef]
49. Liu, C.J.; Zhang, Y.L.; Shang, Y.; Wu, B.; Yang, E.; Luo, Y.Y.; Li, X.R. Intestinal bacteria detected in cancer and adjacent tissue from patients with colorectal cancer. *Oncol. Lett.* **2019**, *17*, 1115–1127. [CrossRef]
50. Murphy, C.L.; Barrett, M.; Pellanda, P.; Killeen, S.; McCourt, M.; Andrews, E.; O'Riordain, M.; Shanahan, F.; O'Toole, P. Mapping the colorectal tumor microbiota. *Gut Microbes* **2021**, *13*, 1920657. [CrossRef]
51. Phipps, O.; Quraishi, M.N.; Dickson, E.A.; Steed, H.; Kumar, A.; Acheson, A.G.; Beggs, A.D.; Brookes, M.J.; Al-Hassi, H.O. Differences in the On- and Off-Tumor Microbiota between Right- and Left-Sided Colorectal Cancer. *Microorganisms* **2021**, *9*, 1108. [CrossRef] [PubMed]
52. Horiuchi, A.; Kokubu, E.; Warita, T.; Ishihara, K. Synergistic biofilm formation by Parvimonas micra and Fusobacterium nucleatum. *Anaerobe* **2020**, *62*, 102100. [CrossRef] [PubMed]
53. Mirzaei, R.; Mirzaei, H.; Alikhani, M.Y.; Sholeh, M.; Arabestani, M.R.; Saidijam, M.; Karampoor, S.; Ahmadyousefi, Y.; Moghadam, M.S.; Irajian, G.R.; et al. Bacterial biofilm in colorectal cancer: What is the real mechanism of action? *Microb. Pathog.* **2020**, *142*, 104052. [CrossRef] [PubMed]
54. Raskov, H.; Kragh, K.N.; Bjarnsholt, T.; Alamili, M.; Gogenur, I. Bacterial biofilm formation inside colonic crypts may accelerate colorectal carcinogenesis. *Clin. Transl. Med.* **2018**, *7*, 30. [CrossRef]
55. Jin, Y.; Geng, R.; Liu, Y.; Liu, L.; Jin, X.; Zhao, F.; Feng, J.; Wei, Y. Prediction of Postoperative Ileus in Patients With Colorectal Cancer by Preoperative Gut Microbiota. *Front. Oncol.* **2020**, *10*, 526009. [CrossRef]
56. Koliarakis, I.; Athanasakis, E.; Sgantzos, M.; Mariolis-Sapsakos, T.; Xynos, E.; Chrysos, E.; Souglakos, J.; Tsiaoussis, J. Intestinal Microbiota in Colorectal Cancer Surgery. *Cancers* **2020**, *12*, 3011. [CrossRef]
57. Liu, Y.; He, W.; Yang, J.; He, Y.; Wang, Z.; Li, K. The effects of preoperative intestinal dysbacteriosis on postoperative recovery in colorectal cancer surgery: A prospective cohort study. *BMC Gastroenterol.* **2021**, *21*, 446. [CrossRef] [PubMed]
58. Fadrosh, D.W.; Ma, B.; Gajer, P.; Sengamalay, N.; Ott, S.; Brotman, R.M.; Ravel, J. An improved dual-indexing approach for multiplexed 16S rRNA gene sequencing on the Illumina MiSeq platform. *Microbiome* **2014**, *2*, 6. [CrossRef]
59. Edgar, R.C. Search and clustering orders of magnitude faster than BLAST. *Bioinformatics* **2010**, *26*, 2460–2461. [CrossRef]
60. Martin, M. Cutadapt removes adapter sequences from high-throughput sequencing reads. *EMBnet. J.* **2011**, *17*, 10. [CrossRef]
61. Edgar, R.C. UPARSE: Highly accurate OTU sequences from microbial amplicon reads. *Nat. Methods* **2013**, *10*, 996–998. [CrossRef] [PubMed]
62. Edgar, R.C. SINTAX: A simple non-Bayesian taxonomy classifier for 16S and ITS sequences. *bioRxiv* **2016**, 074161. [CrossRef]
63. Chong, J.; Liu, P.; Zhou, G.; Xia, J. Using MicrobiomeAnalyst for comprehensive statistical, functional, and meta-analysis of microbiome data. *Nat. Protoc.* **2020**, *15*, 799–821. [CrossRef] [PubMed]
64. Dhariwal, A.; Chong, J.; Habib, S.; King, I.L.; Agellon, L.B.; Xia, J. MicrobiomeAnalyst: A web-based tool for comprehensive statistical, visual and meta-analysis of microbiome data. *Nucleic Acids Res.* **2017**, *45*, W180–W188. [CrossRef] [PubMed]

Disclaimer/Publisher's Note: The statements, opinions and data contained in all publications are solely those of the individual author(s) and contributor(s) and not of MDPI and/or the editor(s). MDPI and/or the editor(s) disclaim responsibility for any injury to people or property resulting from any ideas, methods, instructions or products referred to in the content.

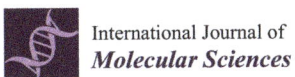

Review

Microbiome and Metabolomics in Liver Cancer: Scientific Technology

Raja Ganesan [†], Sang Jun Yoon [†] and Ki Tae Suk *

Institute for Liver and Digestive Diseases, College of Medicine, Hallym University, Chuncheon 24253, Republic of Korea
* Correspondence: ktsuk@hallym.ac.kr; Tel.: +82-33-240-5826
† These authors equally contributed to this work.

Abstract: Primary liver cancer is a heterogeneous disease. Liver cancer metabolism includes both the reprogramming of intracellular metabolism to enable cancer cells to proliferate inappropriately and adapt to the tumor microenvironment and fluctuations in regular tissue metabolism. Currently, metabolomics and metabolite profiling in liver cirrhosis, liver cancer, and hepatocellular carcinoma (HCC) have been in the spotlight in terms of cancer diagnosis, monitoring, and therapy. Metabolomics is the global analysis of small molecules, chemicals, and metabolites. Metabolomics technologies can provide critical information about the liver cancer state. Here, we review how liver cirrhosis, liver cancer, and HCC therapies interact with metabolism at the cellular and systemic levels. An overview of liver metabolomics is provided, with a focus on currently available technologies and how they have been used in clinical and translational research. We also list scalable methods, including chemometrics, followed by pathway processing in liver cancer. We conclude that important drivers of metabolomics science and scientific technologies are novel therapeutic tools and liver cancer biomarker analysis.

Keywords: liver cancer; microbiome; metabolomics; metabolites; scientific technology

1. Introduction

Hepatocellular carcinoma (HCC) is the second most common cancer-related cause of death worldwide, and, both domestically and internationally, incidence rates are rising. HCC is globally caused by two conditions: alcoholic liver disease (ALD) and non-alcoholic fatty liver disease (NAFLD) [1,2]. Every year, approximately 750,000 novel instances of liver cancer are recorded worldwide. According to population-based interventions, the liver cancer proliferation rate continues to be close to death, meaning that the majority of patients who develop HCC die from it. According to data, the five-year survival rates in the United States have increased slightly to approximately 26%. This expansion is thought to be a result of better surveillance in high-risk patients who can be identified (those who have hepatitis B and C viruses), as well as clinical intervention (resection or transplant) for patients with early-stage disease [3].

Guidelines have been published by a number of organizations, including the National Comprehensive Cancer Network (NCCN), the European Association for the Study of the Liver (EASL), and the American Association for the Study of Liver Disease (AASLD), to normalize the approaches to judgment and treatment [4–6]. The earlier that HCC is detected and treated, the better the prognosis, as is true for the majority of disease processes. The observation of patients who are known to be at a high risk provides the best opportunity for an early diagnosis. Both people who have cirrhosis from any cause and hepatitis B carriers fall under this category [5]. According to the 2012 NCCN guidelines, high-risk patients should receive liver ultrasonography and AFP screenings every six to twelve months. A hepatic nodule larger than 1 cm accompanied by an increasing AFP should be evaluated.

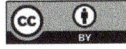

Over the past ten years, the criteria for the diagnosis of HCC have changed. The AASLD, NCCN, and EASL working groups have developed imaging criteria that effectively predict malignancy so as to reduce the necessity for a percutaneous biopsy and its accompanying risks in patients with underlying liver conditions (tract seeding, hemorrhage, etc.) [4,6]. On contrast-enhanced computed tomography (CT) or magnetic resonance imaging (MRI) images, early arterial enhancement and venous phase washout, which are related to the fact that these hypervascular lesions are primarily supplied by branches of the hepatic artery, are imaging markers of HCC. In the context of chronic liver disease, HCC refers to tumors larger than 1 cm in size that have certain imaging characteristics on triple-phase CT or contrast-enhanced MRI.

Escherichia, Pseudomonas, Lactobacillus and other gut bacteria are crucial to the 'gut origin of sepsis' theory. The dominant signs of the gut microbial imbalance are significant increases in gram-negative bacteria such as *Escherichia coli* and the *Atopobium cluster*, which includes the genera *Atopobium, Coriobacterium, Collinsella*, and *Eggerthella*, as well as significant decreases in *Bifidobacterium, Enterococcus,* and *Lactobacillus* species [7]. Moreover, it was discovered that *Fusobacterium nucleatum* was prevalent and abundant in patients with cancer [8].

The previous recommendations required typical enhancement on both imaging modalities (CT and MRI) for lesions between 1 cm and 2 cm to define HCC. Although the imaging standards have changed, only lesions larger than 2 cm and exhibiting typical enhancement qualify as Model for End-Stage Liver Disease (MELD) exemption points for liver transplantation. To more accurately characterize lesions that do not fulfill these criteria on standard arterial and venous phase imaging alone, some facilities have utilized MRI with new contrast agents, such as gadoxetic acid. On T1-weighted (hepatocyte phase) imaging, lesions that could be HCC are darker than the surrounding liver [9]. Despite indications of a better diagnosis accuracy, gadoxetic acid-enhanced MR imaging has not yet altered the paradigm used to determine therapy eligibility. Thus, despite an increased imaging specificity, gadoxetic acid-enhanced MR imaging has not yet altered the diagnostic pattern used to establish clinical prevention [10].

2. Enabling Technologies for Metabolomics Research and Engineering

Microbiome-derived metabolomics or metabolomics profiling refers to the detection of metabolites or small molecules in gut microbial communities that are related to alcoholic liver disease (ALD) and non-alcoholic fatty liver disease (NAFLD) [11,12]. Metabolomics science, a targeted and untargeted profiling method, involves the large-scale study of the metabolic complements of the cells and has the ability to provide adequate coverage of the metabolome. Accurate quantitative information can be provided with wide-spanning technical care for its use in the analysis of metabolic oscillations in the gut microbial environment [13,14]. Metabolomics is a promising platform for the identification of potential responses to stimuli, molecular signatures, and organic compounds that are closely related to metabolic phenotype and therapeutic biomarker discoveries [15,16]. The isotopes of ^{1}H-, ^{13}C-, ^{14}N-, ^{19}F-, ^{31}P-, and ^{43}Ca-rich metabolites in liver cells have led to the development of therapeutic screening applications [11,17].

The metabolomics profiling of microbial metabolites and their computational technologies act as a high-throughput global analytical platform. Metabolomics can illustrate small molecules (molecular weight < 1 kDa) [18–20]. Figure 1A shows the long history of metabolomics. Metabolites, or small molecules, are the fundamental output of combined microbiome and host interactions that may provide signatures of gut-microbiome-mediated ALD conditions.

In Figure 1B, and Figure 1C, the guiding principles of genomics, transcriptomics, proteomics, and metabolomics are listed with targeted and untargeted profiling methods, each with their own benefits and limitations [21–23]. Untargeted metabolomics is focused on the examination of recognizable metabolites and/or metabolomes in biological mixtures, including unknown chemicals. The metabolome is the set of metabolites within a given cell. Metabolome concentrations are widely connected with phenotypic expression [17,24].

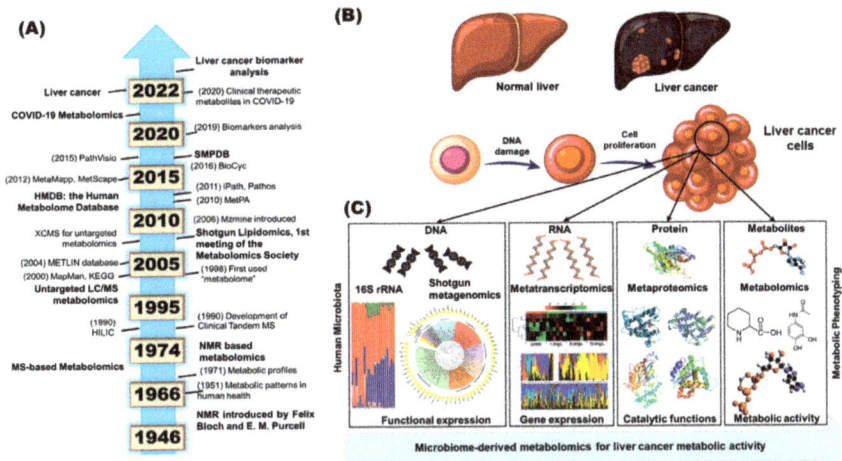

Figure 1. (A) The long history of metabolomics; timeline of major research and development milestones related to metabolomics and their medical applications. (B) Normal liver and liver cancer cells. (C) A schematic representation showing the multiomics cascade of systems biology. The multiomics analysis is influenced by epigenetics, toxicity, disease, and other environmental exposures. Here, metabolic communication within cells is carried out by DNA (metagenomics), RNA (metatranscriptomics), protein (metaproteomics), and metabolites (metabolomics).

In omics sciences, gut-microbiota-based liver therapeutic candidate metabolome screening and metabolomic profiling are significant. Technically, metabolomics has already entered the clinic, with applications in various liver disease screenings. Many metabolomic-signature-based clinical tests can be used to quantitatively analyze low-molecular-weight metabolites in cells, tissue, and/or biofluids [11,25]. Metabolomic signatures have been connected to phenotype expression, which acts as a functional endpoint of a biochemical reaction. The metabolome is the quantification of metabolites that result from the interplay between many domains [26–28]. Microbial metabolomic signature-based liver cancer represents the most 'cutting-edge' example of metabolomics, enabling precision medicine.

Mass spectrometry (MS)-based data analysis and peak identification have been used to explore the regulation of the biological actions of the gut microbiota and host–microbiome relationships by utilizing metabolomics methods [29,30]. The quantitative analysis of microbiome-derived small molecules delivers a functional read-out of cells. MS is a more prominent platform in metabolomics than nuclear magnetic resonance (NMR). MS has become more extensive in host-microbiota analysis because of its high sensitivity, high-throughput discovery, and wide variety of metabolome analyses [31–34]. While NMR can evaluate metabolites in the micromolar range, the utilization of MS licenses the discovery of up to nanomolar concentrations. MS is likewise effectively connected with chromatographic partition, decreasing the impacts of biological samples as well as restricting the complexity of analytes at the time of identification [35–38].

Gas/liquid chromatography (GC/LC) has become the most applied chromatography-MS device for the investigation of both polar and nonpolar metabolites [39,40]. GC/LC-MS has been applied for the examination of various volatile and nonvolatile compounds and for important metabolites after derivatization. Capillary electrophoresis (CE)-MS (CE-MS) is also used for the examination of polar, charged metabolites, as explored in the previous literature [41,42]. LC/GC-MS focuses on changes in mass-to-charge (m/z), with NMR spectroscopy providing the spectral intensities. The analytical characteristics of NMR, MS, Raman micro spectroscopy, immunochemistry, and enzymatic assays are briefly discussed in Table 1. Currently, the NMR and LC/GC-MS methods offer high-quality metabolomic datasets.

In metabolomics investigations, NMR operates with a lower sensitivity than MS-based methods. NMR spectroscopy can quantify and target the metabolites in biofluids, with rapid sample preparation. When the sample complexity can be mitigated, NMR delivers valuable structural information. NMR is valuable for identifying gut microbiota-derived compounds (i.e., amino acids, lipids, fatty acids, organic and inorganic metabolites) [43–46]. However, both MS and NMR allow for small-molecule profiling and the identification of the high diversity of microbial products.

Table 1. Application, analytes, detection, and comparison of top analytical devices for metabolomics scientific technology.

Analytical Devices	Scientific Instruments	Key Functions	Metabolic Applications	Ref
MS		High throughput, high sensitivity/resolution, capable of quickly examining, reduces complexity, improves resolution, specificity, and quantification, allows for isotopic labeling, offers structural information, performed under ambient environmental conditions with the preservation of tissue morphology (DESI-MS).	GC-MS: SCFAs and ketones, carbohydrate metabolites, amino acids. LC-MS: amino acids and their byproducts, bile acids, lipids and fatty acids, sugar metabolites, vitamins, and related compounds. Imaging MS: MALDI/DESI-IMS and nano SIMS.	[31–34,36–38,43,47].
NMR		Affords structural evidence, low-sensitivity compared to MS, high-throughput, permits the quantification of isotopic labeling, delivers spatial data (NMR imaging or MRI).	Sugar metabolites, amino acids and amino acid byproducts SCFAs, vitamins, untargeted analysis, and metabolome finger printing.	[22,23,44,45,48]
Raman MS		3D info, high-throughput, structural data, non-destructive methods, lower sensitivity versus MS and NMR.	This can be united with fluorescent probes and isotopic labeling for the single-cell-resolved assessment of nutrient assimilation.	[43]
UHPLC		High-sensitivity detection	Detection and identification of a broad range of metabolites	[49,50]
Immunochemistry and enzymatic assays	–	Low-throughput, high specificity, may provide spatial information (immunohistochemistry or immunofluorescence).	Eicosanoids, uric acid, serotonin, neurotransmitters, lipopolysaccharide, some vitamins, sugar metabolites.	[51,52]

Abbreviations: DESI-MS, desorption electrospray ionization mass spectrometry; GC-MS, gas chromatography–mass spectrometry; LC-MS, liquid chromatography–mass spectrometry; Raman MS, Raman micro spectroscopy; UHPLC, Ultra-High-Performance Liquid Chromatography; MALDI, matrix-assisted laser desorption; nano SIMS, nanoscale secondary ion mass spectrometry; SCFA, short-chain fatty acid; Ref, References.

Both NMR and MS-based metabolomics have been applied to study the gut microbiota via isotope tracing in nutrient accommodation. Metabolic alterations using isotope labeling remain challenging because of their structural exchange in hosts and various microorganisms and the difficulty of identifying the paths of small molecules and/or metabolites [43,44]. The topographies of MS, nanoscale secondary ion MS, and Raman spectroscopy deliver high-throughput three-dimensional data, which are shared with fluorescent probes and stable isotope tracing to achieve a single-cell resolution within host and gut microbial cells [43,44].

Targeted metabolomics profiling and lipidomic profiling have been used to measure defined groups of metabolites. The methodologies can be defined by the quantity of notable metabolites and the reliability of the quantification of a specific approach. Here, reliability is introduced either as the exactness of entire quantifications, normally transferred in micromolar units, or as accuracy, given by semiquantitative judgments in normalized units [11,24,25]. The best-accuracy approach could be hypothetically accomplished when an isotopically considered internal standard of a specific metabolite is spiked in biofluids during extraction at different concentrations (isotope dilution mass spectrometry). A slightly less reliable technique utilizes an alignment curve of a specific standard spiked at various concentrations, standardized to a spiked constant concentration of an internal standard [26,53]. Table 2 shows the computational tools used for NMR- and MS-based metabolomics analysis in biological samples, focusing on the main breakthroughs in this field.

Table 2. Computational tools used for metabolomic technologies in biological samples.

Platforms	Invention	Ref
MetaboAnalyst	Web-based analytical pipeline tool, all-in-one metabolomics profiling, data collection, pathway enrichments, data analysis.	[24,54,55]
SIMCA-P+	Pattern recognition of PCA, PLS-DA, OPLS-DA, S-plot, and loading plot, multivariate tool, data mining, interactive graphics.	[11,13,56–58]
Chenomx Inc.,	Correction of the spectral data, metabolite profiling, and quantification.	[58–60]
MetExplore	Picturing of biological reaction systems and paths, simplifying the analysis of omics data in the biochemical background, and pathways improvement.	[61,62]
HMDB	Data bank of NMR, LC-MS, and GC-MS packs, metabolites information, structures, and biological properties.	[63–65]
KEGG	Databank of genes and genomes; KEGG ortholog for genes and proteins.	[66]
Reactome	Information base of biomolecular paths: free/open-source data, curated, and peer-reviewed.	[67,68]
Cyc databases	Largest curated collection of metabolic pathways. A wide range of model organisms' data.	[69]
Virtual Metabolic Human	255 diseases, microbial genes, and human and gut microbiome metabolism database.	[70,71]
WikiPathways	Browsable, editable database curated by the research community.	[72]
Metabox	Toolbox for integrating proteomics and transcriptomics data for metabolomics data processing and interpretation.	[73]
Metscape	Cytoscape plugin, metabolomics correlation networks and KEGG-based metabolic networks integrating gene expression and metabolomics.	[74]
ChemRICH	Alternative to biochemical pathway mapping for metabolomic datasets. Not based on biochemistry directly but on structural similarity. The enrichment test is based on the Kolmogorov−Smirnov test (not the hypergeometric test or Fisher's exact test).	[75]
PathBank	Comprehensive, user-friendly resource for metabolic pathways in 10 different model organisms.	[76]
OmicsNet	Multi-omics data integration, biological networks (genes, proteins, microRNAs, transcription factors, metabolites).	[77]
GEM-Vis	The use of metabolic network maps to visualize time-course metabolomic data.	[78]
FEMTO	Combining metabolomic time-series analysis with network data.	[79]

Notes and abbreviations: SIMCA, Soft Independent Modeling of Class Analogy; HMDB, Human Metabolome Database; KEGG, Kyoto Encyclopedia of Genes and Genomics; ChemRICH, Chemical Similarity Enrichment Analysis; GEM-Vis, Genome-Scale Metabolic Model Visualization; FEMTO, Functional Evaluation of Metabolic Time Series Observations; Ref, References.

3. Diagnostics Test of Liver Cancer

Various types of medical testing can be performed to identify liver cancer tumors. However, the following common diagnostic exams are performed:

I. Physical examination: A general practitioner or gastroenterologist can examine the patient to learn about their health history and identify general risk factors for the development of liver cancer. Examinations include those of the skin, eyes, and areas of the abdomen (signs of jaundice). Additional tests could be necessary to identify the cause of symptoms, depending on the results of the initial physical exam [80,81].
II. Radiology tests and imaging: As the name suggests, imaging findings use X-rays, magnetic fields (MRI), or sound waves to provide precise visual scans of internal body regions (ultrasound). Other common tests used to assess liver cancer include CT scans, bone scans, and angiography [82,83].
III. Laparoscopy: For the improved viewing of the liver tissue and adjacent organs, laparoscopic surgeries use a small tube with a camera introduced into the abdomen. Diagnostic laparoscopy is a minimally invasive, low-risk surgical treatment that calls for tiny incisions [84]. An improved understanding of the liver cancer's current stage, assistance in developing a personalized stem cell treatment strategy, or confirmation of an earlier diagnosis can all be achieved with laparoscopy [85].
IV. Liver biopsy: A surgical procedure called a liver biopsy uses a sample of the patient's liver tissue to identify the presence of cancer cells [86].
V. Lab tests and blood panels: Lab tests and blood panels are relatively affordable and efficient tools for checking the health of the body and internal organs, monitoring the success of therapy, looking for cancer indicators, or checking for cancer recurrence [87,88].
VI. Genetic screening for cancer: Circulating tumor DNA (ctDNA) analysis is distinct from previously known conventional diagnostic techniques. Cancer biomarker tests such as ctDNA analysis only need small saliva samples or cheek swabs, as opposed to invasive tissue biopsies [89]. Rapid screening is a reliable method of prognostic marker detection. This method can detect potential metastatic disease very early, monitor treatment, and identify genetic and epigenetic changes resulting from primary tumors [90].

4. Microbiome Research and Engineering in HCC Metabolism

Physiological responses in the host are maintained and coordinated by metabolites produced by the microbiota. The liver cancer processes that HCC may impact through bacterial metabolism, such as these metabolic transportation pathways and their efficacy, must be understood [91]. It is important to comprehend and describe the variety of metabolites that the gut microbiota excretes. Metabolomics has been widely used to illustrate the metabolites produced by gut microbes, particularly in relation to the disease states of the host that they may affect. Metabolomics generally no longer needs to be defined, as we have thoroughly examined this technology [92–94].

In an early study, Nicholson's team discovered significant metabolic differences between germ-free mice and their healthy counterparts for so-called 'cometabolites' such as hippuric acid, which is produced when benzoic acid and glycine are conjugated [95,96]. The gut bacteria produce benzoic acid by converting chlorogenic acid into quinic acid, which is then aromatized [97]. The liver receives benzoic acid via the portal supply, where it is conjugated in the mitochondria by first forming a CoA intermediate and then adding glycine [98].

Phenylacetylglutamine is another instance of a metabolism in which phenyl acetic acid is formed from phenylalanine by the gut microbiota [36] and conjugated with glutamine in the host's hepatic mitochondria [99]. It has been documented that the three aromatic amino acids phenylacetic acid, tyrosine, and tryptophan are all converted into nine aromatic acids via the gut symbiont *Clostridium sporogenes* and circulate in human plasma. These compounds, such as tryptophan-derived indol-3-ylacetic acid, are almost certainly co-metabolized by the host [99].

Dietary flavan3-ol polyphenols, epigallocatechin gallate, epigallocatechin, epicatechin, and catechin may also be sources of aromatic acid metabolites by gut microbiota through intricate oxidation and dihydroxylation pathways that ultimately result in phenylacetic acid, benzoic acid, and catechol [100]. An examination of 143 organic acids frequently found in the urine of healthy individuals revealed that a sizable portion of these were created by the host's microbiota, with some of them being further digested by the host [101]. Figure 2 shows the three-way relationship between the host, the tumor microenvironment, and the microbiota.

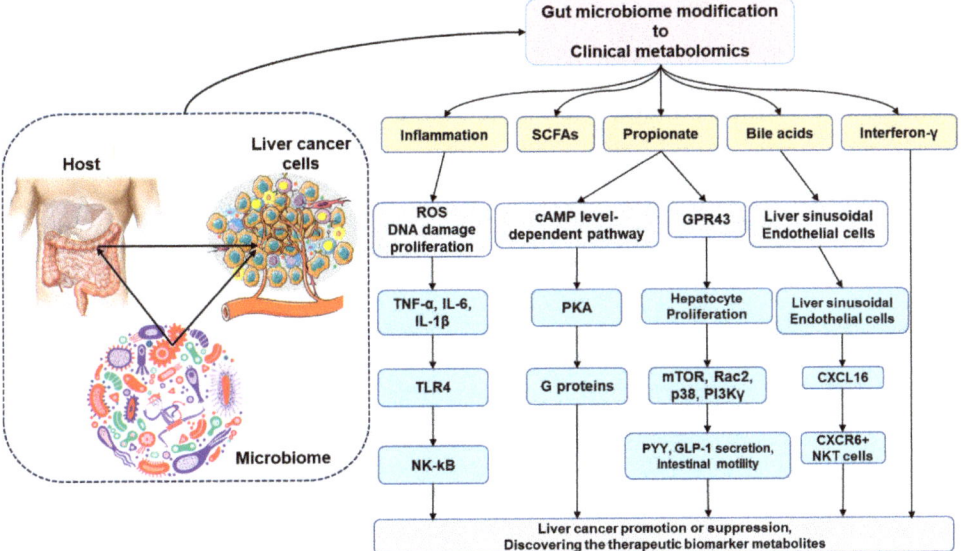

Figure 2. A three-way relationship between the host, tumor microenvironment, and microbiota. The gut microbiome-derived metabolomics target in HCC has been summarized. The host microbiome and metabolic reprogramming for cancer cells and their microenvironment may be related. An altering gut microbiota may boost propionate synthesis, which may reduce the risk of HCC both through a cAMP level-dependent mechanism and by interacting with GPR43. The gut microbiota alteration may result in an anti-HCC impact by boosting the amount of hepatic CXCR6+, NKT cells, and IFN-γ production. Primary-to-secondary bile acid conversion, which is controlled by the gut microbiota, influenced the CXCL16 expression of liver sinusoidal endothelial cells, which in turn affected the accumulation of CXCR6+ and NKT cells. cAMP, cyclic adenosine monophosphate; GPR, G protein-coupled receptor; IFN, interferon; IL, interleukin.

An important group of acidic metabolites generated by the gut microbiota is short-chain fatty acids (SCFAs: acetate, propionate, and butyrate), which are created by gut bacteria during the anaerobic fermentation of plant structural polysaccharides such as cellulose or fiber [102]. The lipopolysaccharide (LPS)-producing genera (*Neisseria*, *Enterobacteriaceae*, and *Veillonella*) were more abundant among liver cancer–HCC, and butyrate-producing genera (*Clostridium*, *Ruminococcus*, and *Coprococcus*) were less abundant. Three more biomarkers—*Enterococcus*, *Phyllobacterium*, and *Limnobacter*—can also be used to reliably detect liver cancer.

In cellular environments, SCFAs represent a sizable proportion of energy metabolites, as it is estimated that they provide 60–85% of an animal's energy needs [102]. In HCC patients with dysregulated fatty acid metabolism, the β-oxidation process of fatty acids is associated with a worse prognosis. The proximal colon of a human contains the largest concentration of SCFAs, where they are both absorbed into the bloodstream and utilized locally by enterocytes [103,104].

In mice with altered gut commensal bacteria, the increase in NKT cells and the suppression of liver tumor growth may both be reversed by colonizing bile acid-metabolizing bacteria (*Clostridium scindens*) and supplementing with secondary bile acids (lithocholic acid or muricholic acid).

The G-protein-coupled receptors GPR41 and GPR43 (free fatty acid receptors) and the niacin receptor GPR109A are only a few of the receptors that can recognize SCFAs, which are present in the colon at concentrations of 50–200 mM. SCFAs can regulate gene expression by inhibiting histone deacetylases in this location and act as signaling molecules that are recognized by particular receptors [105].

5. Microbiome Metabolism for Therapeutic Applications in HCC

Table 3 has summarized the microbiome in HCC. The third most common cause of cancer-related deaths globally is HCC, which carries a heavy disease burden [106]. HCC is notorious for being highly aggressive and is associated with frequent progression and recurrence. Numerous immune checkpoint inhibitors, mainly anti-PD-1/anti-PD-L1 monoclonal antibodies, have been studied and approved for HCC over the past few years. However, only a small portion of patients (20%) benefit [107–109]. To date, there are no known indicators that can accurately predict the clinical outcome of anti-PD-1/anti-PD-L1 immunotherapy [110].

Table 3. HCC-related changes in the microbiota's regulation in animal, rat, and human models. Predominant microbiota present on various sites and their regulation with HCC.

Models	Disease	Implicated Microbiota	Ref
Mice	DEN-induced HCC	Changing gut microbiome	[111]
	DEN-CCL4-induced HCC	Changing gut microbiome	[112]
	STZ-HFD-induced NASH-HCC	*Atopobium* spp. ↑, *Bacteroides* spp. ↑, *Bacteroides vulgatus*↑, *B. acidifaciens*↑, *B. uniformis*↑, *Clostridium cocleatum*↑, *C. xylanolyticum*↑, *Desulfovibrio* spp. ↑ *Mucispirillum*↑, *Desulfovibrio*↑, *Anaerotruncus*↑,	[113]
	HFHC-induced NAFLD-HCC	*Desulfovibrionaceae*↑, *Bifidobacterium*↓, *Bacteroides*↓	[114]
	DMBA-HFD-induced HCC	Changing gut microbiome	[115]
	MYC transgenic spontaneous HCC	Gram-positive bacteria ↑, Bacteria mediating primary-to-secondary bile acid conversion ↑, *Clostridium scindens* ↑	[38]
Rat	DMBA- or DMBA-HFD-induced HCC	Gram-positive bacteria	[116]
	DEN-induced HCC	*Lactobacillus species*↓, *Escherichia coli*↑, *Atopobium cluster*↑, *Atopobium*↑, *Collinsella*↑, *Coriobacterium*↑, *Eggerthella*↑, *Enterococcus species*↓, *Bifidobacterium species*↓,	[117]
Human	HCC	*Escherichia coli*↑	[118]
	HCC	*Cetobacterium*↓, *Proteobacteria*↑, *Desulfococcus*↑, *Enterobacter*↑, *Prevotella*↑, *Veillonella*↑,	[119]
	HCC	*Bifidobacterium*↓, *Bacteroides*↑, *Akkermansia*↓, *Neisseria*↑, *Enterobacteriaceae*↑, *Veillonella*↑, *Limnobacter*↑, *Enterococcus*↓, *Phyllobacterium*↓, *Clostridium*↓, *Ruminococcus*↓, *Coprococcus*↓	[120]
	HCC	Gut microbial α-diversity↓, *Proteobacteria*↑, *Enterobacteriaceae*↑, *Bacteroides xylanisolvens*↑, *B. caecimuris*↑, *Ruminococcus gnavus*↑, *Clostridium bolteae*↑, *Veillonella parvula*↑, *Oscillospiraceae*↓, *Erysipelotrichaceae*↓	[121]
	HCC	*Klebsiella*↑, *Haemophilus*↑, *Alistipes*↓, *Phascolarctobacterium*↓, *Ruminococcus*↓	[122]

Notes and abbreviations: ↑, increased bacterial metabolism; ↓, decreased bacterial metabolism; HCC, hepatocellular carcinoma; DEN, Diethyl nitrosamine; HFD, high-fat diet; NASH, nonalcoholic steatohepatitis; Ref, Reference.

Additional changes to the microbiome occur during the cirrhosis–HCC transition period. The microbial bacteria of *Veillonella, Streptococcus, Clostridium,* and *Prevotella* were more prominent in the cirrhosis patients. *Eubacterium, Alistipes,* and *Faecalibacterium praus-*

nitzii were comfortable in the healthy gut–liver axis [123]. The probiotics are lactic acid bacteria, including species of *Lactobacillus, Streptococcus,* and *Enterococcus,* as well as yeast, *Bifidobacterium, Propionibacterium, Bacillus, Escherichia coli,* and *Bifidobacterium,* which can both encourage the growth of helpful bacteria and inhibit the growth of harmful bacteria [124]. *Actinobacteria* were shown to be more prominent in early HCC vs. cirrhosis [125]. The correct diagnosis of liver cancer may be achieved by using three biomarkers (*Enterococcus, Phyllobacterium,* and *Limnobacter*). Among HCC patients, the abundances of the genera that produce butyrate (*Clostridium, Ruminococcus,* and *Coprococcus*) decreased, while the abundances of the genera that produce LPS (*Neisseria, Enterobacteriaceae,* and *Veillonella*) increased [121]. Figure 3 explains the principal mechanisms of liver cancer and liver damage and the metabolic alterations involved.

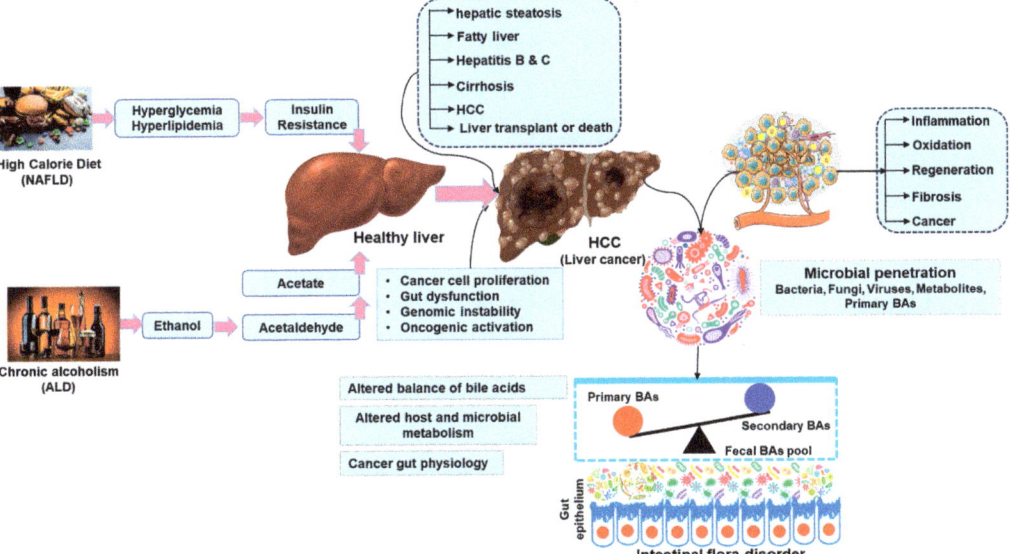

Figure 3. Molecular processes connected to both alcoholic and nonalcoholic HCC. The main risk factors for the development of NAFLD and AFLD, respectively, are a high-calorie diet and excessive alcohol intake. The clinical spectra of liver damage in supporting HCC development in NAFLD and AFLD have comparable molecular mechanisms despite the diverse pathogenic genesis. Within the intestinal tract, microbe-dependent reactions transform primary bile acids into secondary bile acids.

An initial piece of evidence that a gut microbe may influence liver cancer was discovered in mice that had spontaneously acquired *Helicobacter hepaticus* (*H. hepaticus*) infections. The *H. hepaticus* infection has been linked to chronic hepatitis and fibrosis in male BALB/c mice. The *H. hepaticus* is a spiral bacterium that also lives in the bile *canaliculi*, the cecal mucosa, and the colonic mucosa and causes chronic active hepatitis and liver tumors. The *H. hepaticus* is the prototypical carcinogenic bacteria for mice, and experimental infection has already been employed as a model of microbial tumor promotion in the liver [126–128]. Later, it was revealed that *H. hepaticus* intestinal colonization was sufficient to produce aflatoxin B1 (AFB1)- and HCV transgene-induced HCC. This information prompted crucial research. In addition to activating Wnt/-catenin, hepatocyte turnover, and the impaired phagocytic clearance of injured cells, the processes also implicated stimulated NF-B-regulated networks linked to innate and adaptive immunity [129].

6. Liver Transplantation for HCC

The best treatment for both malignancies and the underlying liver condition that most cases of HCC emerge from is generally thought to be liver transplantation. The size and number of tumors determine whether a patient is eligible for a transplant, and standards have been set up to improve outcomes for people with particular types of cancer. The Milan criteria [130], which allow patients with up to three foci of HCC that are less than 3 cm in diameter or one tumor that is less than 5 cm in diameter to receive a liver transplant, are the most often utilized standards globally.

The five-year survival percentage for these patients (75%) was comparable to the survival rate seen in transplant patients at the time who were not cancer patients [130]. The University of California at San Francisco (UCSF) has released its guidelines for liver tumor size regarding tumors measuring less than 6.5 cm, which are observed in one to three tumors. The total tumor diameter should not exceed 8 cm in light of outcome-based evidence with less stringent criteria. There is no negative effect on overall survival in liver cancer [131,132].

Downstaging patients into Milan or UCSF criteria has become a viable method of patient selection as a result of advancements in liver-directed therapy for HCC. What has become clear is that malignancies with a high risk of recurrence after a transplant are those with disease progression despite liver-directed therapy. Scenters can choose patients with better biology and increase patient eligibility without compromising cancer-specific survival by requiring proof of a response to liver-directed therapy prior to the transplant in conjunction with long-term surveillance before deciding to undergo a transplant [133].

7. Systemic Chemotherapy Drugs and Approaches to Improving HCC

The US Food and Drug Administration has approved sorafenib, sunitinib, brivanib, linifanib, sorafenib plus erlotinib, vandetanib, nintedanib, dovitinib, and sorafenib plus doxorubicin for treating HCC. These chemotheraputic drugs act as first-line chemotherapy. Numerous chemotherapeutic drugs have been examined as first-line treatments for patients with advanced HCC. Since its approval, the number of HCC patients receiving treatment with the medicine has increased significantly, irrespective of their tumor stage. Phase 2 findings in patients with advanced metastatic HCC support the use of sorafenib, with the treated group demonstrating a nearly three-month survival advantage over the untreated group. The phase 2 chemotheraputic drugs of brivanib, everolimus, S-1, axitinib, GC33, and tigatuzumab act as valuble drugs for liver cancer. The objective response rate is currently at around 2%, with the majority of the benefit being attributed to the stable disease rate, which was observed in phase 2 and 3 trials to range from 35% to 71%. In the phase 3 study, more than 80% of the participants had previously undergone liver-directed therapy (chemoembolization). Phase 3 chemotheraputic drugs such as lenvatinib, sorafenib plus resminostat, regorafenib, cabozantinib, ramucirumab, and tivantinib (ARQ 197) are promising drugs for HCC [134–136].

Sorafenib is a currently available therapeutic option because the response rate to liver-directed treatment is still around 70%. Sorafenib is a protein kinase inhbiter, including VEGFR, PDGFR, and RAF kinase. When combined with liver-directed therapy, sorafenib was found to show acceptable safety profiles and marginally improved efficacy. The great majority of patients required dose delays and/or reductions [137].

Less persuasive are the most recent phase 3 findings examining sorafenib's advantages in the adjuvant situation following embolization [138]. Sorafenib has not been researched in the neoadjuvant situation before either liver-directed therapy, resection, or transplant. This adds potential periprocedural or postoperative problems that could jeopardize the successful administration of therapy, the life of the patient, or the graft, according to the lessons learnt from the use of various antiangiogenic substances in the neoadjuvanttherapy. For instance, with catheter-based procedures, arterial pruning brought on by antiangiogenic drugs may have an effect on how the small micron particle is delivered into the tumor bed.

There are a number of reasons to refrain from administering sorafenib prior to surgery when liver transplantation is involved. Due to nutritional deficiencies, transplant patients are frequently at a higher baseline risk of wound-healing complications; arterial complications are devastating and frequently fatal, and the nearly 70% stable disease rate seen in phase 3 trials may conceal the underlying metastatic disease, which could make a transplant inappropriate. In other cancer subtypes, antiangiogenic medications and radiation have been successfully combined. Therefore, research examining the combination of stereotactic body radiation therapy plus sorafenib or internal radiation (yttrium-90) plus sorafenib appear appropriate, and information on these combination regimens should become available over the next several years.

8. Conclusions and Challenges for the Future

HCC primarily develops from cirrhosis, and these two diseases cause more than two million fatalities annually around the world. Since liver cirrhosis and HCC have limited available treatments, it is crucial to stop the spread of these diseases as early as possible. In recent years, it has become evident that the gut microbiota, via the gut–liver axis, significantly contributes to the development of HCC. Dysbiosis can be caused by a variety of lifestyle variables, and it has been shown in numerous human trials and animal studies that short-term treatment with probiotics or synbiotics can reverse dysbiosis and consequently enhance liver health. Fatty liver disease is one instance where this is especially accurate. As a means to interfere with the effects of dysbiosis, TLR4 inhibitors are expected to enter clinical development. A possible method of lowering the occurrence of HCC is to prevent the early onset of progressive liver disease through the microbiome. Probiotics and synbiotics, as well as dietary changes, are possible methods for achieving this. As addressed above, the technological advances in liver cancer biomarker profiling have provided a breakthrough in liver metabolomics research.

In addition, challenges connected to HCC metabolism, cellular interfaces, metabolomics, and metabolic changes have been addressed. Future review research initiatives are proposed for improving HCC performances with clinical metabolomics:

- Our review indicates a unique liver cancer–metabolomics connection for therapeutic biomarker invention in HCC.
- Liver cancer remains one of the most difficult disease to treat; however, finding the therapeutic biomarker is possible.
- In single-cell studies of liver cancer, the phenomenon of extensive tumor heterogeneity has been noticed, which creates a major barrier for effective cancer interventions.
- Exploiting scientific systems to disrupt these interactions could establish a viable therapeutic strategy for targeting HCC and stopping HCC evolution, thereby improving treatment efficacy.
- We propose that clinical metabolomics may reflect the evolution of therapeutic biomarkers in a successful liver cancer treatment.

Author Contributions: Conceptualization, R.G.; writing—original draft preparation, R.G.; writing—review and editing, R.G., S.J.Y., and K.T.S.; supervision, K.T.S.; project administration, K.T.S.; funding acquisition, K.T.S. All authors have read and agreed to the final version of the manuscript.

Funding: This research was funded by the Hallym University Research Fund and the Basic Science Research Program through the National Research Foundation (NRF) of Korea, funded by the Ministry of Education, Science, and Technology (NRF-2018M3A9F3020956, NRF-2019R1I1A3A01060447, NRF-2020R1I1A3073530, and NRF-2020R1A6A1A03043026). This work was also supported by the Promotion of Innovative Businesses for Regulation-Free Special Zones, funded by the Ministry of SMEs and Startups (MSS, Korea) (P0020622).

Institutional Review Board Statement: Not applicable.

Informed Consent Statement: Not applicable.

Data Availability Statement: Data are contained within the article.

Acknowledgments: Ki Tae Suk would like to thank the NRF of Korea, the Ministry of Education, Science, and Technology, and the Ministry of SMEs and Startups (MSS) for the funding support. R.G. specially thanks Ki Tae Suk for his support.

Conflicts of Interest: The authors declare no conflict of interest.

References

1. Jemal, A.; Bray, F.; Center, M.M.; Ferlay, J.; Ward, E.; Forman, D. Global cancer statistics. *CA Cancer J. Clin.* **2011**, *61*, 69–90. [CrossRef] [PubMed]
2. Siegel, R.; Naishadham, D.; Jemal, A. Cancer statistics, 2012. *CA Cancer J. Clin.* **2012**, *62*, 10–29. [CrossRef] [PubMed]
3. Simard, E.P.; Ward, E.M.; Siegel, R.; Jemal, A. Cancers with increasing incidence trends in the united states: 1999 through 2008. *CA Cancer J. Clin.* **2012**, *62*, 118–128. [CrossRef] [PubMed]
4. Bruix, J.; Sherman, M. Management of hepatocellular carcinoma: An update. *Hepatology* **2011**, *53*, 1020–1022. [CrossRef] [PubMed]
5. Benson, A.B., 3rd; Abrams, T.A.; Ben-Josef, E.; Bloomston, P.M.; Botha, J.F.; Clary, B.M.; Covey, A.; Curley, S.A.; D'Angelica, M.I.; Davila, R.; et al. Nccn clinical practice guidelines in oncology: Hepatobiliary cancers. *J. Natl. Compr. Cancer Netw. JNCCN* **2009**, *7*, 350–391. [CrossRef] [PubMed]
6. European Association for Study of Liver; European Organisation for Research and Treatment of Cancer. Easl-eortc clinical practice guidelines: Management of hepatocellular carcinoma. *Eur. J. Cancer* **2012**, *48*, 599–641. [CrossRef] [PubMed]
7. MacFie, J.; O'Boyle, C.; Mitchell, C.J.; Buckley, P.M.; Johnstone, D.; Sudworth, P. Gut origin of sepsis: A prospective study investigating associations between bacterial translocation, gastric microflora, and septic morbidity. *Gut* **1999**, *45*, 223–228. [CrossRef]
8. Castellarin, M.; Warren, R.L.; Freeman, J.D.; Dreolini, L.; Krzywinski, M.; Strauss, J.; Barnes, R.; Watson, P.; Allen-Vercoe, E.; Moore, R.A.; et al. Fusobacterium nucleatum infection is prevalent in human colorectal carcinoma. *Genome Res.* **2012**, *22*, 299–306. [CrossRef]
9. Sano, K.; Ichikawa, T.; Motosugi, U.; Sou, H.; Muhi, A.M.; Matsuda, M.; Nakano, M.; Sakamoto, M.; Nakazawa, T.; Asakawa, M.; et al. Imaging study of early hepatocellular carcinoma: Usefulness of gadoxetic acid-enhanced mr imaging. *Radiology* **2011**, *261*, 834–844. [CrossRef]
10. Kudo, M. Early hepatocellular carcinoma: Definition and diagnosis. *Liver Cancer* **2013**, *2*, 69–72. [CrossRef]
11. Raja, G.; Jung, Y.; Jung, S.H.; Kim, T.-J. 1h-nmr-based metabolomics for cancer targeting and metabolic engineering—A review. *Process Biochem.* **2020**, *99*, 112–122. [CrossRef]
12. Dumas, M.E.; Kinross, J.; Nicholson, J.K. Metabolic phenotyping and systems biology approaches to understanding metabolic syndrome and fatty liver disease. *Gastroenterology* **2014**, *146*, 46–62. [CrossRef] [PubMed]
13. Raja, G.; Gupta, H.; Gebru, Y.A.; Youn, G.S.; Choi, Y.R.; Kim, H.S.; Yoon, S.J.; Kim, D.J.; Kim, T.-J.; Suk, K.T. Recent advances of microbiome-associated metabolomics profiling in liver disease: Principles, mechanisms, and applications. *Int. J. Mol. Sci.* **2021**, *22*, 1160. [CrossRef] [PubMed]
14. Xie, G.; Wang, L.; Chen, T.; Zhou, K.; Zhang, Z.; Li, J.; Sun, B.; Guo, Y.; Wang, X.; Wang, Y.; et al. A metabolite array technology for precision medicine. *Anal. Chem.* **2021**, *93*, 5709–5717. [CrossRef]
15. Belhaj, M.R.; Lawler, N.G.; Hoffman, N.J. Metabolomics and lipidomics: Expanding the molecular landscape of exercise biology. *Metabolites* **2021**, *11*, 151. [CrossRef]
16. Zhang, A.; Sun, H.; Yan, G.; Wang, P.; Wang, X. Metabolomics for biomarker discovery: Moving to the clinic. *BioMed Res. Int.* **2015**, *2015*, 354671. [CrossRef]
17. Raja, G.; Cao, S.; Kim, D.-H.; Kim, T.-J. Mechanoregulation of titanium dioxide nanoparticles in cancer therapy. *Mater. Sci. Eng. C* **2020**, *107*, 110303. [CrossRef]
18. Blow, N. Metabolomics: Biochemistry's new look. *Nature* **2008**, *455*, 697–700. [CrossRef]
19. Guijas, C.; Montenegro-Burke, J.R.; Warth, B.; Spilker, M.E.; Siuzdak, G. Metabolomics activity screening for identifying metabolites that modulate phenotype. *Nat. Biotechnol.* **2018**, *36*, 316–320. [CrossRef]
20. Raja, G.; Selvaraj, V.; Suk, M.; Suk, K.T.; Kim, T.-J. Metabolic phenotyping analysis of graphene oxide nanosheets exposures in breast cancer cells: Metabolomics profiling techniques. *Process Biochem.* **2021**, *104*, 39–45. [CrossRef]
21. Roberts, L.D.; Souza, A.L.; Gerszten, R.E.; Clish, C.B. Targeted metabolomics. *Curr. Protoc. Mol. Biol.* **2012**, *98*, 30–32. [CrossRef] [PubMed]
22. Lamichhane, S.; Yde, C.C.; Schmedes, M.S.; Jensen, H.M.; Meier, S.; Bertram, H.C. Strategy for nuclear-magnetic-resonance-based metabolomics of human feces. *Anal. Chem.* **2015**, *87*, 5930–5937. [CrossRef] [PubMed]
23. Paul, H.A.; Bomhof, M.R.; Vogel, H.J.; Reimer, R.A. Diet-induced changes in maternal gut microbiota and metabolomic profiles influence programming of offspring obesity risk in rats. *Sci. Rep.* **2016**, *6*, 20683. [CrossRef] [PubMed]
24. Ganesan, R.; Vasantha-Srinivasan, P.; Sadhasivam, D.R.; Subramanian, R.; Vimalraj, S.; Suk, K.T. Carbon nanotubes induce metabolomic profile disturbances in zebrafish: Nmr-based metabolomics platform. *Front. Mol. Biosci.* **2021**, *8*, 688827. [CrossRef] [PubMed]

25. Angamuthu, S.; Ramaswamy, C.R.; Thangaswamy, S.; Sadhasivam, D.R.; Nallaswamy, V.D.; Subramanian, R.; Ganesan, R.; Raju, A. Metabolic annotation, interactions and characterization of natural products of mango (*Mangifera indica* L.): 1h nmr based chemical metabolomics profiling. *Process Biochem.* **2021**, *108*, 18–25. [CrossRef]
26. Raja, G.; Jang, Y.K.; Suh, J.S.; Prabhakaran, V.S.; Kim, T.J. Advanced understanding of genetic risk and metabolite signatures in construction workers via cytogenetics and metabolomics analysis. *Process Biochem.* **2019**, *86*, 117–126. [CrossRef]
27. Nicholson, J.K.; Lindon, J.C. Systems biology: Metabonomics. *Nature* **2008**, *455*, 1054–1056. [CrossRef]
28. Cavill, R.; Keun, H.C.; Holmes, E.; Lindon, J.C.; Nicholson, J.K.; Ebbels, T.M. Genetic algorithms for simultaneous variable and sample selection in metabonomics. *Bioinformatics* **2009**, *25*, 112–118. [CrossRef]
29. Blanksby, S.J.; Mitchell, T.W. Advances in mass spectrometry for lipidomics. *Annu. Rev. Anal. Chem.* **2010**, *3*, 433–465. [CrossRef]
30. DeBerardinis, R.J.; Thompson, C.B. Cellular metabolism and disease: What do metabolic outliers teach us? *Cell* **2012**, *148*, 1132–1144. [CrossRef]
31. Krautkramer, K.A.; Fan, J.; Bäckhed, F. Gut microbial metabolites as multi-kingdom intermediates. *Nat. Rev. Microbiol.* **2021**, *19*, 77–94. [CrossRef] [PubMed]
32. Lourenço, C.; Kelly, D.; Cantillon, J.; Cauchi, M.; Yon, M.A.; Bentley, L.; Cox, R.D.; Turner, C. Monitoring type 2 diabetes from volatile faecal metabolome in cushing's syndrome and single afmid mouse models via a longitudinal study. *Sci. Rep.* **2019**, *9*, 18779. [CrossRef] [PubMed]
33. Robinson, J.I.; Weir, W.H.; Crowley, J.R.; Hink, T.; Reske, K.A.; Kwon, J.H.; Burnham, C.D.; Dubberke, E.R.; Mucha, P.J.; Henderson, J.P. Metabolomic networks connect host-microbiome processes to human clostridioides difficile infections. *J. Clin. Investig.* **2019**, *129*, 3792–3806. [CrossRef] [PubMed]
34. Zhang, X.-S.; Li, J.; Krautkramer, K.A.; Badri, M.; Battaglia, T.; Borbet, T.C.; Koh, H.; Ng, S.; Sibley, R.A.; Li, Y.; et al. Antibiotic-induced acceleration of type 1 diabetes alters maturation of innate intestinal immunity. *eLife* **2018**, *7*, e37816. [CrossRef] [PubMed]
35. Dettmer, K.; Aronov, P.A.; Hammock, B.D. Mass spectrometry-based metabolomics. *Mass Spectrom. Rev.* **2007**, *26*, 51–78. [CrossRef]
36. Dodd, D.; Spitzer, M.H.; Van Treuren, W.; Merrill, B.D.; Hryckowian, A.J.; Higginbottom, S.K.; Le, A.; Cowan, T.M.; Nolan, G.P.; Fischbach, M.A.; et al. A gut bacterial pathway metabolizes aromatic amino acids into nine circulating metabolites. *Nature* **2017**, *551*, 648–652. [CrossRef]
37. Fujisaka, S.; Avila-Pacheco, J.; Soto, M.; Kostic, A.; Dreyfuss, J.M.; Pan, H.; Ussar, S.; Altindis, E.; Li, N.; Bry, L.; et al. Diet, genetics, and the gut microbiome drive dynamic changes in plasma metabolites. *Cell Rep.* **2018**, *22*, 3072–3086. [CrossRef]
38. Ma, C.; Han, M.; Heinrich, B.; Fu, Q.; Zhang, Q.; Sandhu, M.; Agdashian, D.; Terabe, M.; Berzofsky, J.A.; Fako, V.; et al. Gut microbiome-mediated bile acid metabolism regulates liver cancer via nkt cells. *Science* **2018**, *360*, eaan5931. [CrossRef] [PubMed]
39. Jeon, B.K.; Jang, Y.; Lee, E.M.; Jung, D.W.; Moon, J.H.; Lee, H.J.; Lee, D.Y. A systematic approach to metabolic characterization of thyroid-disrupting chemicals and their in vitro biotransformants based on prediction-assisted metabolomic analysis. *J. Chromatogr. A* **2021**, *1649*, 462222. [CrossRef]
40. Raja, G.; Jang, Y.-K.; Suh, J.-S.; Kim, H.-S.; Ahn, S.H.; Kim, T.-J. Microcellular environmental regulation of silver nanoparticles in cancer therapy: A critical review. *Cancers* **2020**, *12*, 664. [CrossRef]
41. Wolfender, J.L.; Marti, G.; Thomas, A.; Bertrand, S. Current approaches and challenges for the metabolite profiling of complex natural extracts. *J. Chromatogr. A* **2015**, *1382*, 136–164. [CrossRef] [PubMed]
42. Theodoridis, G.A.; Gika, H.G.; Want, E.J.; Wilson, I.D. Liquid chromatography-mass spectrometry based global metabolite profiling: A review. *Anal. Chim. Acta* **2012**, *711*, 7–16. [CrossRef] [PubMed]
43. Berry, D.; Loy, A. Stable-isotope probing of human and animal microbiome function. *Trends Microbiol.* **2018**, *26*, 999–1007. [CrossRef] [PubMed]
44. Röth, D.; Chiang, A.J.; Hu, W.; Gugiu, G.B.; Morra, C.N.; Versalovic, J.; Kalkum, M. Two-carbon folate cycle of commensal lactobacillus reuteri 6475 gives rise to immunomodulatory ethionine, a source for histone ethylation. *FASEB J.* **2019**, *33*, 3536–3548. [CrossRef]
45. Bui, T.P.N.; Ritari, J.; Boeren, S.; de Waard, P.; Plugge, C.M.; de Vos, W.M. Production of butyrate from lysine and the amadori product fructoselysine by a human gut commensal. *Nat. Commun.* **2015**, *6*, 10062. [CrossRef] [PubMed]
46. Nagana Gowda, G.A.; Raftery, D. Recent Advances in NMR-Based Metabolomics. *Anal. Chem.* **2017**, *89*, 490–510. [CrossRef]
47. Rath, C.M.; Alexandrov, T.; Higginbottom, S.K.; Song, J.; Milla, M.E.; Fischbach, M.A.; Sonnenburg, J.L.; Dorrestein, P.C. Molecular analysis of model gut microbiotas by imaging mass spectrometry and nanodesorption electrospray ionization reveals dietary metabolite transformations. *Anal. Chem.* **2012**, *84*, 9259–9267. [CrossRef]
48. Lin, Y.; Ma, C.; Liu, C.; Wang, Z.; Yang, J.; Liu, X.; Shen, Z.; Wu, R. Nmr-based fecal metabolomics fingerprinting as predictors of earlier diagnosis in patients with colorectal cancer. *Oncotarget* **2016**, *7*, 29454–29464. [CrossRef]
49. de Souza, L.P.; Alseekh, S.; Scossa, F.; Fernie, A.R. Ultra-high-performance liquid chromatography high-resolution mass spectrometry variants for metabolomics research. *Nat. Methods* **2021**, *18*, 733–746. [CrossRef]
50. Reher, R.; Aron, A.T.; Fajtová, P.; Stincone, P.; Wagner, B.; Pérez-Lorente, A.I.; Liu, C.; Shalom, I.Y.B.; Bittremieux, W.; Wang, M.; et al. Native metabolomics identifies the rivulariapeptolide family of protease inhibitors. *Nat. Commun.* **2022**, *13*, 4619. [CrossRef]
51. Yano, J.M.; Yu, K.; Donaldson, G.P.; Shastri, G.G.; Ann, P.; Ma, L.; Nagler, C.R.; Ismagilov, R.F.; Mazmanian, S.K.; Hsiao, E.Y. Indigenous bacteria from the gut microbiota regulate host serotonin biosynthesis. *Cell* **2015**, *161*, 264–276. [CrossRef] [PubMed]

52. Kim, M.; Qie, Y.; Park, J.; Kim, C.H. Gut microbial metabolites fuel host antibody responses. *Cell Host Microbe* **2016**, *20*, 202–214. [CrossRef] [PubMed]
53. Raja, G.; Kim, S.; Yoon, D.; Yoon, C.; Kim, S. H-1 nmr based metabolomics studies of the toxicity of titanium dioxide nanoparticles in zebrafish (danio rerio). *Bull. Korean Chem. Soc.* **2018**, *39*, 33–39. [CrossRef]
54. Chong, J.; Soufan, O.; Li, C.; Caraus, I.; Li, S.; Bourque, G.; Wishart, D.S.; Xia, J. Metaboanalyst 4.0: Towards more transparent and integrative metabolomics analysis. *Nucleic Acids Res.* **2018**, *46*, W486–W494. [CrossRef]
55. Pang, Z.; Chong, J.; Zhou, G.; de Lima Morais, D.A.; Chang, L.; Barrette, M.; Gauthier, C.; Jacques, P.-É.; Li, S.; Xia, J. Metaboanalyst 5.0: Narrowing the gap between raw spectra and functional insights. *Nucleic Acids Res.* **2021**, *49*, W388–W396. [CrossRef] [PubMed]
56. Eilers, P. Chemometrics. Data analysis for the laboratory and chemical plant. *J. Chemom.* **2003**, *17*, 360–361. [CrossRef]
57. Tistaert, C.; Thierry, L.; Szandrach, A.; Dejaegher, B.; Fan, G.; Frédérich, M.; Vander Heyden, Y. Quality control of citri reticulatae pericarpium: Exploratory analysis and discrimination. *Anal. Chim. Acta* **2011**, *705*, 111–122. [CrossRef] [PubMed]
58. Raja, G.; Kim, S.; Yoon, D.; Yoon, C.; Kim, S. 1h-nmr-based metabolomics studies of the toxicity of mesoporous carbon nanoparticles in zebrafish (danio rerio). *Bull. Korean Chem. Soc.* **2017**, *38*, 271–277. [CrossRef]
59. Weljie, A.M.; Newton, J.; Mercier, P.; Carlson, E.; Slupsky, C.M. Targeted profiling: Quantitative analysis of 1h nmr metabolomics data. *Anal. Chem.* **2006**, *78*, 4430–4442. [CrossRef]
60. Chang, D.; Banack, C.D.; Shah, S.L. Robust baseline correction algorithm for signal dense nmr spectra. *J. Magn. Reson.* **2007**, *187*, 288–292. [CrossRef]
61. Cottret, L.; Wildridge, D.; Vinson, F.; Barrett, M.P.; Charles, H.; Sagot, M.F.; Jourdan, F. Metexplore: A web server to link metabolomic experiments and genome-scale metabolic networks. *Nucleic Acids Res.* **2010**, *38*, W132–W137. [CrossRef] [PubMed]
62. Cottret, L.; Frainay, C.; Chazalviel, M.; Cabanettes, F.; Gloaguen, Y.; Camenen, E.; Merlet, B.; Heux, S.; Portais, J.C.; Poupin, N.; et al. Metexplore: Collaborative edition and exploration of metabolic networks. *Nucleic Acids Res.* **2018**, *46*, W495–W502. [CrossRef]
63. Wishart, D.S.; Tzur, D.; Knox, C.; Eisner, R.; Guo, A.C.; Young, N.; Cheng, D.; Jewell, K.; Arndt, D.; Sawhney, S.; et al. Hmdb: The human metabolome database. *Nucleic Acids Res.* **2007**, *35*, D521–D526. [CrossRef] [PubMed]
64. Wishart, D.S.; Feunang, Y.D.; Marcu, A.; Guo, A.C.; Liang, K.; Vázquez-Fresno, R.; Sajed, T.; Johnson, D.; Li, C.; Karu, N.; et al. Hmdb 4.0: The human metabolome database for 2018. *Nucleic Acids Res.* **2017**, *46*, D608–D617. [CrossRef] [PubMed]
65. Yogarajalakshmi, P.; Poonguzhali, T.V.; Ganesan, R.; Karthi, S.; Senthil-Nathan, S.; Krutmuang, P.; Radhakrishnan, N.; Mohammad, F.; Kim, T.-J.; Vasantha-Srinivasan, P. Toxicological screening of marine red algae champia parvula (c. Agardh) against the dengue mosquito vector aedes aegypti (linn.) and its non-toxicity against three beneficial aquatic predators. *Aquat. Toxicol.* **2020**, *222*, 105474. [CrossRef] [PubMed]
66. Kanehisa, M.; Furumichi, M.; Tanabe, M.; Sato, Y.; Morishima, K. Kegg: New perspectives on genomes, pathways, diseases and drugs. *Nucleic Acids Res.* **2017**, *45*, D353–D361. [CrossRef]
67. Bohler, A.; Wu, G.; Kutmon, M.; Pradhana, L.A.; Coort, S.L.; Hanspers, K.; Haw, R.; Pico, A.R.; Evelo, C.T. Reactome from a wikipathways perspective. *PLoS Comput. Biol.* **2016**, *12*, e1004941. [CrossRef]
68. Fabregat, A.; Korninger, F.; Viteri, G.; Sidiropoulos, K.; Marin-Garcia, P.; Ping, P.; Wu, G.; Stein, L.; D'Eustachio, P.; Hermjakob, H. Reactome graph database: Efficient access to complex pathway data. *PLoS Comput. Biol.* **2018**, *14*, e1005968. [CrossRef]
69. Caspi, R.; Billington, R.; Fulcher, C.A.; Keseler, I.M.; Kothari, A.; Krummenacker, M.; Latendresse, M.; Midford, P.E.; Ong, Q.; Ong, W.K.; et al. The metacyc database of metabolic pathways and enzymes. *Nucleic Acids Res.* **2018**, *46*, D633–D639. [CrossRef]
70. Noronha, A.; Danielsdottir, A.D.; Gawron, P.; Johannsson, F.; Jonsdottir, S.; Jarlsson, S.; Gunnarsson, J.P.; Brynjolfsson, S.; Schneider, R.; Thiele, I.; et al. Reconmap: An interactive visualization of human metabolism. *Bioinformatics* **2017**, *33*, 605–607. [CrossRef]
71. Noronha, A.; Modamio, J.; Jarosz, Y.; Guerard, E.; Sompairac, N.; Preciat, G.; Danielsdottir, A.D.; Krecke, M.; Merten, D.; Haraldsdottir, H.S.; et al. The virtual metabolic human database: Integrating human and gut microbiome metabolism with nutrition and disease. *Nucleic Acids Res.* **2019**, *47*, D614–D624. [CrossRef] [PubMed]
72. Slenter, D.N.; Kutmon, M.; Hanspers, K.; Riutta, A.; Windsor, J.; Nunes, N.; Melius, J.; Cirillo, E.; Coort, S.L.; Digles, D.; et al. Wikipathways: A multifaceted pathway database bridging metabolomics to other omics research. *Nucleic Acids Res.* **2018**, *46*, D661–D667. [CrossRef] [PubMed]
73. Wanichthanarak, K.; Fan, S.; Grapov, D.; Barupal, D.K.; Fiehn, O. Metabox: A toolbox for metabolomic data analysis, interpretation and integrative exploration. *PLoS ONE* **2017**, *12*, e0171046. [CrossRef] [PubMed]
74. Karnovsky, A.; Weymouth, T.; Hull, T.; Tarcea, V.G.; Scardoni, G.; Laudanna, C.; Sartor, M.A.; Stringer, K.A.; Jagadish, H.V.; Burant, C.; et al. Metscape 2 bioinformatics tool for the analysis and visualization of metabolomics and gene expression data. *Bioinformatics* **2012**, *28*, 373–380. [CrossRef] [PubMed]
75. Barupal, D.K.; Fiehn, O. Chemical similarity enrichment analysis (chemrich) as alternative to biochemical pathway mapping for metabolomic datasets. *Sci. Rep.* **2017**, *7*, 14567. [CrossRef] [PubMed]
76. Wishart, D.S.; Li, C.; Marcu, A.; Badran, H.; Pon, A.; Budinski, Z.; Patron, J.; Lipton, D.; Cao, X.; Oler, E.; et al. Pathbank: A comprehensive pathway database for model organisms. *Nucleic Acids Res.* **2020**, *48*, D470–D478. [CrossRef] [PubMed]
77. Zhou, G.; Xia, J. Omicsnet: A web-based tool for creation and visual analysis of biological networks in 3d space. *Nucleic Acids Res.* **2018**, *46*, W514–W522. [CrossRef] [PubMed]

78. Buchweitz, L.F.; Yurkovich, J.T.; Blessing, C.; Kohler, V.; Schwarzkopf, F.; King, Z.A.; Yang, L.; Johannsson, F.; Sigurjonsson, O.E.; Rolfsson, O.; et al. Visualizing metabolic network dynamics through time-series metabolomic data. *BMC Bioinform.* **2020**, *21*, 130. [CrossRef]
79. Nagele, T.; Furtauer, L.; Nagler, M.; Weiszmann, J.; Weckwerth, W. A strategy for functional interpretation of metabolomic time series data in context of metabolic network information. *Front. Mol. Biosci.* **2016**, *3*, 6. [CrossRef]
80. Sakaue, M.; Sugimura, K.; Masuzawa, T.; Takeno, A.; Katsuyama, S.; Shinnke, G.; Ikeshima, R.; Kawai, K.; Hiraki, M.; Katsura, Y.; et al. Long-term survival of her2 positive gastric cancer patient with multiple liver metastases who obtained pathological complete response after systemic chemotherapy: A case report. *Int. J. Surg. Case Rep.* **2022**, *94*, 107097. [CrossRef]
81. Xu, M.; Xie, L.-T.; Xiao, Y.-Y.; Liang, P.; Zhao, Q.-Y.; Wang, Z.-M.; Chai, W.-L.; Wei, Y.-T.; Xu, L.-F.; Hu, X.-K.; et al. Chinese clinical practice guidelines for ultrasound-guided irreversible electroporation of liver cancer (version 2022). *Hepatobiliary Pancreat. Dis. Int.* **2022**, *21*, 462–471. [CrossRef] [PubMed]
82. Şahin, E.; Elboğa, U.; Çelen, Y.Z.; Sever, Ö.N.; Çayırlı, Y.B.; Çimen, U. Comparison of 68ga-dota-fapi and 18fdg pet/ct imaging modalities in the detection of liver metastases in patients with gastrointestinal system cancer. *Eur. J. Radiol.* **2021**, *142*, 109867. [CrossRef] [PubMed]
83. Bekki, Y.; Mahamid, A.; Lewis, S.; Ward, S.C.; Simpson, W.; Argiriadi, P.; Kamath, A.; Facciuto, L.; Patel, R.S.; Kim, E.; et al. Radiological and pathological assessment with eob-mri after y90 radiation lobectomy prior to liver resection for hepatocellular carcinoma. *HPB* **2022**, *24*, 2185–2192. [CrossRef] [PubMed]
84. Pedrazzani, C.; Kim, H.J.; Park, E.J.; Turri, G.; Zagolin, G.; Foppa, C.; Baik, S.H.; Spolverato, G.; Spinelli, A.; Choi, G.S. Does laparoscopy increase the risk of peritoneal recurrence after resection for pt4 colon cancer? Results of a propensity score-matched analysis from an international cohort. *Eur. J. Surg. Oncol.* **2022**, *48*, 1823–1830. [CrossRef]
85. Borgstein, A.B.J.; Keywani, K.; Eshuis, W.J.; van Berge Henegouwen, M.I.; Gisbertz, S.S. Staging laparoscopy in patients with advanced gastric cancer: A single center cohort study. *Eur. J. Surg. Oncol.* **2022**, *48*, 362–369. [CrossRef]
86. Hagström, H.; Thiele, M.; Sharma, R.; Simon, T.G.; Roelstraete, B.; Söderling, J.; Ludvigsson, J.F. Risk of cancer in biopsy-proven alcohol-related liver disease: A population-based cohort study of 3410 persons. *Clin. Gastroenterol. Hepatol.* **2022**, *20*, 918–929.e8. [CrossRef]
87. Listopad, S.; Magnan, C.; Asghar, A.; Stolz, A.; Tayek, J.A.; Liu, Z.-X.; Morgan, T.R.; Norden-Krichmar, T.M. Differentiating between liver diseases by applying multiclass machine learning approaches to transcriptomics of liver tissue or blood-based samples. *JHEP Rep.* **2022**, *4*, 100560. [CrossRef]
88. Fujiwara, N.; Kobayashi, M.; Fobar, A.J.; Hoshida, A.; Marquez, C.A.; Koneru, B.; Panda, G.; Taguri, M.; Qian, T.; Raman, I.; et al. A blood-based prognostic liver secretome signature and long-term hepatocellular carcinoma risk in advanced liver fibrosis. *Med* **2021**, *2*, 836–850.e10. [CrossRef]
89. Moy, R.H.; Nguyen, A.; Loo, J.M.; Yamaguchi, N.; Kajba, C.M.; Santhanam, B.; Ostendorf, B.N.; Wu, Y.G.; Tavazoie, S.; Tavazoie, S.F. Functional genetic screen identifies itpr3/calcium/relb axis as a driver of colorectal cancer metastatic liver colonization. *Dev. Cell* **2022**, *57*, 1146–1159.e7. [CrossRef]
90. Calderwood, A.H.; Sawhney, M.S.; Thosani, N.C.; Rebbeck, T.R.; Wani, S.; Canto, M.I.; Fishman, D.S.; Golan, T.; Hidalgo, M.; Kwon, R.S.; et al. American society for gastrointestinal endoscopy guideline on screening for pancreatic cancer in individuals with genetic susceptibility: Methodology and review of evidence. *Gastrointest. Endosc.* **2022**, *95*, 827–854.e8. [CrossRef]
91. McCarville, J.L.; Chen, G.Y.; Cuevas, V.D.; Troha, K.; Ayres, J.S. Microbiota metabolites in health and disease. *Annu. Rev. Immunol.* **2020**, *38*, 147–170. [CrossRef] [PubMed]
92. Beyoğlu, D.; Idle, J.R. Metabolomic insights into the mode of action of natural products in the treatment of liver disease. *Biochem. Pharmacol.* **2020**, *180*, 114171. [CrossRef]
93. Beyoğlu, D.; Idle, J.R. Metabolomic and lipidomic biomarkers for premalignant liver disease diagnosis and therapy. *Metabolites* **2020**, *10*, 50. [CrossRef]
94. Beyoğlu, D.; Idle, J.R. Metabolic rewiring and the characterization of oncometabolites. *Cancers* **2021**, *13*, 2900. [CrossRef] [PubMed]
95. Beyoğlu, D.; Idle, J.R. The glycine deportation system and its pharmacological consequences. *Pharmacol. Ther.* **2012**, *135*, 151–167. [CrossRef] [PubMed]
96. Beyoğlu, D.; Smith, R.L.; Idle, J.R. Dog bites man or man bites dog? The enigma of the amino acid conjugations. *Biochem. Pharmacol.* **2012**, *83*, 1331–1339. [CrossRef]
97. Adamson, R.H.; Bridges, J.W.; Evans, M.E.; Williams, R.T. Species differences in the aromatization of quinic acid in vivo and the role of gut bacteria. *Biochem. J.* **1970**, *116*, 437–443. [CrossRef]
98. Claesson, M.J.; Jeffery, I.B.; Conde, S.; Power, S.E.; O'Connor, E.M.; Cusack, S.; Harris, H.M.; Coakley, M.; Lakshminarayanan, B.; O'Sullivan, O.; et al. Gut microbiota composition correlates with diet and health in the elderly. *Nature* **2012**, *488*, 178–184. [CrossRef]
99. James, M.O.; Smith, R.L.; Williams, R.T.; Reidenberg, M. The conjugation of phenylacetic acid in man, sub-human primates and some non-primate species. *Proc. R. Soc. Lond. Ser. B Biol. Sci.* **1972**, *182*, 25–35.
100. Mosele, J.I.; Macià, A.; Motilva, M.J. Metabolic and microbial modulation of the large intestine ecosystem by non-absorbed diet phenolic compounds: A review. *Molecules* **2015**, *20*, 17429–17468. [CrossRef]
101. Liebich, H.M.; Först, C. Basic profiles of organic acids in urine. *J. Chromatogr.* **1990**, *525*, 1–14. [CrossRef] [PubMed]

102. McNeil, N.I. The contribution of the large intestine to energy supplies in man. *Am. J. Clin. Nutr.* **1984**, *39*, 338–342. [CrossRef] [PubMed]
103. Tan, J.; McKenzie, C.; Potamitis, M.; Thorburn, A.N.; Mackay, C.R.; Macia, L. The role of short-chain fatty acids in health and disease. *Adv. Immunol.* **2014**, *121*, 91–119.
104. Ganesan, R.; Suk, K.T. Therapeutic potential of human microbiome-based short-chain fatty acids and bile acids in liver disease. *Livers* **2022**, *2*, 139–145. [CrossRef]
105. Louis, P.; Flint, H.J. Formation of propionate and butyrate by the human colonic microbiota. *Environ. Microbiol.* **2017**, *19*, 29–41. [CrossRef]
106. Forner, A.; Llovet, J.M.; Bruix, J. Hepatocellular carcinoma. *Lancet* **2012**, *379*, 1245–1255. [CrossRef]
107. El-Khoueiry, A.B.; Sangro, B.; Yau, T.; Crocenzi, T.S.; Kudo, M.; Hsu, C.; Kim, T.-Y.; Choo, S.-P.; Trojan, J.; Welling, T.H.; et al. Nivolumab in patients with advanced hepatocellular carcinoma (checkmate 040): An open-label, non-comparative, phase 1/2 dose escalation and expansion trial. *Lancet* **2017**, *389*, 2492–2502. [CrossRef]
108. Zhu, A.X.; Finn, R.S.; Edeline, J.; Cattan, S.; Ogasawara, S.; Palmer, D.; Verslype, C.; Zagonel, V.; Fartoux, L.; Vogel, A.; et al. Pembrolizumab in patients with advanced hepatocellular carcinoma previously treated with sorafenib (keynote-224): A non-randomised, open-label phase 2 trial. *Lancet Oncol.* **2018**, *19*, 940–952. [CrossRef]
109. Finn, R.S.; Qin, S.; Ikeda, M.; Galle, P.R.; Ducreux, M.; Kim, T.-Y.; Kudo, M.; Breder, V.; Merle, P.; Kaseb, A.O.; et al. Atezolizumab plus bevacizumab in unresectable hepatocellular carcinoma. *N. Engl. J. Med.* **2020**, *382*, 1894–1905. [CrossRef]
110. Kambayashi, Y.; Fujimura, T.; Hidaka, T.; Aiba, S. Biomarkers for predicting efficacies of anti-pd1 antibodies. *Front. Med.* **2019**, *6*, 174. [CrossRef]
111. Yu, L.X.; Yan, H.X.; Liu, Q.; Yang, W.; Wu, H.P.; Dong, W.; Tang, L.; Lin, Y.; He, Y.Q.; Zou, S.S.; et al. Endotoxin accumulation prevents carcinogen-induced apoptosis and promotes liver tumorigenesis in rodents. *Hepatology* **2010**, *52*, 1322–1333. [CrossRef] [PubMed]
112. Dapito, D.H.; Mencin, A.; Gwak, G.Y.; Pradere, J.P.; Jang, M.K.; Mederacke, I.; Caviglia, J.M.; Khiabanian, H.; Adeyemi, A.; Bataller, R.; et al. Promotion of hepatocellular carcinoma by the intestinal microbiota and tlr4. *Cancer Cell* **2012**, *21*, 504–516. [CrossRef] [PubMed]
113. Xie, G.; Wang, X.; Liu, P.; Wei, R.; Chen, W.; Rajani, C.; Hernandez, B.Y.; Alegado, R.; Dong, B.; Li, D.; et al. Distinctly altered gut microbiota in the progression of liver disease. *Oncotarget* **2016**, *7*, 19355–19366. [CrossRef] [PubMed]
114. Zhang, X.; Coker, O.O.; Chu, E.S.; Fu, K.; Lau, H.C.H.; Wang, Y.-X.; Chan, A.W.H.; Wei, H.; Yang, X.; Sung, J.J.Y.; et al. Dietary cholesterol drives fatty liver-associated liver cancer by modulating gut microbiota and metabolites. *Gut* **2021**, *70*, 761–774. [CrossRef] [PubMed]
115. Yoshimoto, S.; Loo, T.M.; Atarashi, K.; Kanda, H.; Sato, S.; Oyadomari, S.; Iwakura, Y.; Oshima, K.; Morita, H.; Hattori, M.; et al. Obesity-induced gut microbial metabolite promotes liver cancer through senescence secretome. *Nature* **2013**, *499*, 97–101. [CrossRef]
116. Loo, T.M.; Kamachi, F.; Watanabe, Y.; Yoshimoto, S.; Kanda, H.; Arai, Y.; Nakajima-Takagi, Y.; Iwama, A.; Koga, T.; Sugimoto, Y.; et al. Gut microbiota promotes obesity-associated liver cancer through pge(2)-mediated suppression of antitumor immunity. *Cancer Discov.* **2017**, *7*, 522–538. [CrossRef]
117. Zhang, H.L.; Yu, L.X.; Yang, W.; Tang, L.; Lin, Y.; Wu, H.; Zhai, B.; Tan, Y.X.; Shan, L.; Liu, Q.; et al. Profound impact of gut homeostasis on chemically-induced pro-tumorigenic inflammation and hepatocarcinogenesis in rats. *J. Hepatol.* **2012**, *57*, 803–812. [CrossRef]
118. Grąt, M.; Wronka, K.M.; Krasnodębski, M.; Masior, Ł.; Lewandowski, Z.; Kosińska, I.; Grąt, K.; Stypułkowski, J.; Rejowski, S.; Wasilewicz, M.; et al. Profile of gut microbiota associated with the presence of hepatocellular cancer in patients with liver cirrhosis. *Transplant. Proc.* **2016**, *48*, 1687–1691. [CrossRef]
119. Ni, J.; Huang, R.; Zhou, H.; Xu, X.; Li, Y.; Cao, P.; Zhong, K.; Ge, M.; Chen, X.; Hou, B.; et al. Analysis of the relationship between the degree of dysbiosis in gut microbiota and prognosis at different stages of primary hepatocellular carcinoma. *Front. Microbiol.* **2019**, *10*, 1458. [CrossRef]
120. Zheng, R.; Wang, G.; Pang, Z.; Ran, N.; Gu, Y.; Guan, X.; Yuan, Y.; Zuo, X.; Pan, H.; Zheng, J.; et al. Liver cirrhosis contributes to the disorder of gut microbiota in patients with hepatocellular carcinoma. *Cancer Med.* **2020**, *9*, 4232–4250. [CrossRef]
121. Behary, J.; Amorim, N.; Jiang, X.-T.; Raposo, A.; Gong, L.; McGovern, E.; Ibrahim, R.; Chu, F.; Stephens, C.; Jebeili, H.; et al. Gut microbiota impact on the peripheral immune response in non-alcoholic fatty liver disease related hepatocellular carcinoma. *Nature Commun.* **2021**, *12*, 187. [CrossRef] [PubMed]
122. Ferrarini, A.; Di Poto, C.; He, S.; Tu, C.; Varghese, R.S.; Kara Balla, A.; Jayatilake, M.; Li, Z.; Ghaffari, K.; Fan, Z.; et al. Metabolomic Analysis of Liver Tissues for Characterization of Hepatocellular Carcinoma. *J. Proteome Res.* **2019**, *18*, 3067–3076. [CrossRef] [PubMed]
123. Qin, N.; Yang, F.; Li, A.; Prifti, E.; Chen, Y.; Shao, L.; Guo, J.; Le Chatelier, E.; Yao, J.; Wu, L.; et al. Alterations of the human gut microbiome in liver cirrhosis. *Nature* **2014**, *513*, 59–64. [CrossRef]
124. Sanders, M.E.; Akkermans, L.M.; Haller, D.; Hammerman, C.; Heimbach, J.; Hörmannsperger, G.; Huys, G.; Levy, D.D.; Lutgendorff, F.; Mack, D.; et al. Safety assessment of probiotics for human use. *Gut Microbes* **2010**, *1*, 164–185. [CrossRef]
125. Ren, Z.; Li, A.; Jiang, J.; Zhou, L.; Yu, Z.; Lu, H.; Xie, H.; Chen, X.; Shao, L.; Zhang, R.; et al. Gut microbiome analysis as a tool towards targeted non-invasive biomarkers for early hepatocellular carcinoma. *Gut* **2019**, *68*, 1014–1023. [CrossRef]

126. Fox, J.G.; Dewhirst, F.E.; Tully, J.G.; Paster, B.J.; Yan, L.; Taylor, N.S.; Collins, M.J., Jr.; Gorelick, P.L.; Ward, J.M. Helicobacter hepaticus sp. Nov., a microaerophilic bacterium isolated from livers and intestinal mucosal scrapings from mice. *J. Clin. Microbiol.* **1994**, *32*, 1238–1245. [CrossRef] [PubMed]
127. Ward, J.M.; Anver, M.R.; Haines, D.C.; Benveniste, R.E. Chronic active hepatitis in mice caused by helicobacter hepaticus. *Am. J. Pathol.* **1994**, *145*, 959–968. [PubMed]
128. Ward, J.M.; Fox, J.G.; Anver, M.R.; Haines, D.C.; George, C.V.; Collins, M.J., Jr.; Gorelick, P.L.; Nagashima, K.; Gonda, M.A.; Gilden, R.V.; et al. Chronic active hepatitis and associated liver tumors in mice caused by a persistent bacterial infection with a novel helicobacter species. *J. Natl. Cancer Inst.* **1994**, *86*, 1222–1227. [CrossRef]
129. Fox, J.G.; Feng, Y.; Theve, E.J.; Raczynski, A.R.; Fiala, J.L.; Doernte, A.L.; Williams, M.; McFaline, J.L.; Essigmann, J.M.; Schauer, D.B.; et al. Gut microbes define liver cancer risk in mice exposed to chemical and viral transgenic hepatocarcinogens. *Gut* **2010**, *59*, 88–97. [CrossRef]
130. Mazzaferro, V.; Regalia, E.; Doci, R.; Andreola, S.; Pulvirenti, A.; Bozzetti, F.; Montalto, F.; Ammatuna, M.; Morabito, A.; Gennari, L. Liver transplantation for the treatment of small hepatocellular carcinomas in patients with cirrhosis. *N. Engl. J. Med.* **1996**, *334*, 693–699. [CrossRef]
131. Yao, F.Y.; Ferrell, L.; Bass, N.M.; Bacchetti, P.; Ascher, N.L.; Roberts, J.P. Liver transplantation for hepatocellular carcinoma: Comparison of the proposed ucsf criteria with the milan criteria and the pittsburgh modified tnm criteria. *Liver Transplant.* **2002**, *8*, 765–774. [CrossRef] [PubMed]
132. Duffy, J.P.; Vardanian, A.; Benjamin, E.; Watson, M.; Farmer, D.G.; Ghobrial, R.M.; Lipshutz, G.; Yersiz, H.; Lu, D.S.; Lassman, C.; et al. Liver transplantation criteria for hepatocellular carcinoma should be expanded: A 22-year experience with 467 patients at ucla. *Ann. Surg.* **2007**, *246*, 502–509. [CrossRef] [PubMed]
133. Hanje, A.J.; Yao, F.Y. Current approach to down-staging of hepatocellular carcinoma prior to liver transplantation. *Curr. Opin. Organ Transplant.* **2008**, *13*, 234–240. [CrossRef]
134. Abou-Alfa, G.K.; Schwartz, L.; Ricci, S.; Amadori, D.; Santoro, A.; Figer, A.; De Greve, J.; Douillard, J.Y.; Lathia, C.; Schwartz, B.; et al. Phase ii study of sorafenib in patients with advanced hepatocellular carcinoma. *J. Clin. Oncol.* **2006**, *24*, 4293–4300. [CrossRef] [PubMed]
135. Llovet, J.M.; Ricci, S.; Mazzaferro, V.; Hilgard, P.; Gane, E.; Blanc, J.F.; de Oliveira, A.C.; Santoro, A.; Raoul, J.L.; Forner, A.; et al. Sorafenib in advanced hepatocellular carcinoma. *N. Engl. J. Med.* **2008**, *359*, 378–390. [CrossRef]
136. Cheng, A.L.; Kang, Y.K.; Chen, Z.; Tsao, C.J.; Qin, S.; Kim, J.S.; Luo, R.; Feng, J.; Ye, S.; Yang, T.S.; et al. Efficacy and safety of sorafenib in patients in the asia-pacific region with advanced hepatocellular carcinoma: A phase iii randomised, double-blind, placebo-controlled trial. *Lancet Oncol.* **2009**, *10*, 25–34. [CrossRef] [PubMed]
137. Pawlik, T.M.; Reyes, D.K.; Cosgrove, D.; Kamel, I.R.; Bhagat, N.; Geschwind, J.F. Phase ii trial of sorafenib combined with concurrent transarterial chemoembolization with drug-eluting beads for hepatocellular carcinoma. *J. Clin. Oncol.* **2011**, *29*, 3960–3967. [CrossRef]
138. Kudo, M.; Imanaka, K.; Chida, N.; Nakachi, K.; Tak, W.Y.; Takayama, T.; Yoon, J.H.; Hori, T.; Kumada, H.; Hayashi, N.; et al. Phase iii study of sorafenib after transarterial chemoembolisation in japanese and korean patients with unresectable hepatocellular carcinoma. *Eur. J. Cancer* **2011**, *47*, 2117–2127. [CrossRef]

Disclaimer/Publisher's Note: The statements, opinions and data contained in all publications are solely those of the individual author(s) and contributor(s) and not of MDPI and/or the editor(s). MDPI and/or the editor(s) disclaim responsibility for any injury to people or property resulting from any ideas, methods, instructions or products referred to in the content.

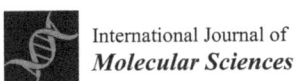

Article

Analysis of 16S rRNA Gene Sequence of Nasopharyngeal Exudate Reveals Changes in Key Microbial Communities Associated with Aging

Sergio Candel [1,2,3,*,†], Sylwia D. Tyrkalska [1,2,3,†], Fernando Pérez-Sanz [2], Antonio Moreno-Docón [4,5], Ángel Esteban [2], María L. Cayuela [2,3] and Victoriano Mulero [1,2,3,*,‡]

1. Grupo de Inmunidad, Inflamación y Cáncer, Departamento de Biología Celular e Histología, Facultad de Biología, Universidad de Murcia, 30100 Murcia, Spain
2. Instituto Murciano de Investigación Biosanitaria (IMIB)-Arrixaca, 30120 Murcia, Spain
3. Centro de Investigación Biomédica en Red de Enfermedades Raras (CIBERER), Instituto de Salud Carlos III, 28029 Madrid, Spain
4. Servicio de Microbiología, Hospital Clínico Universitario Virgen de la Arrixaca, 30120 Murcia, Spain
5. Grupo de Telomerasa, Cáncer y Envejecimiento, Servicio de Cirugía, Hospital Clínico Universitario Virgen de la Arrixaca, 30120 Murcia, Spain
* Correspondence: scandel@um.es (S.C.); vmulero@um.es (V.M.)
† These authors contributed equally to this work.
‡ Lead contact.

Abstract: Functional or compositional perturbations of the microbiome can occur at different sites of the body and this dysbiosis has been linked to various diseases. Changes in the nasopharyngeal microbiome are associated to patient's susceptibility to multiple viral infections, supporting the idea that the nasopharynx may be playing an important role in health and disease. Most studies on the nasopharyngeal microbiome have focused on a specific period in the lifespan, such as infancy or the old age, or have other limitations such as low sample size. Therefore, detailed studies analyzing the age- and sex-associated changes in the nasopharyngeal microbiome of healthy people across their whole life are essential to understand the relevance of the nasopharynx in the pathogenesis of multiple diseases, particularly viral infections. One hundred twenty nasopharyngeal samples from healthy subjects of all ages and both sexes were analyzed by 16S rRNA sequencing. Nasopharyngeal bacterial alpha diversity did not vary in any case between age or sex groups. Proteobacteria, Firmicutes, Actinobacteria, and Bacteroidetes were the predominant phyla in all the age groups, with several sex-associated. *Acinetobacter, Brevundimonas, Dolosigranulum, Finegoldia, Haemophilus, Leptotrichia, Moraxella, Peptoniphilus, Pseudomonas, Rothia,* and *Staphylococcus* were the only 11 bacterial genera that presented significant age-associated differences. Other bacterial genera such as *Anaerococcus, Burkholderia, Campylobacter, Delftia, Prevotella, Neisseria, Propionibacterium, Streptococcus, Ralstonia, Sphingomonas,* and *Corynebacterium* appeared in the population with a very high frequency, suggesting that their presence might be biologically relevant. Therefore, in contrast to other anatomical areas such as the gut, bacterial diversity in the nasopharynx of healthy subjects remains stable and resistant to perturbations throughout the whole life and in both sexes. Age-associated abundance changes were observed at phylum, family, and genus levels, as well as several sex-associated changes probably due to the different levels of sex hormones present in both sexes at certain ages. Our results provide a complete and valuable dataset that will be useful for future research aiming for studying the relationship between changes in the nasopharyngeal microbiome and susceptibility to or severity of multiple diseases.

Keywords: nasopharyngeal microbiome; age differences; sex differences; aging; human microbiome; 16S rRNA sequencing

Citation: Candel, S.; Tyrkalska, S.D.; Pérez-Sanz, F.; Moreno-Docón, A.; Esteban, Á.; Cayuela, M.L.; Mulero, V. Analysis of 16S rRNA Gene Sequence of Nasopharyngeal Exudate Reveals Changes in Key Microbial Communities Associated with Aging. *Int. J. Mol. Sci.* **2023**, *24*, 4127. https://doi.org/10.3390/ijms24044127

Academic Editor: Maria Teresa Mascellino

Received: 9 January 2023
Revised: 13 February 2023
Accepted: 14 February 2023
Published: 18 February 2023

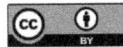

Copyright: © 2023 by the authors. Licensee MDPI, Basel, Switzerland. This article is an open access article distributed under the terms and conditions of the Creative Commons Attribution (CC BY) license (https://creativecommons.org/licenses/by/4.0/).

1. Background

Among the remaining challenges in biomedical sciences, one of the most important is to fully understand the effect of aging on human biological processes, health, and wellness. In recent years, solid evidence has been collected to support the idea that the microbial communities that inhabit the different anatomical areas of the human body could play a key role in these processes, and there has been much speculation about possible medical interventions [1–6]. Although most research has focused on the well-studied gut microbiome, there is growing evidence that variations in microbial communities in other sites of the body are also responsible for wide-ranging health effects [7–11]. The case of the respiratory tract is curious, since the lungs were long believed to be sterile, despite the fact that they are constantly exposed to microorganisms in inhaled air and the upper respiratory tract [12], which has been the main cause that the respiratory microbiome has barely been studied until very recently [13]. However, new culture-independent microbial identification techniques, such as metagenomics, have revealed that the respiratory tract is a dynamic ecosystem, and this has raised the interest of the scientific community in the role of the respiratory microbiota in health and disease [12,13].

The human upper respiratory tract that comprises the anterior nares, nasal cavity, sinuses, nasopharynx, Eustachian tube, middle ear cavity, oral cavity, oropharynx, and larynx is the major portal of entry for infectious droplet- or aerosol-transmitted microorganisms [14]. Among these different areas, the nasopharynx is anatomically unique because it presents a common meeting place for the ear, nose, and mouth cavities [15], but has not gained special prominence until the outbreak of the current COVID-19 pandemic [16]. Importantly, dozens of studies have already detected unquestionable correlations between the composition of the nasopharyngeal microbiota and susceptibility to different viral infections in humans [13], and some evidence is emerging, although still controversial, that it may be playing a role in the susceptibility to SARS-CoV-2 infection, too [17]. Elucidating this might shed light on the still unexplained fact that some COVID-19 patients, such as the elderly, are more susceptible and present more severe forms of COVID-19 than others [18].

Large cohort studies of human microbiome data with appropriate controls are particularly valuable, especially of all ages and both sexes, as these datasets are difficult to obtain due to multiple factors, including our long lifespans, heterogeneity in consent and other sample access issues, and because of socioeconomic confounds. Therefore, human studies have tended to focus on a specific component of the lifespan, such as infanthood, or studies of the elderly, rather than examining variation across an entire population. Knowledge about the relationships between changes in the nasopharyngeal microbiota and susceptibility to viral infections is a good example of this, since most studies have focused only on children [13].

A crucial factor to consider in studies of variation across the lifespan is sex as a biological variable. For aging research, this includes the understanding that females and males may have different aging trajectories [19–21], including in key systems such as the digestive tract. For example, the gut microbiome and sex hormones may interact to predispose women to autoimmune diseases [22] and dietary interventions are known to have sex-specific effects on gut microbiota [23]. There are no studies analyzing the possible sex-associated differences in the nasopharyngeal microbiome at different life stages.

Here, we analyze, for the first time, the diversity and relative abundance of the nasopharyngeal microbiota across the whole lifespan in 120 healthy individuals of all ages and both sexes, the taxonomic changes in the nasopharynx associated to age or sex, and the possible biological relevance of several taxa whose frequency of appearance in the population is high. We therefore provide a very comprehensive and valuable dataset that will be the base for future research aimed at identifying relationships between age- and sex-associated changes in nasopharyngeal microbiome and susceptibility to or severity of the diseases of interest.

2. Results

2.1. Data Annotation and Sample Overview

A total of 120 nasopharyngeal microbiomes from 120 healthy individuals were analyzed. A total of 4,538,196 high-quality 16S rRNA sequences ranging from 10,627 to 256,449 sequences per sample (mean = 37,818.3; median = 33,169) were obtained after quality control analyses and OTU filtering. The 16S rRNA sequences were binned into 128 families, 250 genera and 561 species. The most abundant families were Staphylococcaceae (12.14%), Burkholderiaceae (11.52%), Carnobacteriaceae (11.48%) and Corynebacteriaceae (9.47%). The most abundant genera were *Staphylococcus* (13.06%), *Dolosigranulum* (11.99%), *Corynebacterium* (10.18%) and *Ralstonia* (10.08%). The most abundant species were *Dolosigranulum pigrum* (24.55%), *Ralstonia pickettii* (19.02%), *Corynebacterium pseudodiphtheriticum* (4.87%) and *Propionibacterium acnes* (4.85%). We excluded one sample with an abnormally high proportion of *Chlamydophila*, which is an indication of an abnormal sampling or pathological disorder of this individual 'C_A1_M8'. To reveal age-related progression of nasopharyngeal microbiota, we divided the samples into six age groups, each divided into females and males to be able to also study possible sex-associated differences (Table S1). There were 20 samples in each age group and 10 samples in each sex group within them, except for the first age group (A1: 1–20 years) where one male had to be excluded as indicated above (Table S1).

We sought to determine the ways in which different samples were grouped according to their OTU composition. To that end, we applied nonmetric multidimensional scaling (NMDS), which is a powerful statistical tool that enables complex multivariate data sets to be visualized in a reduced number of dimensions, to determine the clustering patterns of samples according to their Bray–Curtis distances (which were calculated based on the relative abundance matrix of the 250 genera across the 119 samples) (Figure 1). The analysis of similarities (ANOSIM), which is a non-parametric statistical test, was used to analyze whether there were statistically significant differences among the different age groups included in this study. Thus, even though the samples apparently did not form distinct clusters when viewed using this approach as they appeared mostly intermixed and the different confidence ellipses overlapped each other, the differences between the age groups A1–A4 (ANOSIM statistic, 0.1075; significance, 0.016) and A1–A5 (ANOSIM statistic, 0.1075; significance, 0.016) were significant according to ANOSIM (Figure 1). Similar result was obtained when focusing on possible differences between the two sexes, as samples from females and males also appeared completely intermixed and did not form any groups, and significant differences were not detected according to ANOSIM (Figure 1).

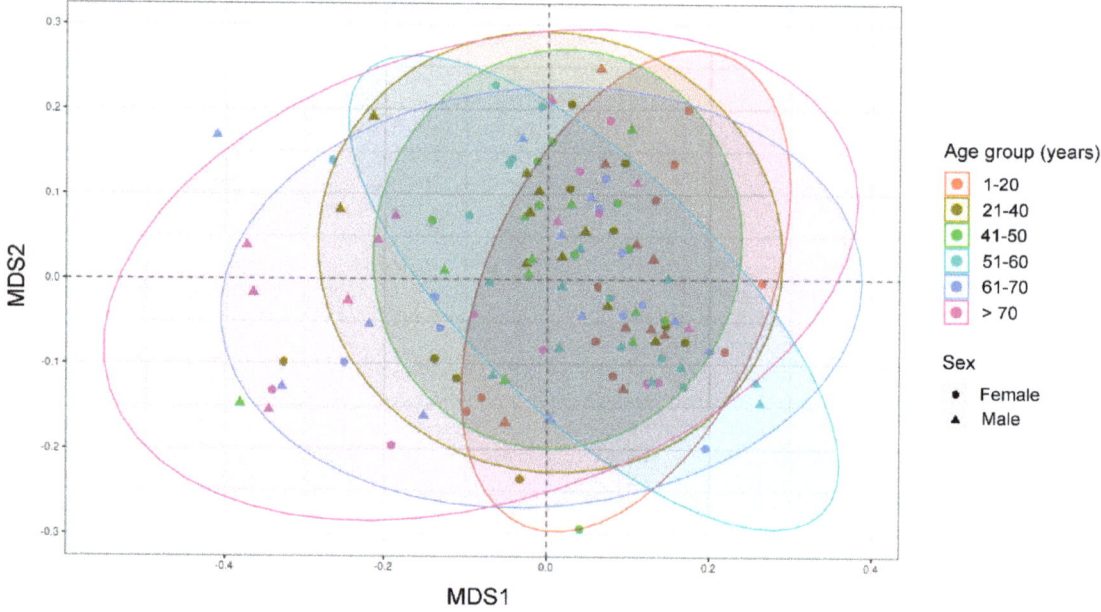

Figure 1. Microbial community composition. Nonmetric multidimensional scaling (NMDS) plot of the Bray–Curtis distances which were calculated using the relative abundance of the 250 genera across the 119 samples as input. Each sample is represented by one dot, colored according to age, and shaped according to sex. The 90% confidence data ellipses are shown for each age group.

2.2. Bacterial Diversity in the Nasopharynx of Healthy Individuals Is Stable throughout Lifespan

The fact that significant changes in bacterial diversity throughout life had previously been described in the well-studied gut microbiota of healthy individuals [24] prompted us to test whether similar changes occur in the nasopharynx by analyzing the alpha diversity, referred to as within-community diversity [25], for the different age and sex groups established for this study (Table S1). However, the Shannon's diversity index, which measures evenness and richness of communities within a sample, did not show any statistically significant changes in bacterial diversity among the different age groups (Figure 2a). Moreover, alpha diversity also did not vary as a function of sex when the Shannon index was calculated considering all individuals of all ages included in this study (Figure 2b), nor when the same analysis was performed comparing females and males within each age group (Figure 2c). The use of other indexes commonly used to measure alpha diversity, such as the inverse Simpson's diversity index, which is an indication of the richness in a community with uniform evenness that would have the same level of diversity (Figure S1), or the Chao1 index, which measures the total richness of communities within a sample (Figure S2), confirmed the absence of any statistically significant differences in bacterial diversity between the different age groups (Figures S1a and S2a) or between females and males (Figures S1b,c and S2b,c). Therefore, all these results together suggest that contrary to what occurs in other anatomical areas, such as the gut where bacterial diversity decreases with aging [24], it remains stable in the nasopharynx of healthy people over time, without notable changes at any stage of life, not even in very young people or in the elderly over 70 years of age (Figure 2a and Figures S1a and S2a). Curiously, another interesting finding provided by this work, for the first time, is that there are no significant differences when comparing bacterial diversity in the nasopharynx of healthy females and males (Figure 2b,c and Figures S1b,c and S2b,c), regardless of the stage of life studied and the important hormonal differences that exist between both sexes at certain ages.

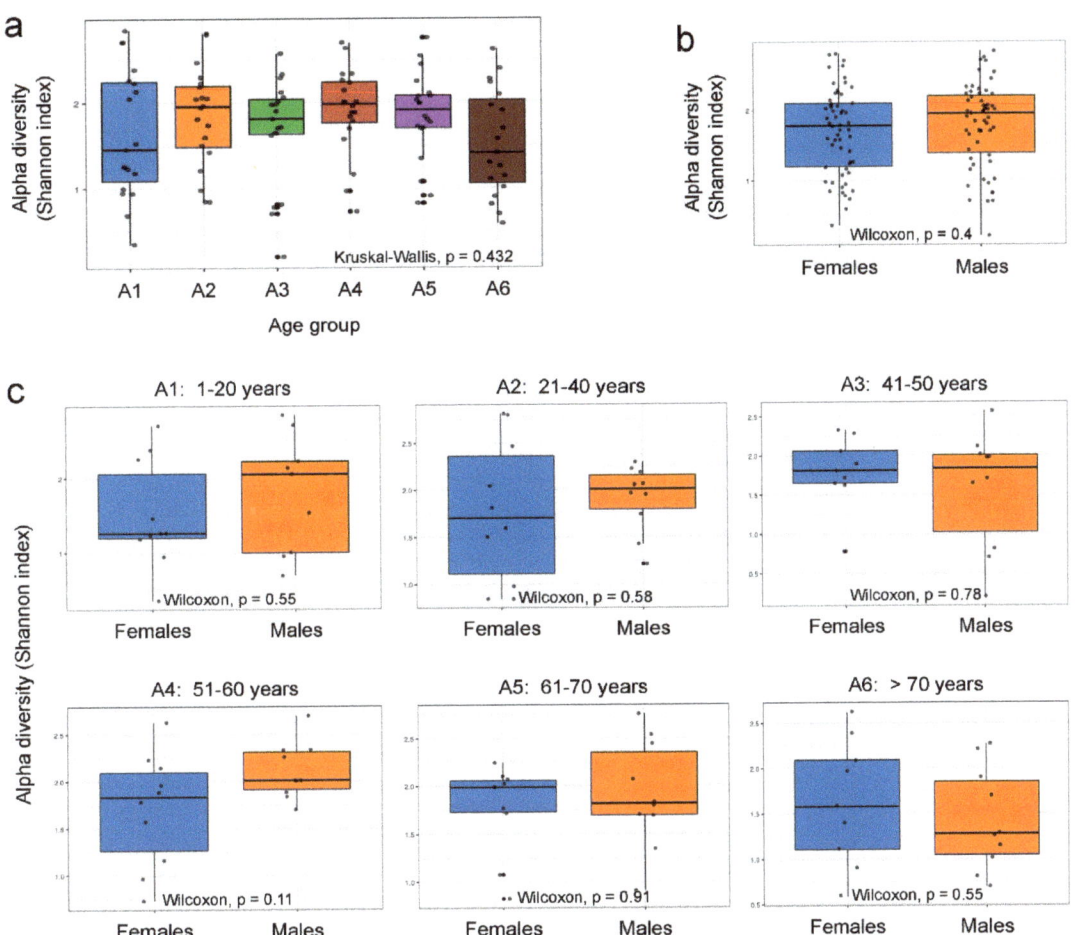

Figure 2. Comparison of alpha diversity parameters across the age and sex groups studied. Box-whisker plots of the alpha diversity Shannon index and its comparison using the Kruskal–Wallis test among the different age groups established for this study (**a**), and the Wilcoxon signed-rank test between females and males (**b**,**c**). Each sample is represented by one dot. The age group A1 includes subjects between 1 and 20 years old, A2 between 21 and 40, A3 between 41 and 50, A4 between 51 and 60, A5 between 61 and 70, and A6 includes individuals over 70 years of age (Table S1).

2.3. Age- and Sex-Associated Changes in Relative Abundance of Bacterial Taxa in the Nasopharynx of Healthy Individuals

To determine differences in nasopharyngeal taxa abundance among age and sex classes, we compared the nasopharyngeal microbiome of healthy women and men in the six different age groups established for this study (Table S1). The first general analysis at the phylum level revealed that Firmicutes and Proteobacteria relative abundances showed opposite kinetics with aging (Figure 3a–f), while the relative abundance of Firmicutes, which is the majority phylum in the youngest individuals (50%) (Figure 3a), clearly decreased with aging reaching its lowest values in subjects in their 50s and 60s (21% and 27%, respectively) (Figure 3d,e). The relative abundance of Proteobacteria presented its lowest value in the youngest people (24%) (Figure 3a) and increased in older individuals, peaking in subjects who were in their 50s (53%) (Figure 3d). The relative abundance of other phyla, such as Actinobacteria, Bacteroidetes, Tenericutes, or Cyanobateria, remained more stable throughout life (Figure 3a–f). Moreover, when we continued working at the phylum level and searched for any abundance differences between the nasopharyngeal microbiota of females and males, we determined that, interestingly, the results were almost identical for both sexes within the two age groups containing the youngest (1–20 years) (Figure S3a) and oldest (>70 years) (Figure S3f) individuals. However, several differences between females and males were observed in other age groups, notably a higher relative abundance of Actinobacteria in males in their 20s and 30s compared to females of the same age group (20% vs. 7%) (Figure S3b), a higher relative abundance of Proteobacteria in males in their 40s compared to females of the same age group (46% vs. 29%) (Figure S3c), a higher relative abundance of Proteobacteria in females in their 50s compared to males of the same age group (57% vs. 47%) (Figure S3d), and a higher relative abundance of Firmicutes and lower of Actinobacteria in females in their 60s compared to males of the same age group (37% vs. 20% and 10% vs. 22%, respectively) (Figure S3e). Therefore, the fact that there were differences in taxa abundance when comparing the nasopharyngeal microbiota of females and males in most of the age groups studied (individuals between 21 and 70 years of age) (Figure S3b–e), but not within the two age groups containing the youngest and oldest individuals (people between 1 and 20 and older than 70 years of age) (Figure S3a,f), suggests that the different levels of sex hormones present in both sexes at different life stages might be modulating the nasopharyngeal microbiome.

Next, we proceeded further in this study and moved to the family level, finding that 24 distinct bacterial families presented an average abundance of >1% in at least one of the age groups studied (Figure 3g). Our analyses revealed the dominant family in each of the age groups: Staphylococcaceae in A1, Carnobacteriaceae in A2, Staphylococcaceae in A3, Burkholderiaceae in A4, Streptococcaceae in A5, and Staphylococcaceae in A6 (Figure 3g). Thus, it is curious that although Proteobacteria was the majority taxa in all the age groups when analyzing the nasopharyngeal microbiota at the phylum level (Figure 3a–f), the dominant family in all the age groups belongs to the Firmicutes phylum, except in the case of age group A4 where the family Burkholderiaceae, which belongs to the Proteobacteria phylum, was the most abundant taxa at family level (Figure 3g). Differences in the relative abundance of some families were detected when compared between age groups, but without following any easily interpretable pattern (Figure 3g). Analysis of differential taxa abundance at the family level between age groups, but separately in females and males, did not show any relevant sex-associated differences between sexes regarding the dominant bacterial families in each age group compared to the results described above for both sexes together (Figure 3g), excepting that Burkholderiaceae was the most abundant family in males of age group A3 instead of Staphylococcaceae, and that Corynebacteriaceae is the dominant family in males of age group A5 instead of Streptococcaceae (Figure S4). As mentioned above when working with females and males together, differences in relative abundance were detected in some families when comparing between different age groups in both sexes, but without following any easily interpretable patterns (Figure S4). Visualization of taxa abundance at the family level in all the individuals included in this study showed that most of them had a very diverse microbiome, with a high number of families with relative abundance of >1% (Figure S5). However, a few individuals had one dominant family that represented the majority of their nasopharyngeal microbiomes; these families tended to be Burkholderiaceae, Carnobacteriaceae and Staphylococcaceae (Figure S5).

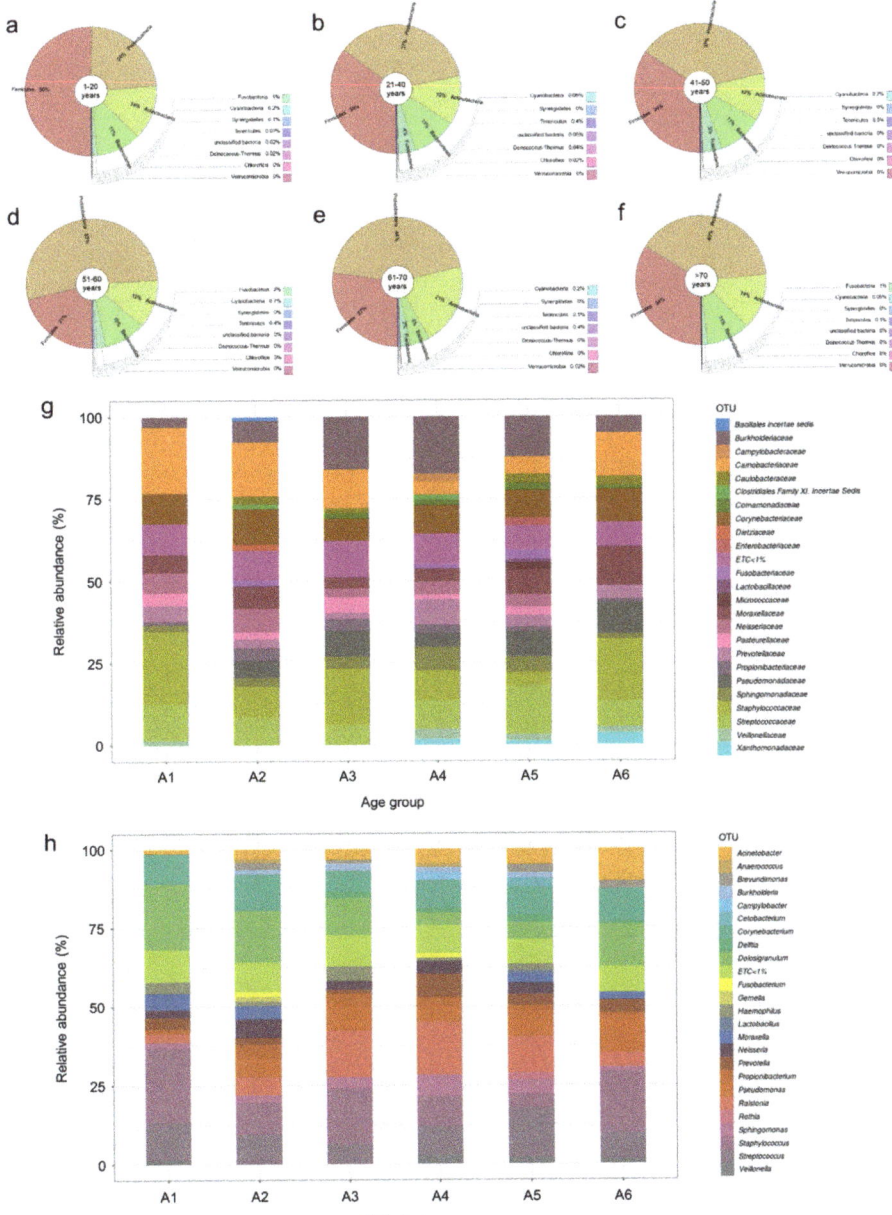

Figure 3. Taxonomic composition and age-associated metagenomic changes in the nasopharynx of healthy individuals. (**a–f**) Krona charts showing the bacterial community composition at the phylum level in the indicated age groups. Stacked bar charts showing the relative abundance (%) of bacterial phyla. (**g**) Stacked bar charts showing the relative abundance (%) of bacterial families in the indicated age groups. (**h**) Stacked bar charts showing the relative abundance (%) of bacterial genera in the indicated age groups. For clarity, only bacterial families (**g**) and genera (**h**) with average abundance >1% at each age group are shown.

Working at the genus level, we determined that 24 bacterial genera presented an average abundance of >1% in at least one of the age groups studied (Figure 3h). Moreover, our results showed that *Staphylococcus* was the dominant genus in age group A1, *Dolosigranulum* in A2, *Staphylococcus* in A3 and A6, *Ralstonia* in A4, and *Streptococcus* in A5 (Figure 3h). No relevant differences were detected when comparing taxa abundance in the nasopharynx of females and males at the genus level within the age groups studied (Figure S6). Similar to what was described above at the family level, visualization of taxa abundance at the genus level in all the individuals included in this study showed that most of them had a high number of genera with relative abundance of >1%, with a few individuals presenting one dominant genus (mostly *Dolosigranulum* or *Staphylococcus*) that represented the majority of their nasopharyngeal microbiomes (Figure S7). Next, we focused on those genera whose relative abundance were significantly different between the different age groups established in this study, as this could help us to identify changes in the nasopharyngeal microbiota that are characteristic of aging. Thus, our analyses revealed that there were statistically significant differences (adjusted p-value < 0.05) in relative abundance between the distinct age groups in 11 bacterial genera: *Acinetobacter*, *Brevundimonas*, *Dolosigranulum*, *Finegoldia*, *Haemophilus*, *Leptotrichia*, *Moraxella*, *Peptoniphilus*, *Pseudomonas*, *Rothia* and *Staphylococcus* (Figure 4a and Table S2). Interestingly, most of these statistically significant differences in relative abundance between the age groups for the 11 mentioned genera were between age groups A1 or A6, which include individuals between 1 and 20 years of age and over 70 years old, respectively, and the rest of age groups (18 out of 37 cases for the age group A1 and 16 out of 37 cases for the age group A6) (Table S2). Among these statistically significant changes detected, it should be noted that *Acinetobacter* was the only genus whose relative abundance in the nasopharynx clearly increased progressively throughout life, peaking in individuals older than 70 years of age (Figure 4a and Table S2). In the cases of *Dolosigranulum* and *Rothia*, their relative abundance drastically increased and decreased, respectively, in individuals over 70 years of age, compared to middle-aged people in their 50s and 60s (Figure 4a and Table S2). Changes among the different age groups of *Finegoldia*, *Leptotrichia* and *Haemophilus* were also interesting, as their relative abundance was markedly reduced in elderly people over 70 years of age, even though they were present at other ages throughout life, mainly during middle age (Figure 4a and Table S2). The case of *Haemophilus* was particularly intriguing, as while its relative abundance was at least 10% of the nasopharyngeal microbiota composition in age groups A1-A5 (if we consider only these 11 genera that present statistically significant differences between age groups), it dramatically decreased in the group of individuals over 70 years old (Figure 4a and Table S2). Furthermore, it is noteworthy that the bacterial genera *Brevundimonas*, *Finegoldia*, *Leptotrichia* and *Peptoniphilus* presented a very low relative abundance in the youngest individuals, who are between 1 and 20 years old, compared to other age groups (Figure 4a and Table S2). Finally, although *Moraxella* and *Staphylococcus* showed significant differences in relative abundance between the distinct age groups in several cases, these differences did not seem to follow any easily interpretable pattern relating relative abundance levels to a particular life stage (Figure 4a and Table S2). Next, we wondered whether the significant differences in relative abundance between age groups observed for these 11 bacterial genera were due to sex-associated differences. Visualization of taxa abundance in females and males separately, considering only these 11 genera, showed no notable differences between both sexes (Figure S8). The only exception was a higher relative abundance of *Dolosigranulum* in males in their 20s and 30s compared to females of the same age, because this genus was clearly dominant in five males from that age group while only in one female of the same age (Figure S9). Besides this observation regarding *Dolosigranulum*, analyzing the taxa abundance in all the individuals included in this study also revealed that in most people, 1 out of these 11 genera was dominant compared to the relative abundance of the other 10 genera (Figure S9). Interestingly, 8 out of the 11 genera, excepting *Bevundimonas*, *Finegoldia* and *Peptoniphilus*, were determined to be the dominant genus in at least one individual, demonstrating that nasopharyngeal taxonomic composition at this level can be very variable between different individuals, even if they belong to the same age or sex groups (Figures S9 and S10).

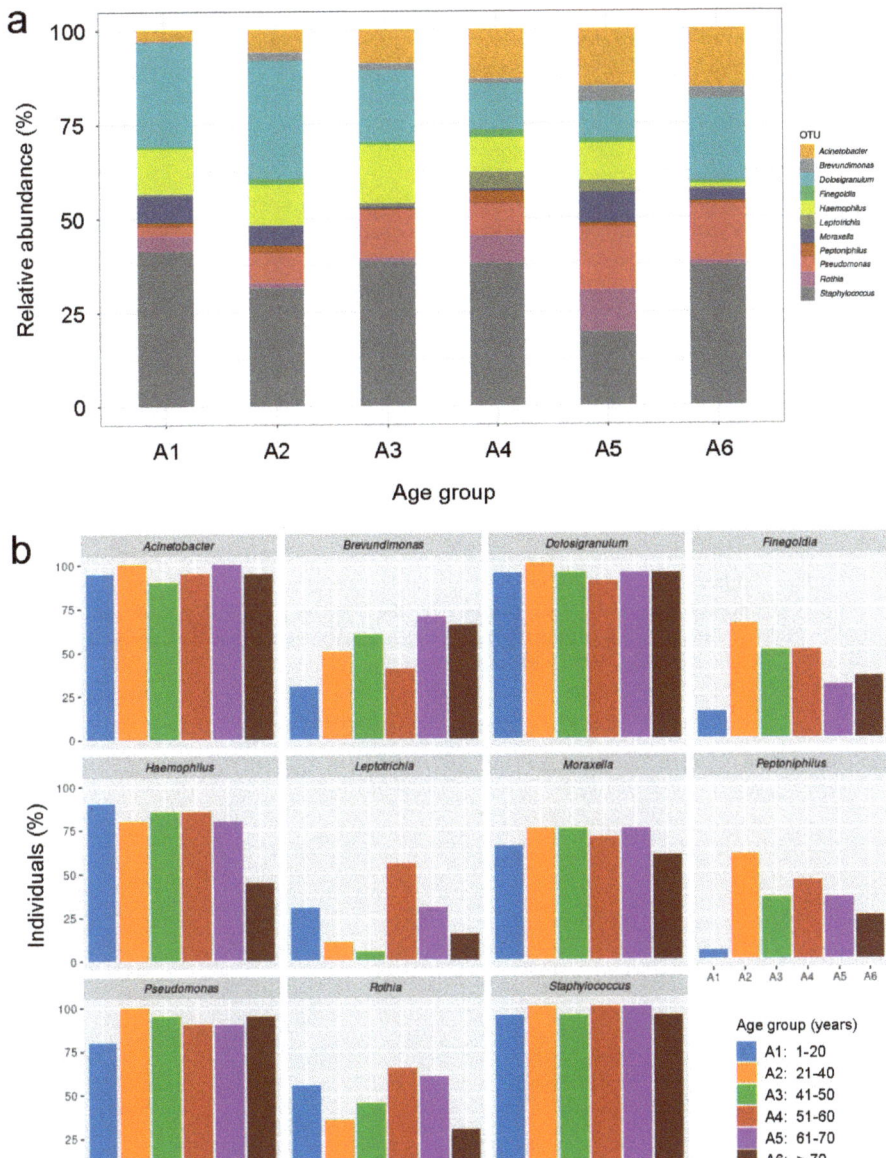

Figure 4. Taxonomic composition and frequency of appearance of the 11 bacterial genera which show significant differences between age groups. (**a**) Stacked bar charts showing the relative abundance (%) of the 11 bacterial genera indicated in the age groups established for this study. (**b**) Percentage of individuals, of the total included in this study, in which the indicated genera are present in the indicated age groups.

2.4. Identification of Potentially Biologically Relevant Bacterial Genera by Analyzing Their Frequency of Appearance in the Nasopharynx of Healthy Individuals

After analyzing taxa abundance at the phylum, family, and genus levels, looking for differences between age and sex groups, we decided to apply another strategy to attempt to identify bacterial genera whose presence in the nasopharynx might be characteristic of a certain life stage, independently on their abundance levels. Thus, based on the idea that in some cases the presence of a genus within a certain sex or age group but not in others can be biologically relevant, even if its abundance is low, we studied the frequency with which each genus appeared in the individuals included in this study by visualizing, for each genus, the percentage of people from each age group in which it is present. Firstly, we analyzed this in the 11 genera that presented significant differences between the distinct age groups, with the aim of checking whether these genera were present in a high percentage of individuals and, therefore, that the relative abundance results previously shown in Figure 4a were reliable. Indeed, our results showed that these 11 genera appeared with a high frequency in the individuals included in this study, especially in the cases of *Acinetobacter, Dolosigranulum, Haemophilus, Moraxella, Pseudomonas* and *Staphylococcus* (Figure 4b). These data also revealed that several genera, such as *Brevundimonas, Finegoldia* and *Peptoniphilus*, appeared less frequently in the youngest people than in the other age groups, while the frequency of appearance of others, such as *Rothia*, decreases in the oldest people (Figure 4b). Interestingly, it coincides that these genera that appear most frequently in the individuals included in this study are also the ones that appear most often as the dominant genus in the taxonomic composition of individuals (Figures S9 and S10). Next, we identified several bacterial genera that could be biologically relevant as part of the nasopharyngeal microbiota, although they did not show any significant differences in relative abundance between age or sex groups. This was (i) because their frequency of appearance in the nasopharynx of the healthy population was very high, as in the case of *Anaerococcus, Burkholderia, Campylobacter, Delftia, Prevotella, Neisseria, Propionibacterium, Streptococcus, Ralstonia, Sphingomonas* and *Corynebacterium* (Figure 5a); (ii) because their frequency of appearance drastically increased with age, such as the cases of *Faecalibacterium, Stenotrophomonas* and *Phascolarctobacterium* (Figure 5b); or (iii) because their frequency of appearance drastically decreased with age, such as the cases of *Aggregatibacter, Gemella* and *Fusobacterium* (Figure 5c).

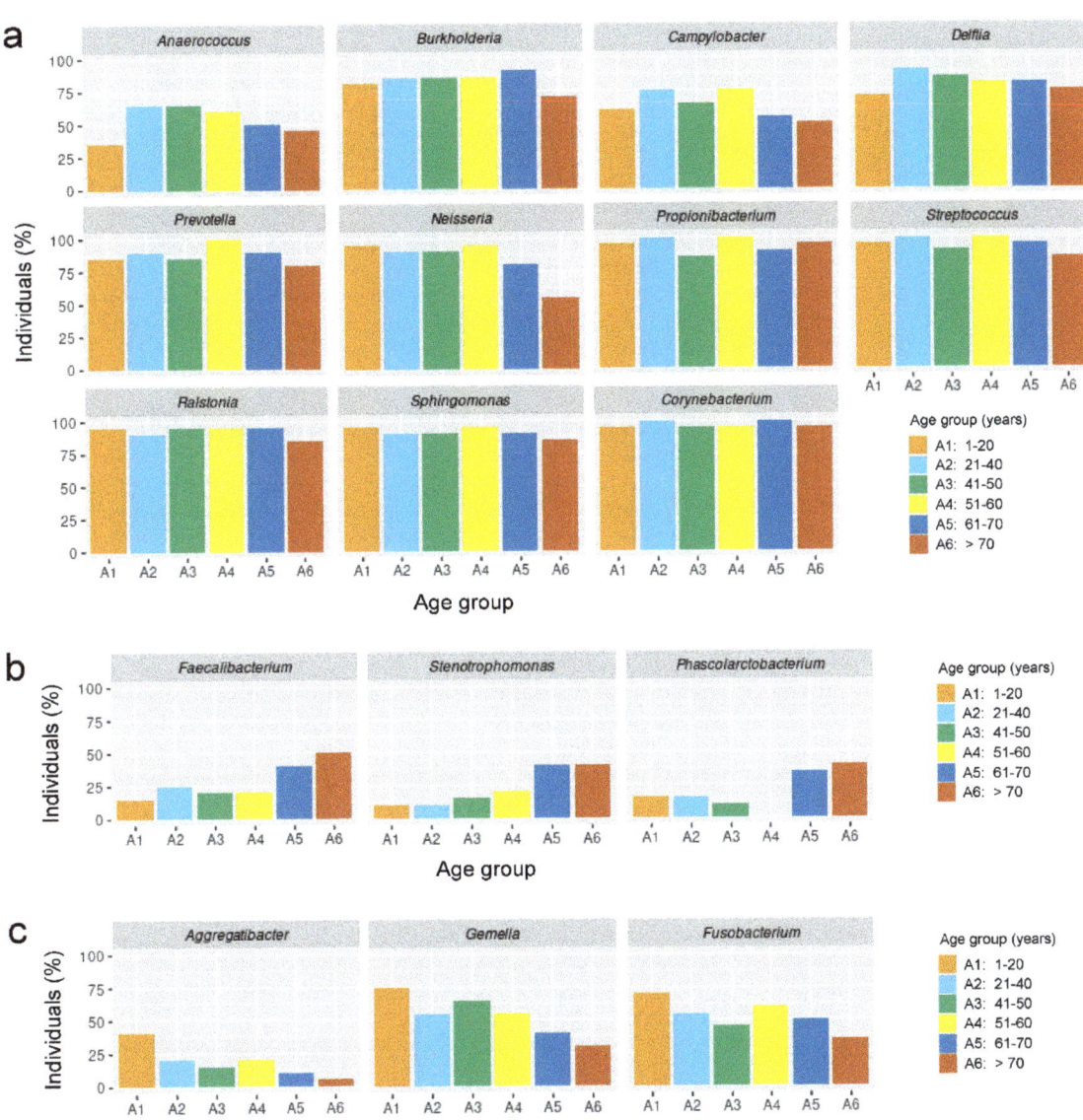

Figure 5. Frequency of appearance of potential biologically relevant bacterial genera. (**a**–**c**) Percentage of individuals, of the total included in this study, in which the indicated genera are present in the indicated age groups.

3. Discussion

Comparing bacterial species richness in the nasopharynx of healthy individuals in the different age groups established for this study and between females and males revealed no age- or sex-associated significant differences in alpha diversity. These results, which were confirmed by using three of the most reliable and commonly used alpha diversity indexes, such as the Shannon's diversity index, the inverse Simpson's diversity index, and the Chao1 diversity index, indicate that the nasopharyngeal microbiome is highly stable and robust to perturbations throughout life as well as between sexes within each of the different age groups in healthy subjects. Alpha diversity could be expected to be lower in the youngest individuals compared to older individuals in all the anatomical areas, as the fetus is sterile until the moment of birth, when the newborn begins to be progressively colonized by microorganisms until its definitive microbiota is established [26]. This is exactly what happens, for example, with the gut microbiome of infants, whose alpha diversity is consistently determined to be lower than in adults [27,28], probably due to the introduction of new diversity from food, which increases with the consumption of foods other than breast milk [29]. Detailed metagenomic studies, which should include samples collected at multiple time points during childhood and during adulthood, would be needed to determine whether something similar occurs in the nasopharynx. In the case of the present study, we would not be able to detect such differences in diversity between the youngest individuals and the rest of age groups, if they exist, for two reasons: (i) because our first age group, which includes the youngest individuals, is very broad and encompasses individuals up to 20 years old, so any differences from young children could be diluted; (ii) because as we were not interested specifically in children, but in broader age groups spanning all stages of life, we excluded children younger than 1 year of age from this study, as their highly changing microbiota in formation could bias the analyses we were interested in. Interestingly, although it is known that there are relevant sex-associated differences in diversity in other anatomical areas such as the gut, and that such differences are probably due to the different levels of sex hormones between both sexes [30], we did not observe any significant diversity differences between females and males, even in the age groups where sex hormones levels should be quite different. It is also curious that, contrary to what occurs in the gut where the alpha diversity of the microbiota decreases with aging [24], we did not observe a similar reduction in diversity in the nasopharynx of older individuals. This difference between both anatomical areas might be explained by the fact that decreased microbial diversity of the gut in older subjects is associated with chronological age, number of concomitant diseases, number of medications used, increasing coliform numbers, and changes in diet [31], and although chronological age affects both anatomical areas in a similar way, it seems probable that other of these factors might affect the gut microbiota in a more intense way compared to the nasopharyngeal microbiota. In summary, we can say that the diversity of the nasopharyngeal community is very stable throughout life and between sexes.

Our analyses of taxa abundance in the nasopharynx at the phylum level revealed the existence of sex-associated differences within the age groups including individuals between 21 and 70 years of age, but not in the youngest and oldest people. As previously mentioned for the alpha diversity results, multiple sex-associated differences in taxonomic composition have also been described for the human gut microbiome [30], and numerous studies have reported evidence to support the idea that levels of sex hormones, such as progesterone [32], androgen [33], and estrogen [34], regulate its composition [35,36]. The effects of sex hormones on other microbial niches, such as the human vaginal microbiota, have also recently been demonstrated [37]. Although it has been shown that estrogen stimulation (hormone/gender effect) in the upper respiratory tract mucosa could reduce virus virulence by improving both nasal clearance and local immune response [38], the relationship between sex hormone levels and the nasopharyngeal microbiota has so far not been directly observed in clinical studies. However, the fact that our results reveal differences between females and males at the phylum level in all the age groups, except for those where differences in sex hormones levels do not exist or are not so strong (>70 years and 1–20 years old), suggests that sex hormones might be modulating the taxonomic composition of the healthy human nasopharynx. Note that although differences in sex hormones could be expected to be relevant in the age group that includes individuals between 1 and 20 years of age since pubescents and adolescents are part of this group, we assumed that such differences should not be so significant in our case because 70% of individuals in this age group are prepubescent in our study.

We might be tempted to think that the microbiota of nearby anatomical sites that are closely related in terms of structure and function should be practically identical. However, the reality seems to be much more complex. A good example of this is that although nasopharynx and nose are adjacent, and previous metagenomic studies comparing the microbiome of both anatomical areas have revealed a clear continuity, there are important differences between the two sites and even niche-specific bacteria [39]. Furthermore, this study also reported an evident heterogeneity among participants, since the nasopharyngeal microbiome of half of them was dominated by *Moraxella*, *Streptococcus*, *Fusobacterium*, *Neisseria*, *Alloprevotella* or *Haemophilus*, while in the other half it contained an intermixed bacterial profile where *Staphylococcus*, *Corynebacterium*, and *Dolosigranulum* seemed to be important bacterial members with varying relative abundances [39]. Our taxa abundance analyses at the genus level only detected statistically significant relative abundance differences between the different age groups for 11 bacterial genera: *Acinetobacter*, *Brevundimonas*, *Dolosigranulum*, *Finegoldia*, *Haemophilus*, *Leptotrichia*, *Moraxella*, *Peptoniphilus*, *Pseudomonas*, *Rothia*, and *Staphylococcus*. Interestingly, most of the 37 statistically significant differences detected between the different age groups for these 11 genera appear when comparing age groups A1 and A6 with the rest of the age groups (18 out of 37 and 16 out of 37, respectively). Therefore, these results reveal that, in terms of relative abundance of bacterial genera, the nasopharyngeal microbiota of the youngest and oldest subjects is more different from that of the other age groups than that of any other age group. Among these age-associated changes, from a clinical perspective, it is particularly concerning that *Dolosigranulum*, which is an opportunistic pathogen that causes pneumonia in elderly patients [40], is overrepresented in the nasopharynx of individuals over 70 years of age compared to middle-aged subjects. This suggests that the relative abundance of *Dolosigranulum* may be higher in elderly people due to the process of immunosenescence that occurs in them [41,42], or that its higher abundance may be due to other unidentified age-related factors. Nevertheless, the relevance of *Dolosigranulum* in the nasopharynx deserved further investigation, since nasal administration *Dolosigranulum pigrum* 040417 to mice increased the resistance against respiratory syncytial virus (RSV) and *Streptococcus pneumoniae* [43,44]. However, other strains of the same species failed to protect mice against these pathogens [43,44]. Another interesting observation of our study is that *Haemophilus* that causes pneumonia mainly in elderly people [45] is underrepresented precisely in individuals over 70 years of age. This suggests that their lower relative abundance in elderly subjects is due to other unidentified age-related factors, and that the elderly are much more susceptible to opportunistic infections caused by this bacterium, probably due to the previously mentioned process of immunosenescence. Further research will be necessary to elucidate the precise reason for this. Something similar could be said for *Rothia*, as its relative abundance also decreases drastically in people over 70 years of age while it is known to cause pneumonia mostly in aged individuals [46]. It is worth noting that, regardless of their relative abundance or whether they show statistically significant differences between age or sex groups, those bacterial genera that are present in most individuals or whose frequency of appearance changes drastically throughout life could be relevant from a biomedical and ecological point of view. Based on this idea, we highlight *Anaerococcus*, *Burkholderia*, *Campylobacter*, *Delftia*, *Prevotella*, *Neisseria*, *Propionibacterium*, *Streptococcus*, *Ralstonia*, *Sphingomonas* and *Corynebacterium* as candidate bacterial genera that could be playing an important role as they are present in the nasopharynx of most healthy individuals. In addition, we propose *Faecalibacterium*, *Stenotrophomonas* and *Phascolarctobacterium* as candidate bacterial genera that could be playing a relevant role, as their frequency of appearance in the nasopharynx of healthy subjects increases progressively throughout life, and *Aggregatibacter*, *Gemella* and *Fusobacterium* because their frequency of appearance in the nasopharynx decreases drastically and progressively as healthy people age. Elucidating the biomedical relevance of all these bacterial genera which are part of the healthy nasopharyngeal microbiota and determining their potential involvement in health and disease at different stages of life is certainly an exciting topic for future work.

Our study has several limitations. This was an observational, retrospective study, and collection of data was not standardized in advance. The 16S rRNA gene sequencing approach to study the microbiota could introduce bias in the obtained data because this method does not allow the study of the whole microbiome, but only the genera amplified by PCR. The taxonomic assignment at the species level may not be fully accurate. Nevertheless, it is the most common technique to study microbiota in clinical samples. Moreover, it was not possible to obtain serial samples. Furthermore, the groups are small, particularly the sex groups within each age group, so the study may have been underpowered to detect certain associations. Finally, we could not access any sociodemographic, environmental, lifestyle, or medical information of subjects enrolled in this study, which would have been helpful to better understand the characteristics of the cohort.

Although multiple studies have analyzed the microorganisms present in the nasopharynx in different contexts before this work, the characteristics of the healthy and mature human nasopharyngeal microbiota was largely unknown since (i) most studies focused on children or elderly people, (ii) confounding factors such as external drivers that alter it are not well known to date, and (iii) focus is generally shifted to its variation in diseases. With this work, we fill this important gap in knowledge. However, further research will be necessary to elucidate the effects of the nasopharyngeal taxonomic composition as well as the age- and sex-associated changes described here on the susceptibility of certain individuals to infectious diseases. Studying the case of the elderly people in detail will be particularly interesting from a biomedical and clinical perspective, since their nasopharyngeal microbiota is significantly different from that of younger subjects, and they are known to be much more susceptible to multiple infectious diseases, most notably COVID-19 [47]. Therefore, we hypothesize that there may be some correlation between the taxonomic composition in the nasopharynx of the elderly and their increased susceptibility to COVID-19, but this will be a challenge for future metagenomic studies that should include different age groups, both sexes, and patients infected with SARS-CoV-2 who have developed the disease with different severity.

4. Methods and Materials

4.1. Sample Selection, Collection, and Classification

Due to the available economic resources, we randomly selected 120 nasopharyngeal samples from a cohort of 6354 healthy subjects belonging to the Health Area I of the Region of Murcia (Spain) who voluntarily provided their samples between 27 August 2020 and 8 September 2020 for diagnostic purposes and tested negative for SARS-CoV-2 infection. Nasopharyngeal swabs were obtained by approaching the nasopharynx transnasally and stored in Universal Transport Medium (UTM): Viral Transport medium (COPAN Diagnostics Inc., Murrieta, CA, USA). Nucleic acid extraction was performed using the automatized system Nuclisens EasymaG (bioMérieux, Madrid, Spain) based on the ability of silica to bind DNA and RNA in high salt concentrations (Boom technology). The polymerase chain reaction (PCR) kit used to verify that all the samples were negative for SARS-CoV-2 infection was Novel Coronavirus (2019-nCoV) Real Time Multiplex RT-PCR kit (Detection for 3 Genes), manufactured by Shanghai ZJ Bio-Tech Co., Ltd. (Liferiver Biotech, la Jolla, CA, USA) and the CFX96 Touch Real-Time PCR Detection System (BioRad, Madrid, Spain).

To facilitate the study of age- and sex-associated changes in the nasopharyngeal microbiota throughout life, and to ensure that the sample size of all the age and sex groups were homogeneous, we decided on an experimental design that distributed the 120 nasopharyngeal samples that we could analyse into six age groups with 20 individuals each, of which 10 were females and the other 10 were males (Table S1). For this, the 6354 healthy subjects of our parent cohort were divided into their age matched groups and numbered, and then randomly obtained numbers were used to select 10 females and 10 males from each of the age groups. Random numbers were generated in RANDOM.ORG, which is a True Random Number Generator (TRNG) that generates true randomness via atmospheric noise, unlike the most common and less trustworthy Pseudo-Random

Number Generators (PRNGs) [RANDOM.ORG: True Random Number Service. Available at: https://www.random.org]. According to the exclusion criteria we established for this study, (1) individuals younger than 1 year of age were disqualified because the microbiome of infants is known to be highly fluctuating with age, and (2) subjects who were tested for SARS-CoV-2 infection because they had respiratory or any other kind of symptoms were also excluded to avoid the enrolment of individuals who could have any infection or disease that could alter their nasopharyngeal microbiota although they were not infected by SARS-CoV-2.

4.2. Amplification, Library Preparation, and Sequencing

Bacterial identification was performed by sequencing the 16S rRNA gene's hypervariable regions. The 16S rRNA gene was amplified by multiplex PCR using Ion Torrent 16S Metagenomics kit (Ion Torrent, Thermo Fisher Scientific Inc., Alcobendas, Spain), with two sets of primers, which targets regions V2, V4, and V8, and V3, V6–7, and V9, respectively. Amplification was carried out in a SimpliAmp thermal cycler (Thermo Fisher Scientific Inc., Alcobendas, Spain) running the following program: denaturation at 95 °C for 10 min, followed by a 3-step cyclic stage consisting of 25 cycles of denaturation at 95 °C for 30 s, annealing at 58 °C for 30 s, and extension at 72 °C for 20 s; at the end of this stage, the program concludes with an additional extension period at 72 °C for 7 min and the reaction is stopped by cooling at 4 °C. The resulting amplicons were tested by electrophoresis through 2% agarose gels in tris-acetate-EDTA (TAE) buffer, purified with AMPure® XP Beads (Beckman Coulter, Inc, Atlanta, GA, USA), and quantified using QubitTM dsDNA HS Assay Kit in a Qubit 3 fluorometer (Thermo Fisher Scientific Inc., Alcobendas, Spain).

A library was generated from each sample using the Ion Plus Fragment Library Kit (Ion Torrent), whereby each library is indexed by ligating Ion Xpress™ Barcode Adapters (Ion Torrent) to the amplicons. Libraries were purified with AMPure® XP Beads and quantified using the Ion Universal Library Quantitation Kit (Ion Torrent, Thermo Fisher Scientific Inc., Alcobendas, Spain) in a QuantStudio 5 Real-Time PCR Instrument (Thermo Fisher Scientific Inc., Alcobendas, Spain). The libraries were then pooled and clonally amplified onto Ion Sphere Particles (ISPs) by emulsion PCR in an Ion OneTouch™ 2 System (Ion Torrent) according to the manufacturer´s instructions. Sequencing of the amplicon libraries was carried on an Ion 530™ Kit (Ion Torrent) on an Ion S5™ System (Ion Torrent). After sequencing, the individual sequence reads were filtered by the Torrent Suite™ Software v5.12.1 to remove low quality and polyclonal sequences.

4.3. Bioinformatics and Statistical Analysis

The obtained sequences were analyzed and annotated with the Ion Reporter 5.18.2.0 software (Thermo Fisher Scientific Inc., Alcobendas, Spain) using the 16S rRNA Profiling workflow 5.18. Clustering into OTUs and taxonomic assignment were performed based on the Basic Local Alignment Search Tool (BLAST) using two reference libraries, MicroSEQ® 16S Reference Library v2013.1 and the Greengenes v13.5 database. For an OTU to be accepted as valid, at least ten reads with an alignment coverage of ≥90% between hit and query were required. Identifications were accepted at the genus and species level with sequence identity of >97% and >99%, respectively. Annotated OTUs were then exported for analysis with R (v.4.1.2) (https://www.R-project.org/), where data were converted to phyloseq object [48] and abundance bar plots were generated. Data were converted to DESeq2 object [49] that uses a generalized linear model based on a negative binomial distribution to calculate differential abundance between groups. Thus, the differential abundance analysis was conducted according to the phyloseq package vignette with bioconductor DESeq2 (https://bioconductor.org/packages/devel/bioc/vignettes/phyloseq/inst/doc/phyloseq-mixture-models.html#import-data-with-phyloseq-convert-to-deseq2, accessed on 10 January 2022). The raw abundance matrix was imported into phyloseq object (as specified in the documentation of phyloseq with DESeq2) and subsequently converted to DESeq2 object. Then, estimated size factors were used with the DESeq2 function to obtain the differential abundance. DESeq automatically searches for outliers and, if possible, replaces the outlier values estimating mean-dispersion relationship. If it is not possible to replace, *p*-values are replaced by NA. R (v.4.1.2) was also used to perform a non-metric multidimensional scaling (NMDS) analysis on Bray–Curtis dissimilarity measures among samples based on relative OTU abundances (i.e., percentages). The relative abundances of OTUs were also used to test for statistically significant differences among age and sex groups. Group OTU compositions were compared through the non-parametric statistical tool ANOSIM. The 90% confidence data ellipses for each of the age groups were plotted. Alpha diversity was estimated based on Chao1, Shannon, and Inverse-Simpson indices by using the phyloseq package. To test for statistically significant differences between pairwise groups in alpha diversity, the non-parametric Wilcoxon test was used. Frequency of appearance was obtained by calculating the percentage of individuals in each age group in which that taxon occurs. The bar plots aggregated by groups (age and/or gender) show the aggregated relative abundance (sum of relative abundances). Krona charts that aid in the estimation of relative abundances even within complex metagenomic classifications were generated as previously described [50]. All the other graphs were generated with the R package ggplot2 version 3.3.3., including the confidence data ellipses which were plotted using the 'stat_ellipse' function, also from this package [51].

5. Conclusions

Our study shows that bacterial diversity in the nasopharynx of healthy subjects remains very stable and resistant to perturbations throughout the whole life and in both sexes. Age-associated changes in taxa abundance were observed at phylum, family, and genus levels, as well as several sex-associated changes probably due to the different levels of sex hormones present in both sexes at certain ages. We provide a complete and valuable dataset that will be useful for future research aiming for studying the relationship between changes in the nasopharyngeal microbiome and susceptibility to or severity of multiple diseases.

Supplementary Materials: The supporting information can be downloaded at: https://www.mdpi.com/article/10.3390/ijms24044127/s1.

Author Contributions: The authors offer the following declarations about their contributions: Conceived and designed the experiments: S.C., S.D.T., M.L.C., V.M. Performed the experiments: S.C., F.P.-S. Analyzed the data: S.C., S.D.T, F.P.-S., Á.E., M.L.C., V.M. Provided essential samples: A.M.-D. Writing—original draft: S.C. Writing—review & editing;: S.C., V.M. All authors have read and agreed to the published version of the manuscript.

Funding: This work was supported by the grant 00006/COVI/20 to VM and MLC funded by Fundación Séneca-Murcia, the Saavedra Fajardo contract 21118/SF/19 to SC funded by Fundación Séneca-Murcia, the Juan de la Cierva-Incorporación contract to SDT funded by Ministerio de Ciencia y Tecnología/AEI/FEDER. The funders had no role in the study design, data collection and analysis, decision to publish, or preparation of the manuscript.

Institutional Review Board Statement: All procedures in this work were carried out following the principles expressed in the Declaration of Helsinki, as well as in all the other applicable international, national, and/or institutional guidelines for the use of samples and data, and have been approved by the Comité de Ética de la Investigación (CEIm) at Hospital Clínico Universitario Virgen de la Arrixaca (protocol number 2020-10-12-HCUVA—Effects of aging in the susceptibility to SARS-CoV-2).

Informed Consent Statement: Nasopharyngeal swabs were collected for diagnosis of SARS-CoV-2 infection before this study was conceived, without the need of any informed consent as the collection procedure was non-invasive and risk-free. However, when the COVID-19 pandemic spread out of control, samples were kept at the Microbiology Service instead of destroyed after diagnosis as it was considered that they might be extremely relevant for research. This, together with the facts that (i) the retrospective use of these samples did not affect donor health or treatment at all, (ii) all data has been treated anonymously, and (iii) movement was limited due to the exceptional circumstances of the pandemic meant that it was not possible to obtain informed consent for the use of these samples in research. Moreover, none of the subjects expressly objected to their samples being used for research.

Data Availability Statement: Raw sequencing data of all 16S rRNA sequences, metadata, and abundance tables are available at the open access repository Figshare under the accession numbers 10.6084/m9.figshare.19785991 and 10.6084/m9.figshare.19786147, respectively.

Acknowledgments: We thank I. Fuentes, P. Martinez for their excellent technical assistance, Anabel Antón for 16S rRNA sequencing, and the staff of the Microbiology Service of HCUVA for sample collection and processing.

Conflicts of Interest: The authors declare no competing interest.

References

1. Heintz, C.; Mair, W. You are what you host: Microbiome modulation of the aging process. *Cell* **2014**, *156*, 408–411. [CrossRef] [PubMed]
2. Kim, M.; Benayoun, B.A. The microbiome: An emerging key player in aging and longevity. *Transl. Med. Aging* **2020**, *4*, 103–116. [CrossRef] [PubMed]
3. Mossad, O.; Batut, B.; Yilmaz, B.; Dokalis, N.; Mezö, C.; Nent, E.; Nabavi, L.S.; Mayer, M.; Maron, F.J.M.; Buescher, J.M.; et al. Gut microbiota drives age-related oxidative stress and mitochondrial damage in microglia via the metabolite N^6-carboxymethyllysine. *Nat. Neurosci.* **2022**, *25*, 295–305. [CrossRef] [PubMed]
4. Warman, D.J.; Jia, H.; Kato, H. The Potential Roles of Probiotics, Resistant Starch, and Resistant Proteins in Ameliorating Inflammation during Aging (Inflammaging). *Nutrients* **2022**, *14*, 747. [CrossRef]
5. Gates, E.J.; Bernath, A.K.; Klegeris, A. Modifying the diet and gut microbiota to prevent and manage neurodegenerative diseases. *Rev. Neurosci.* **2022**, *33*, 767–787. [CrossRef]
6. Murray, E.R.; Kemp, M.; Nguyen, T.T. The Microbiota-Gut-Brain Axis in Alzheimer's Disease: A Review of Taxonomic Alterations and Potential Avenues for Interventions. *Arch. Clin. Neuropsychol.* **2022**, *37*, 595–607. [CrossRef]
7. Das, S.; Bhattacharjee, M.J.; Mukherjee, A.K.; Khan, M.R. Recent advances in understanding of multifaceted changes in the vaginal microenvironment: Implications in vaginal health and therapeutics. *Crit. Rev. Microbiol.* **2022**, 1–27. [CrossRef]
8. Aleti, G.; Kohn, J.N.; Troyer, E.A.; Weldon, K.; Huang, S.; Tripathi, A.; Dorrestein, P.C.; Swafford, A.D.; Knight, R.; Hong, S. Salivary bacterial signatures in depression-obesity comorbidity are associated with neurotransmitters and neuroactive dipeptides. *BMC Microbiol.* **2022**, *22*, 75. [CrossRef]
9. Song, H.; Xiao, K.; Min, H.; Chen, Z.; Long, Q. Characterization of Conjunctival Sac Microbiome from Patients with Allergic Conjunctivitis. *J. Clin. Med.* **2022**, *11*, 1130. [CrossRef]
10. Saud Hussein, A.; Ibraheem Salih, N.; Hashim Saadoon, I. Effect of Microbiota in the Development of Breast Cancer. *Arch. Razi Inst.* **2021**, *76*, 761–768. [CrossRef]
11. Costantini, C.; Nunzi, E.; Spolzino, A.; Merli, F.; Facchini, L.; Spadea, A.; Melillo, L.; Codeluppi, K.; Marchesi, F.; Marchesini, G.; et al. A High-Risk Profile for Invasive Fungal Infections Is Associated with Altered Nasal Microbiota and Niche Determinants. *Infect. Immun.* **2022**, *90*, e0004822. [CrossRef] [PubMed]
12. Dickson, R.P.; Erb-Downward, J.R.; Martinez, F.J.; Huffnagle, G.B. The Microbiome and the Respiratory Tract. *Annu. Rev. Physiol.* **2016**, *78*, 481–504. [CrossRef]
13. Dubourg, G.; Edouard, S.; Raoult, D. Relationship between nasopharyngeal microbiota and patient's susceptibility to viral infection. *Expert Rev. Anti. Infect. Ther.* **2019**, *17*, 437–447. [CrossRef] [PubMed]
14. Sahin-Yilmaz, A.; Naclerio, R.M. Anatomy and physiology of the upper airway. *Proc. Am. Thorac. Soc.* **2011**, *8*, 31–39. [CrossRef]
15. Bluestone, C.D.; Doyle, W.J. Anatomy and physiology of eustachian tube and middle ear related to otitis media. *J. Allergy Clin. Immunol.* **1988**, *81*, 997–1003. [CrossRef]
16. Zhou, P.; Yang, X.L.; Wang, X.G.; Hu, B.; Zhang, L.; Zhang, W.; Si, H.R.; Zhu, Y.; Li, B.; Huang, C.L.; et al. A pneumonia outbreak associated with a new coronavirus of probable bat origin. *Nature* **2020**, *579*, 270–273. [CrossRef]
17. Candel, S.; Tyrkalska, S.D.; Alvarez-Santacruz, C.; Mulero, V. The nasopharyngeal microbiome in COVID-19. *Emerg. Microbes Infect.* **2023**, *12*, e2165970. [CrossRef]
18. Mueller, A.L.; McNamara, M.S.; Sinclair, D.A. Why does COVID-19 disproportionately affect older people? *Aging (Albany N. Y.)* **2020**, *12*, 9959–9981. [CrossRef]
19. Jašarević, E.; Morrison, K.E.; Bale, T.L. Sex differences in the gut microbiome-brain axis across the lifespan. *Philos. Trans. R. Soc. Lond. B Biol. Sci.* **2016**, *371*, 20150122. [CrossRef] [PubMed]
20. Ji, H.; Kim, A.; Ebinger, J.E.; Niiranen, T.J.; Claggett, B.L.; Bairey Merz, C.N.; Cheng, S. Sex Differences in Blood Pressure Trajectories Over the Life Course. *JAMA Cardiol.* **2020**, *5*, 19–26. [CrossRef]
21. Scheinost, D.; Finn, E.S.; Tokoglu, F.; Shen, X.; Papademetris, X.; Hampson, M.; Constable, R.T. Sex differences in normal age trajectories of functional brain networks. *Hum. Brain. Mapp.* **2015**, *36*, 1524–1535. [CrossRef] [PubMed]

22. Markle, J.G.; Frank, D.N.; Mortin-Toth, S.; Robertson, C.E.; Feazel, L.M.; Rolle-Kampczyk, U.; von Bergen, M.; McCoy, K.D.; Macpherson, A.J.; Danska, J.S. Sex differences in the gut microbiome drive hormone-dependent regulation of autoimmunity. *Science* 2013, *339*, 1084–1088. [CrossRef] [PubMed]
23. Bolnick, D.I.; Snowberg, L.K.; Hirsch, P.E.; Lauber, C.L.; Org, E.; Parks, B.; Lusis, A.J.; Knight, R.; Caporaso, J.G.; Svanbäck, R. Individual diet has sex-dependent effects on vertebrate gut microbiota. *Nat. Commun.* 2014, *5*, 4500. [CrossRef] [PubMed]
24. Claesson, M.J.; Cusack, S.; O'Sullivan, O.; Greene-Diniz, R.; de Weerd, H.; Flannery, E.; Marchesi, J.R.; Falush, D.; Dinan, T.; Fitzgerald, G.; et al. Composition, variability, and temporal stability of the intestinal microbiota of the elderly. *Proc. Natl. Acad. Sci. USA* 2011, *108* (Suppl. 1), 4586–4591. [CrossRef]
25. Lemon, K.P.; Armitage, G.C.; Relman, D.A.; Fischbach, M.A. Microbiota-targeted therapies: An ecological perspective. *Sci. Transl. Med.* 2012, *4*, 137rv135. [CrossRef]
26. Shao, Y.; Forster, S.C.; Tsaliki, E.; Vervier, K.; Strang, A.; Simpson, N.; Kumar, N.; Stares, M.D.; Rodger, A.; Brocklehurst, P.; et al. Stunted microbiota and opportunistic pathogen colonization in caesarean-section birth. *Nature* 2019, *574*, 117–121. [CrossRef]
27. Yatsunenko, T.; Rey, F.E.; Manary, M.J.; Trehan, I.; Dominguez-Bello, M.G.; Contreras, M.; Magris, M.; Hidalgo, G.; Baldassano, R.N.; Anokhin, A.P.; et al. Human gut microbiome viewed across age and geography. *Nature* 2012, *486*, 222–227. [CrossRef]
28. Koenig, J.E.; Spor, A.; Scalfone, N.; Fricker, A.D.; Stombaugh, J.; Knight, R.; Angenent, L.T.; Ley, R.E. Succession of microbial consortia in the developing infant gut microbiome. *Proc. Natl. Acad. Sci. USA* 2011, *108* (Suppl. 1), 4578–4585. [CrossRef]
29. Bokulich, N.A.; Chung, J.; Battaglia, T.; Henderson, N.; Jay, M.; Li, H.; D Lieber, A.; Wu, F.; Perez-Perez, G.I.; Chen, Y.; et al. Antibiotics, birth mode, and diet shape microbiome maturation during early life. *Sci. Transl. Med.* 2016, *8*, 343ra382. [CrossRef]
30. Consortium, H.M.P. Structure, function and diversity of the healthy human microbiome. *Nature* 2012, *486*, 207–214. [CrossRef]
31. Leite, G.; Pimentel, M.; Barlow, G.M.; Chang, C.; Hosseini, A.; Wang, J.; Parodi, G.; Sedighi, R.; Rezaie, A.; Mathur, R. Age and the aging process significantly alter the small bowel microbiome. *Cell Rep.* 2021, *36*, 109765. [CrossRef]
32. Kornman, K.S.; Loesche, W.J. Effects of estradiol and progesterone on Bacteroides melaninogenicus and Bacteroides gingivalis. *Infect. Immun.* 1982, *35*, 256–263. [CrossRef]
33. Org, E.; Mehrabian, M.; Parks, B.W.; Shipkova, P.; Liu, X.; Drake, T.A.; Lusis, A.J. Sex differences and hormonal effects on gut microbiota composition in mice. *Gut Microbes* 2016, *7*, 313–322. [CrossRef]
34. Koren, O.; Goodrich, J.K.; Cullender, T.C.; Spor, A.; Laitinen, K.; Bäckhed, H.K.; Gonzalez, A.; Werner, J.J.; Angenent, L.T.; Knight, R.; et al. Host remodeling of the gut microbiome and metabolic changes during pregnancy. *Cell* 2012, *150*, 470–480. [CrossRef]
35. Neuman, H.; Debelius, J.W.; Knight, R.; Koren, O. Microbial endocrinology: The interplay between the microbiota and the endocrine system. *FEMS Microbiol. Rev.* 2015, *39*, 509–521. [CrossRef]
36. He, S.; Li, H.; Yu, Z.; Zhang, F.; Liang, S.; Liu, H.; Chen, H.; Lü, M. The Gut Microbiome and Sex Hormone-Related Diseases. *Front. Microbiol.* 2021, *12*, 711137. [CrossRef]
37. Wessels, J.M.; Felker, A.M.; Dupont, H.A.; Kaushic, C. The relationship between sex hormones, the vaginal microbiome and immunity in HIV-1 susceptibility in women. *Dis. Model Mech.* 2018, *11*, dmm035147. [CrossRef]
38. Di Stadio, A.; Della Volpe, A.; Ralli, M.; Ricci, G. Gender differences in COVID-19 infection. The estrogen effect on upper and lower airways. Can it help to figure out a treatment? *Eur. Rev. Med. Pharmacol. Sci.* 2020, *24*, 5195–5196. [CrossRef]
39. De Boeck, I.; Wittouck, S.; Wuyts, S.; Oerlemans, E.F.M.; van den Broek, M.F.L.; Vandenheuvel, D.; Vanderveken, O.; Lebeer, S. Comparing the Healthy Nose and Nasopharynx Microbiota Reveals Continuity As Well As Niche-Specificity. *Front. Microbiol.* 2017, *8*, 2372. [CrossRef]
40. Lécuyer, H.; Audibert, J.; Bobigny, A.; Eckert, C.; Jannière-Nartey, C.; Buu-Hoï, A.; Mainardi, J.L.; Podglajen, I. Dolosigranulum pigrum causing nosocomial pneumonia and septicemia. *J. Clin. Microbiol.* 2007, *45*, 3474–3475. [CrossRef]
41. Gruver, A.L.; Hudson, L.L.; Sempowski, G.D. Immunosenescence of ageing. *J. Pathol.* 2007, *211*, 144–156. [CrossRef] [PubMed]
42. Fulop, T.; Larbi, A.; Dupuis, G.; Le Page, A.; Frost, E.H.; Cohen, A.A.; Witkowski, J.M.; Franceschi, C. Immunosenescence and Inflamm-Aging As Two Sides of the Same Coin: Friends or Foes? *Front. Immunol.* 2017, *8*, 1960. [CrossRef] [PubMed]
43. Ortiz Moyano, R.; Raya Tonetti, F.; Tomokiyo, M.; Kanmani, P.; Vizoso-Pinto, M.G.; Kim, H.; Quilodran-Vega, S.; Melnikov, V.; Alvarez, S.; Takahashi, H.; et al. The Ability of Respiratory Commensal Bacteria to Beneficially Modulate the Lung Innate Immune Response Is a Strain Dependent Characteristic. *Microorganisms* 2020, *8*, 727. [CrossRef] [PubMed]
44. Raya Tonetti, F.; Tomokiyo, M.; Ortiz Moyano, R.; Quilodran-Vega, S.; Yamamuro, H.; Kanmani, P.; Melnikov, V.; Kurata, S.; Kitazawa, H.; Villena, J. The Respiratory Commensal Bacterium *Dolosigranulum pigrum* 040417 Improves the Innate Immune Response to *Streptococcus pneumoniae*. *Microorganisms* 2021, *9*, 1324. [CrossRef] [PubMed]
45. Blain, A.; MacNeil, J.; Wang, X.; Bennett, N.; Farley, M.M.; Harrison, L.H.; Lexau, C.; Miller, L.; Nichols, M.; Petit, S.; et al. Invasive Haemophilus influenzae Disease in Adults ≥65 Years, United States, 2011. *Open Forum. Infect. Dis.* 2014, *1*, ofu044. [CrossRef] [PubMed]
46. Maraki, S.; Papadakis, I.S. Rothia mucilaginosa pneumonia: A literature review. *Infect. Dis. (Lond.)* 2015, *47*, 125–129. [CrossRef]
47. Chen, Y.; Klein, S.L.; Garibaldi, B.T.; Li, H.; Wu, C.; Osevala, N.M.; Li, T.; Margolick, J.B.; Pawelec, G.; Leng, S.X. Aging in COVID-19: Vulnerability, immunity and intervention. *Ageing Res. Rev.* 2021, *65*, 101205. [CrossRef]
48. McMurdie, P.J.; Holmes, S. phyloseq: An R package for reproducible interactive analysis and graphics of microbiome census data. *PLoS ONE* 2013, *8*, e61217. [CrossRef]
49. Love, M.I.; Huber, W.; Anders, S. Moderated estimation of fold change and dispersion for RNA-seq data with DESeq2. *Genome Biol.* 2014, *15*, 550. [CrossRef]

50. Ondov, B.D.; Bergman, N.H.; Phillippy, A.M. Interactive metagenomic visualization in a Web browser. *BMC Bioinform.* **2011**, *12*, 385. [CrossRef]
51. Wickham, H. *ggplot2: Elegant Graphics for Data Analysis*; Springer: New York, NY, USA, 2016.

Disclaimer/Publisher's Note: The statements, opinions and data contained in all publications are solely those of the individual author(s) and contributor(s) and not of MDPI and/or the editor(s). MDPI and/or the editor(s) disclaim responsibility for any injury to people or property resulting from any ideas, methods, instructions or products referred to in the content.

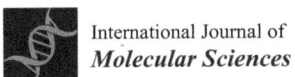

Article

Comparative Analysis of the Placental Microbiome in Pregnancies with Late Fetal Growth Restriction versus Physiological Pregnancies

Aleksandra Stupak [1,*], Tomasz Gęca [1], Anna Kwaśniewska [1], Radosław Mlak [2], Paweł Piwowarczyk [3], Robert Nawrot [4], Anna Goździcka-Józefiak [4] and Wojciech Kwaśniewski [5]

1. Chair and Department of Obstetrics and Pathology of Pregnancy, Medical University of Lublin, 20-059 Lublin, Poland
2. Body Composition Research Laboratory, Department of Preclinical Science, Medical University of Lublin, 20-059 Lublin, Poland
3. 2nd Department of Anesthesiology and Intensive Care Unit, Medical University of Lublin, 20-059 Lublin, Poland
4. Department of Molecular Virology, Institute of Experimental Biology, Adam Mickiewicz University in Poznan, 61-712 Poznań, Poland
5. Department of Gynecologic Oncology and Gynecology, Medical University of Lublin, 20-059 Lublin, Poland
* Correspondence: aleksandra.stupak@umlub.pl

Abstract: A comparative analysis of the placental microbiome in pregnancies with late fetal growth restriction (FGR) was performed with normal pregnancies to assess the impact of bacteria on placental development and function. The presence of microorganisms in the placenta, amniotic fluid, fetal membranes and umbilical cord blood throughout pregnancy disproves the theory of the "sterile uterus". FGR occurs when the fetus is unable to follow a biophysically determined growth path. Bacterial infections have been linked to maternal overproduction of pro-inflammatory cytokines, as well as various short- and long-term problems. Proteomics and bioinformatics studies of placental biomass allowed the development of new diagnostic options. In this study, the microbiome of normal and FGR placentas was analyzed by LC-ESI-MS/MS mass spectrometry, and the bacteria present in both placentas were identified by analysis of a set of bacterial proteins. Thirty-six pregnant Caucasian women participated in the study, including 18 women with normal pregnancy and eutrophic fetuses (EFW > 10th percentile) and 18 women with late FGR diagnosed after 32 weeks of gestation. Based on the analysis of the proteinogram, 166 bacterial proteins were detected in the material taken from the placentas in the study group. Of these, 21 proteins had an exponentially modified protein abundance index (emPAI) value of 0 and were not included in further analysis. Of the remaining 145 proteins, 52 were also present in the material from the control group. The remaining 93 proteins were present only in the material collected from the study group. Based on the proteinogram analysis, 732 bacterial proteins were detected in the material taken from the control group. Of these, 104 proteins had an emPAI value of 0 and were not included in further analysis. Of the remaining 628 proteins, 52 were also present in the material from the study group. The remaining 576 proteins were present only in the material taken from the control group. In both groups, we considered the result of ns prot ≥ 60 as the cut-off value for the agreement of the detected protein with its theoretical counterpart. Our study found significantly higher emPAI values of proteins representative of the following bacteria: *Actinopolyspora erythraea*, *Listeria costaricensis*, *E. coli*, *Methylobacterium*, *Acidobacteria bacterium*, *Bacteroidetes bacterium*, *Paenisporsarcina* sp., *Thiodiazotropha endol oripes* and *Clostridiales bacterium*. On the other hand, in the control group statistically more frequently, based on proteomic data, the following were found: *Flavobacterial bacterium*, *Aureimonas* sp. and *Bacillus cereus*. Our study showed that placental dysbiosis may be an important factor in the etiology of FGR. The presence of numerous bacterial proteins present in the control material may indicate their protective role, while the presence of bacterial proteins detected only in the material taken from the placentas of the study group may indicate their potentially pathogenic nature. This phenomenon is probably important in the development of the immune system in early life, and the placental microbiota and its metabolites may have great potential in the screening, prevention, diagnosis and treatment of FGR.

Citation: Stupak, A.; Gęca, T.; Kwaśniewska, A.; Mlak, R.; Piwowarczyk, P.; Nawrot, R.; Goździcka-Józefiak, A.; Kwaśniewski, W. Comparative Analysis of the Placental Microbiome in Pregnancies with Late Fetal Growth Restriction versus Physiological Pregnancies. *Int. J. Mol. Sci.* 2023, 24, 6922. https://doi.org/10.3390/ijms24086922

Academic Editor: Maria Teresa Mascellino

Received: 6 March 2023
Revised: 3 April 2023
Accepted: 6 April 2023
Published: 7 April 2023

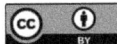

Copyright: © 2023 by the authors. Licensee MDPI, Basel, Switzerland. This article is an open access article distributed under the terms and conditions of the Creative Commons Attribution (CC BY) license (https:// creativecommons.org/licenses/by/ 4.0/).

Keywords: microbiome; bacteria; proteome; pregnancy; FGR; placenta

1. Introduction

The human body is inhabited by numerous microorganisms that constitute a kind of microbiome. The importance of microorganisms inhabiting various parts of the human body is not fully understood. Little is known about their impact on human growth, development and health. There is particularly little data on the impact of bacteria and viruses on the development of the placenta in normal and complicated pregnancies, e.g., with fetal growth disorders.

Fetal growth retardation, observed in approximately 3–10% of pregnancies, is one of the problems of perinatology, whose etiology and pathogenesis are not fully understood [1,2]. FGR is most commonly defined as the estimated fetal weight below the 10th percentile for gestational age based on prenatal ultrasound assessment [3]. This condition is associated with a number of short-term and long-term complications that can seriously affect the quality of life [4].

About 40% of FGR cases are idiopathic with no identifiable cause. In the remaining 60% of cases, 1/3 of intrauterine growth retardation is caused by genetic abnormalities and 2/3 is induced by environmental factors [5]. Factors affecting the development of intrauterine growth retardation can be divided into four groups: maternal factors, placental factors, fetal factors and infectious factors [6–8].

So far, cases of FGR have been documented with bacterial infections such as mycoplasma, listeria and mycobacteria, tuberculosis, and infection with a virulent, pathogenic *E. coli* strain. There are also indications that the composition of the vaginal flora may increase the likelihood of FGR. Studies have shown that the simultaneous presence of *Bacteroides*, *Prevotella*, *Porphyromonas* spp., *M. hominis*, *U. urealyticum* and *T. vaginalis* doubles the likelihood of FGR [9]. The presence of bacterial and viral infections causes overproduction of pro-inflammatory cytokines in the mother's body, such as interferon, tumor necrosis factor (TNF) or interleukins [10]. This causes widespread inflammation and necrosis, which in the case of the placenta can lead to abnormal distribution of nutrients and oxygen.

The state of the microenvironment of the maternal-fetal unit and its impact on the course of pregnancy, delivery and further health of the child and adult has been controversial for many years. They resulted from technical difficulties related to sampling and their analysis (biomass samples with a low content of microorganisms could be dominated by contamination during sampling or DNA isolation). On the other hand, in the studies carried out so far, we observe a very high methodological heterogeneity of the methods used to detect bacteria and viruses in placental tissues. This applies, for example, to the selection of a sequencing platform, DNA isolation kits and the selection of variable regions of the 16sRNA gene, which affects the ambiguity of the analyzed results. The introduction of new generation sequencing (NGS), mass spectrophotometry, proteomics and bioinformatics analysis of the obtained results enabled new diagnostic possibilities, primarily high sensitivity of biomass diagnostics of the tested material, e.g., bearing.

The presence of microorganisms in the placenta, amniotic fluid, fetal membranes and umbilical cord blood in studies using next-generation DNA sequencing technology undermines the sterility of the intrauterine environment during pregnancy and at the same time refutes the "sterile uterus" hypothesis, which was considered formulated in the early 20th century. The consequences of the presence of bacteria in the uterus are far-reaching in medicine and basic sciences and shed new light on the antibiotic treatment of pregnant women. It has been shown that the state of the biomass of the uterine environment later affects the development of atopy, asthma, allergies and obesity [11–13].

There are two working definitions of the "microbiome". The first definition given by *Nature* defines the "microbiome" as *"all the genetic material it contains"* (*microbiota—the entire collection of microorganisms in a specific niche, such as the human gut*). This can also be called the metagenomic microbiome [14]. The second definition proposed by Whipps et al. defines "microbiome" as *"a distinctive microbial community occupying a fairly well-defined habitat that has distinct physicochemical properties"* [15]. So, the term doesn't just refer to the microorganisms involved, it also covers their mechanisms of action. Both definitions are linked by emphasizing the functional capacity of the microbiome and the resulting activity [16].

The best-known microbiome is the microbiome of the digestive system, in which, apart from potentially pathogenic organisms, bacteria beneficial to metabolism and human health have been identified [17–19]. The microbiome is also called our "second genome" because it is the genome of the microorganisms that inhabit our bodies.

Since 2007 the human microbiome has been studied by the *Human Microbiome Project* (*HMP*) [20]. These studies made it possible to characterize the normal flora of the female genital organ [21]. The results of HMP and Sirota show a low diversity of genital micropopulations with a predominance of *Lactobacillus bacteria cillus* with a slight predominance of *Provotella*, *Grdnerella* and *Atopobium* [20–22]. These species form a "physiological flora" and by their presence prepare the endometrium from embryo implantation to the ability to carry a fetus to term [23].

It is now believed that the baby's microbiome is influenced by both the mother's microbiome and the immediate external environment. Given the important role of the microbiome, it is crucial to know and understand the mechanisms of colonization of the newborn. It has been suggested that the first colonization of the fetus occurs via the placental microbiome, but there is no clear evidence for this [24,25]. Hemochorial placentas found in humans are characterized by high permeability to lipophilic substances, contain a protein-mediated transport system for glucose and amino acids, exhibit exocytosis and endocytosis, and are permeable to hydrophilic substances through pores that can be used for bacterial migration [24,26].

2. Results

The aim of the presented study was to analyze and compare the microbiome of normal and FGR placentas using proteomic methods. In our studies, bacteria present in normal and FGR placentas were identified based on the analysis of a set of bacterial proteins (bacterial proteome) present in the examined clinical material.

2.1. Characteristics of the Control and Study Group

The results of the study were obtained from 18 placentas taken from women with fetal growth disorders and from 18 control placentas. The clinical characteristics along with anthropometric measurements of mothers and their newborns are presented in our previous study, as in Table 1 [27].

There were no statistically significant differences between the research groups in terms of age, height, fertility, BMI prior to pregnancy and body weight before pregnancy and at delivery. The only statistically significant difference between the two groups was that the control group gained significantly more weight during pregnancy than the experimental group ($p = 0.032$). In the study group, the mean pulsation index (PI) in the gestational uterine arteries was statistically substantially greater than in the control group ($p = 0.025$), as was the PI in the arterial umbilical cord of fetuses with FGR compared to eutrophic fetuses ($p = 0.0001$). The CPR was substantially greater in the control group than in the study group ($p = 0.0005$). Women in the experimental group gave birth much earlier than those in the control group ($p = 0.001$). Compared to neonates from the control group, infants with FGR had a lower birth weight ($p = 0.0001$), shorter body length ($p = 0.001$), and poorer Apgar score in the first minute of life ($p = 0.002$).

2.2. Analysis of the Bacterial Proteome in the Study and Control Groups

In both groups, we considered an ns prot score ≥ 60 as a cut-off value for the detected protein's agreement with its theoretical equivalent. Based on the analysis of the proteinogram in the material collected from people from the study group (n = 18), 166 bacterial proteins were detected. Of these, 21 proteins had an emPAI value of 0 and were not included in further analysis. Out of the remaining 145 proteins, 52 were also present in the material from the control group (the differences in their content in individual materials are presented in Figures 1 and 2, and Tables 2 and 3). The remaining 93 proteins were present only in the material collected from the study group (their content in the material is shown in Figure 3B,D,F and Supplementary Figure S1B,D).

Table 1. Clinical characteristics and anthropometric measurements of mothers and newborns.

	Control Group N = 18 Median (Range)	Study Group (FGR) N = 18	*p*-Value
	Baseline characteristics		
age (years)	30.2 ± 6.5	28.2 ± 5.6	0.466
height (m)	1.7 ± 0.06	1.67 ± 0.08	0.373
Actual weight (kg)	80.3 ± 11.3	79.5 ± 7	0.854
Weight before pregnancy (kg)	63.6 ± 11.3	66.7 ± 6.3	0.458
BMI before pregnancy (kg/m^2)	22 ± 3.5	23.9 ± 2.1	0.154
weight gain (kg)	14 (12–28)	12.5 (11–15)	0.032 *
weight of the placenta (g)	515 ± 46	328 ± 53	<0.001 *
Parity	2 (1–4)	1 (1–3)	0.504
Gestation	2 (1–4)	1.5 (1–4)	0.699
	Perinatal outcomes		
Gestational age at the delivery (weeks)	39 (38–41)	37 (35/4–40)	0.002 *
Fetal weight at birth (g)	3540 (2910–3890)	2300 (1385–2570)	<0.001 *
neonatal length (cm)	54 (47–57)	48 (35–51)	0.001 *
APGAR 1 min (points)	9 (min. 8–max. 10)	8 (min. 6–max. 9)	0.002 *
APGAR 5 min (points)	10 (min. 9–max. 10)	10 (min. 6–max. 10)	0.597
	Feto-placental Doppler before delivery		
AU PI	0.77 (0.72–0.91)	1.11 (0.98–1.9)	<0.001 *
MCA PI	1.44 ± 0.21	1.31 ± 0.22	0.191
UTA PI	0.79 ± 0.05	0.93 ± 0.17	0.025 *
CPR	1.703 (1.48–2.444)	0.995 (0.737–1.687)	<0.001 *

Values are shown as median (interquartile range) or mean ± standard deviation; statistical analysis was performed using a Mann–Whitney U test. Body mass index (BMI), pulsatility index (PI), umbilical artery (UA), middle cerebral artery (MCA), uterine artery (Ut A), cerebro-placental ratio (CPR), *—statistically significant results.

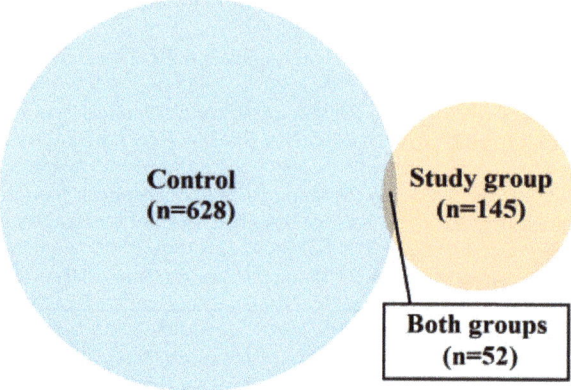

Figure 1. Venn diagram showing the proportion between the number of proteins (for which emPAI values > 0) identified only in the material representing the control or study group and present simultaneously in both types of the samples.

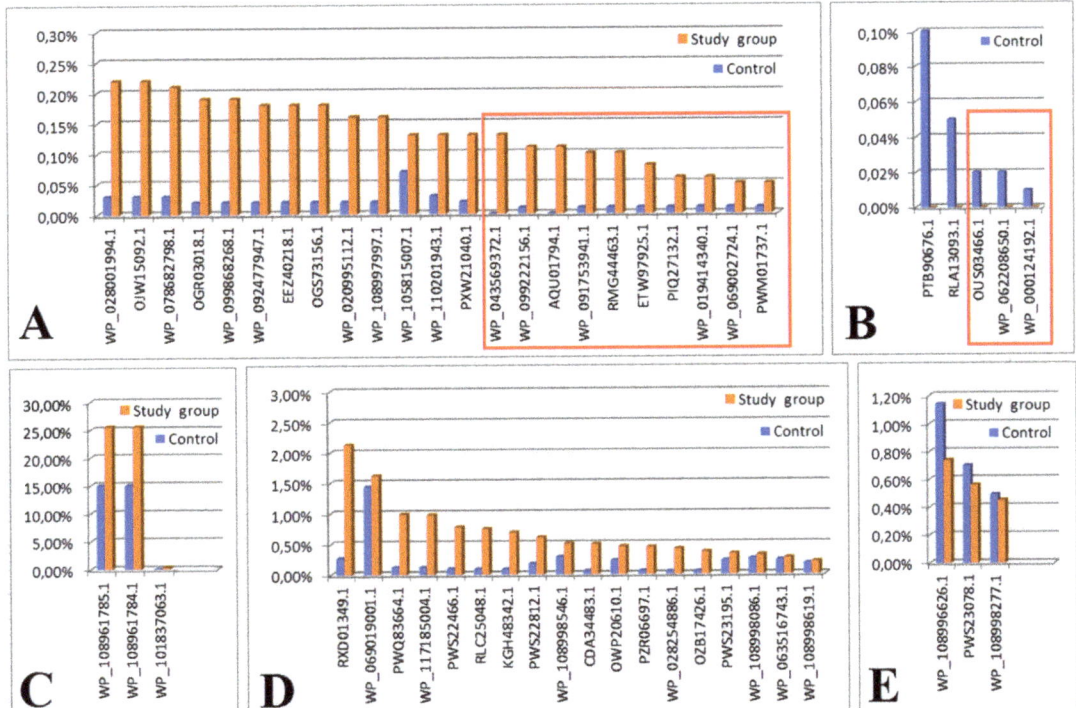

Figure 2. Bar graphs showing the comparison of proteins present in both the test group and the control group. Statistically significant results that remained significant after applying the Bonferroni correction are marked with a red square. Graph showing protein content comparisons for which emPAI values were: significantly higher in the study group compared to control (**A**); significantly higher in control compared to the study group (**B**); not significantly higher in the study group compared to the control (the results, however, trend toward significance) (**C**); not significantly higher in the study group compared to control (**D**); not significantly higher in control compared to study group (**E**). Expressions from Figure 2 are explained in Table 2.

Table 2. Legend to Figure 2.

Accession number	Protein (Bacteria)
WP_043569372.1	catalase (*Actinopolyspora erythraea*)
WP_099222156.1	HTH domain-containing protein (*Listeria costaricensis*)
AQU01794.1	glucose-6-phosphate isomerase (*Escherichia coli*)
WP_091753941.1	AAA family ATPase (*Methylobacterium* sp. ap11)
RMG44463.1	hypothetical protein D6718_10020 (*Acidobacteria bacterium*)
ETW97925.1	hypothetical protein ETSY1_20835, partial (*Candidatus entotheonella* factor)
PIQ27132.1	DNA polymerase I (*Bacteroidetes bacterium* CG18_big_fil_WC_8_21_14_2_50_41_14)
WP_019414340.1	hypothetical protein (*Paenisporosarcina* sp. TG20)
WP_069002724.1	DUF1631 family protein (*Candidatus Thiodiazotropha endoloripes*)
PWM01737.1	hypothetical protein DBY05_04045 (*Clostridiales bacterium*)
WP_28001994.1	shikimate dehydrogenase (*Shinorhizobium arboris*)
GCI 15092.1	phytoene synthase (*Mucilagini bacteria* sp.)
WP_078682797.1	dTDP-4dehydrorramnose reductase (*Lentisphaerae bacteria* GWF-2)
OGR030118.1	hypothetical protein (*Pararhizbium haloflavum*)

Table 2. *Cont.*

WP_92477947.1	A/G-specific adenine glycolase (*Clostridium polysaccharoliticum*)
EEZ40218.1	derythrose-4-phosphate dehygrogenase (*Photobacterium damselae subs daselae*)
OGS73156.1	flagellar biosynthesis protein F1hB (*Gallionellales bacterium* GWAZ)
WP_020995112.1	hypothetical protein (*Oxalobacter formigenes*)
WP_108997997.1	4-hydroxybenzoate-3-monooxygenase (*Salinibacterium* sp.)
WP_105815007.1	hypothetical protein (*Mycobacterium tuberculosis*)
WP_110201943	protein disulfide isomerase (*Kangiella* sp.)
PXW21040	activator of mannose operon (transcriptional terminatol) (*Pantoea* sp.)
	Figure 2B
OUS03466.1	hypothetical protein A9Q86_00710 (*Flavobacteriales bacterium* 33_180_T64)
WP_062208650.1	tryptophan–tRNA ligase (*Aureimonas* sp. AU12)
WP_000124192.1	S8 family peptidase (*Bacillus cereus*)
PTB9-676.1	hypothetical protein (*Marvigra lubricoides*)
RLA13093.1	uracil DNA glucose (*Gammaproteobacteria bacterium*)
	Figure 2C
WP_108961785	hypothetical protein (*E. coli*)
WP_108961784.1	hypothetical protein (*E. coli*)
WP_101837063.1	hypothetical protein (*Klebsiella* sp.)
	Figure 2D
RXD 01349.1	ubiquitin (*Splinomonassp*)
WP_069019000.1	actin cytoplasmic (*Pseudoalteramonas* sp.)
PWQ83644.1	30 Sribosomal oritein S15, partial (*Stenoprophomonas maltophilla*)
WP_1171850004.1	hypothtical protein (*Pseudomonas chorii*)
PWS22466.1	hypothtical protein PKP2260 (*Enterococcus faecium*)
RLC25048.1	hypothetical protein DRX56 (*Dettaproteobacteria bacterium*)
KGH48342.1	hypothetical protein GS19 (*Acinetobacter baumans*)
PWS22812.1	hypothetical protein PKP2260 (*Enterococcus faecium*)
CDA34483.1	Predicted DNA-binding protein withPD1 like DNA binding motif (*Firmicutes bacterium* CAG-536)
OWP2061.01	hypothetical protein CBF 90 (*Microbacterium sp.*)
PZR06697.1	hypothetical protein DI536 (*Archangium gephora*)
WP_028254886.1	BREX-3-SYSTEMP loop-containing protein BrxF (*Vellonella magna*)
OZB17426.1	ribosomal recycling factor (*Hyphomonas* sp.)
PWS233195.1	hypothetical protein DKP78 (*Enterococcus faecium*)
WP_108998086.1	NADP+ isocitrinate dehydrogenase (*Escherichia coli*)
WP_063516743.1	molecular chaperone Htp G (*Lactobacillus harninensis*)
WP_108998619.1	lactate dehydrogenase (*E. coli*)
	Figure 2E
WP_108996626.1	hypothetical protein (*Klebsiella pneumoniae*)
PWS23078.1	hypothetical protein (*Enterococcus faecium*)
WP_108998277.1	malate dehydrogenase (*E. coli*)

Table 3. Legend to Figure 3.

	Protein content > 1%
PWS22997.1	hypothetical protein DKP78_15465, partial (*Enterococcus faecium*)
RCU22074.1	hypothetical protein DVA69_20680, partial (*Acinetobacter baumannii*)
WP_087674330.1	MULTISPECIES: peptidylprolyl isomerase (*Gammaproteobacteria*)
SCV65427.1	Core histone H2A/H2B/H3/H4 (*Anaplasma phagocytophilum*)
WP_110201987.1	actin, cytoplasmic 2 (*Kangiella spongicola*)
PPI78337.1	actin, cytoplasmic 2, partial (*Marinobacter flavimaris*)
WP_108998291.1	50S ribosomal protein P1 (*E. coli*)
WP_108997701.1	F0F1 ATP synthase subunit beta (*E. coli*)
WP_068854620.1	hypothetical protein (*Klebsiella pneumoniae*)
WP_094934562.1	hypothetical protein (*Klebsiella pneumoniae*)
WP_089438650.1	actin, cytoplasmic 2 (*E. coli*)
WP_108997512.1	actin, cytoplasmic 2 (*E. coli*)
WP_125183134.1	hypothetical protein, partial (*Enterobacter hormaechei*)

Table 3. Cont.

	Figure 3B
	Protein content > 1%
PWS20985.1	hypothetical protein DKP78_25965, partial (*Enterococcus faecium*)
WP_087674313.1	hypothetical protein (*Pseudomonas syringae*)
SCH44985.1	Uncharacterized protein (uncultured *Clostridium* sp.)
PCD00708.1	hypothetical protein CO192_04000, partial (*Pseudomonas pelagia*)
ECO79390.1	hypothetical protein LEP1GSC068_2346 (*Leptospira* sp. Fiocruz LV3954)
WP_113909648.1	hypothetical protein (*Arcobacter* sp. FW59)
SKA29821.1	CheW-like domain-containing protein (*Oceanospirillum multiglobuliferum*)
WP_052604738.1	hypothetical protein (*Acidithrix ferrooxidans*)
	Figure 3C
RCU23962.1	Glu/Leu/Phe/Val dehydrogenase, partial (*Acinetobacter baumannii*)
AAB30179.1	p105 = epidermal keratin type 1 intermediate filament protein homolog {29 kda fragment} (*Mycoplasma*, Peptide Partial, 24 aa)
PCD01111.1	actin, cytoplasmic 2, partial (*Pseudomonas pelagia*)
WP_108998557.1	pyruvate kinase, partial (*E. coli*)
WP_081215088.1	hypothetical protein (*Lactococcus lactis*)
WP_081041455.1	hypothetical protein (*Lactococcus lactis*)
WP_081041454.1	hypothetical protein (*Lactococcus lactis*)
WP_1089977856.1	malate dehydrogenase (*E. coli*)
OSR81808.1	hypothetical protein BV331_05659 (*Pseudomonas syringae pv. actinidiae*)
ERM00395.1	hypothetical protein Q644_05090 (*Ochrobactrum intermedium* 229E)
OCR48569.1	hypothetical protein RJ97_26685, partial (*Klebsiella pneumoniae*)
OIE06819.1	hypothetical protein A7L78_18910 (*Acinetobacter baumannii*)
WP_108997697.1	fructose-bisphosphate aldolase class I, partial (*Escherichia coli*)
WP_087674327.1	50S ribosomal protein L10, partial (*Pseudomonas syringae*)
WP_108998140.1	nucleoside-diphosphate kinase, partial (*Escherichia coli*)
RCU28295.1	hypothetical protein DVA69_17570, partial (*Acinetobacter baumannlii*)
WP_108127784.1	tropomyosin (*Saccharospirillum mangrove*)
WP_082849626.1	molecular chaperone DnaK (*Lactobacillus harbinensis*)
WP_071212565.1	30S ribosomal protein S11, partial (*Acinetobacter baumannii*)
PSE04460.1	hypothetical protein C7G98_18875, partial (*Acinetobacter baumannii*)
	Figure 3D engraving
WP_10004729.1	integrase, partial (*E. coli*)
KMV72674.1	hypothetical protein AI28_14165 (bacteria symbiont BFo1 of *Frankliniella occidentalis*)
WP_076541277.1	DUF3833 domain-containing protein (*Shewanella sp*. UCD-KL21)
OFX06156.1	ATP:cob (I) alamine adenosyltransferase (*Alphaproteobacteria bacterium* RIFCSPHIGHO2_12_FULL_63_12)
WP_117453876.1	MULTISPECIES: hypothetical protein (*Absiella*)
PIU07782.1	hydrolase (*Methylobacterium sp*. CG09_land_8_20_14_0_10_71_15)
PIU06397.1	hypothetical protein COT56_11130 (*Methylobacterium sp*. CG09_land_8_20_14_0_10_71_15)
OHB84455.1	hypothetical protein A3J73_04470 (*Planctomycetes bacterium* RIFCSPHIGHO2_02_FULL_38_41)
OGU00202.1	thioredoxin peroxidase (*Geobacteraceae bacterium* GWC2_48_7)
SCD64547.1	transcriptional regulator, TetR family (*Streptomyces* sp. di50b)
SHI22323.1	NlpC/P60 family protein (*Leeuwenhoekiella palythoae*)
PIR74343.1	hypothetical protein COU35_02740 (*Candidatus Magasanikbacteria bacterium* CG10_big_fil_rev_8_21_14_0_10_47_10)
CCY99834.1	putative uncharacterized protein (*Clostridium sp*. CAG:793)
OGP11570.1	metal-dependent hydrolase (*Deltaproteobacteria bacterium* GWA2_43_19)
PCI14785.1	cell division ATP-binding protein FtsE (*Thiotrichales bacterium*)
WP_034753543.1	phosphoglycolate phosphatase (*Janthinobacterium liquid*)
RPG61346.1	lipoyl (octoyl) transferase LipB (*Flavobacteriaceae bacterium* TMED206)
KOX35357.1	HAD family hydrolase (*Saccharothrix* sp. NRRL B-16348)
WP_009284699.1	3-hydroxyacyl-CoA dehydrogenase (*Fibrisoma limit*)
WP_116657611.1	hydroxyacylglutathione hydrolase (*Pseudomonas* sp. NDM)
	Figure 3E
RFC01619.1	hypothetical protein DDJ49_30220, partial (*Klebsiella pneumoniae*)
WP_07280094.1	hypothetical protein (*E. coli*)
WP_077250818.1	hypothetical protein (*E. coli*)
WP_073034642.1	hypothetical protein (*E. coli*)

Table 3. *Cont.*

WP_108998184.1	hypothetical protein (*E. coli*)
WP_072794647.1	hypothetical protein (*E. coli*)
WP_108998612.1	hypothetical protein (*E. coli*)
WP_072794633.1	hypothetical protein (*E. coli*)
WP_072794629.1	hypothetical protein (*E. coli*)
WP_108998509.1	hypothetical protein (*E. coli*)
WP_108998559.1	hypothetical protein (*E. coli*)
WP_126755742.1	hypothetical protein (*E. coli*)
WP_108998635.1	60S ribosomal protein L22 (*E. coli*)
WP_094948604.1	MULTISPECIES: translation elongation factor EF-1 subunit alpha (*Enterobacteriaceae*)
WP_888381079.1	hypothetical protein (*Microbacterium sp.* AISO3)
PWS23168.1	hypothetical protein DKP78_14555, partial (*Enterococcus faecium*)
WP_108998558.1	30S ribosomal protein S19e (*E. coli*)
EHM02625.1	hypothetical protein HMPREF9946_00894 (*Acetobacteraceae bacterium* AT-5844)
WP_114597919.1	tubulin beta chain (*Microbacterium arborescens*)
WP_110201953.1	hypothetical protein (*Kangiella spongicola*)
	Figure 3F
WP_067782112.1	hypothetical protein (*Actinomyces vulturis*)
WP_117305475.1	MinD/ParA family protein (*Bacillus sp.* V59.32a)
WP_078453723.1	molecular chaperone DnaK, partial (*Solemya velum gill symbiont*)
OGV57400.1	hypothetical protein A2X49_01235 (*Lentisphaerae bacteria* GWF2_52_8)
OGV38480.1	transcriptional regulator (*Lentisphaerae bacteria* GWF2_49_21)
REF04934.1	LacI family transcriptional regulator (*Microbacterium chocolate*)
WP_021076726.1	magnesium chelate ATPase subunit I (*Bradyrhizobium sp.* MOS004)
RJP82014.1	MCE family protein (*Desulfobacteraceae bacterium*)
OGT19887.1	histidinol-phosphate transaminase (*Gammaproteobacteria bacterium* RBG_16_57_12)
SDW00717.1	hypothetical protein SAMN04487912_10192 (*Arthrobacter sp.* cf158)
WP_0069060036.1	phage major capsid protein (*Shuttleworthia satelles*)
WP_1193915508.1	pyrophosphate–fructose-6-phosphate 1-phosphotransferase (*Phyllobacteriaceae bacterium* SYSU D60012)
AST06406.1	MFS transporter (*Anoxybacillus flavithermus*)
RKV99493.1	type II secretion system F family protein (*Candidatus Saccharimonas sp.*)
RTF38711.1	hypothetical protein CG399_02610, partial (*Bifidobacteriaceae bacterium* NR015)
WP_106563713.1	ABC transporter permease (*Labedella gwakjiensis*)
GBU15610.1	integrase (*Polaromonas sp.*)
WP_066008415.1	tRNA (guanosine(46)-N7)-methyltransferase TrmB (*Campylobacter ornithocola*)
PYM16032.1	homoserine dehydrogenase (*Verrucomicrobia bacterium*)
WP_088892294.1	polysaccharide pyruvyl transferase family protein (*Leptolyngbya ohadii*)

Based on the proteinogram analysis, 732 bacterial proteins were detected in the material collected from the control group (n = 18). Of these, 104 proteins had an emPAI value of 0 and were not included in the further analysis. Of the remaining 628 proteins, 52 were also present in the material from the study group. The remaining 576 proteins were present only in the material collected from the control group (their content in the material is shown in Figure 3A,C,E and Supplementary Figures S1A,C,E and S2–S5).

Based on proteomic data, the bacteria identified in both groups are presented in Tables 4 and 5.

Based on proteomic data, the bacteria identified in both groups, but significantly higher in the study group, are: *Actinopolyspora erythraea*, *Listeria costaricensis*, *E. coli*, *Methylobacterium*, *Acidobacteria bacterium*, *Bacteroidetes bacterium*, *Paenisporsarcina* sp., *Thiodiazotropha endolloripes* and *Clostridiales bacterium*. The tendency towards statistical significance also concerned *Klebsiella* sp.

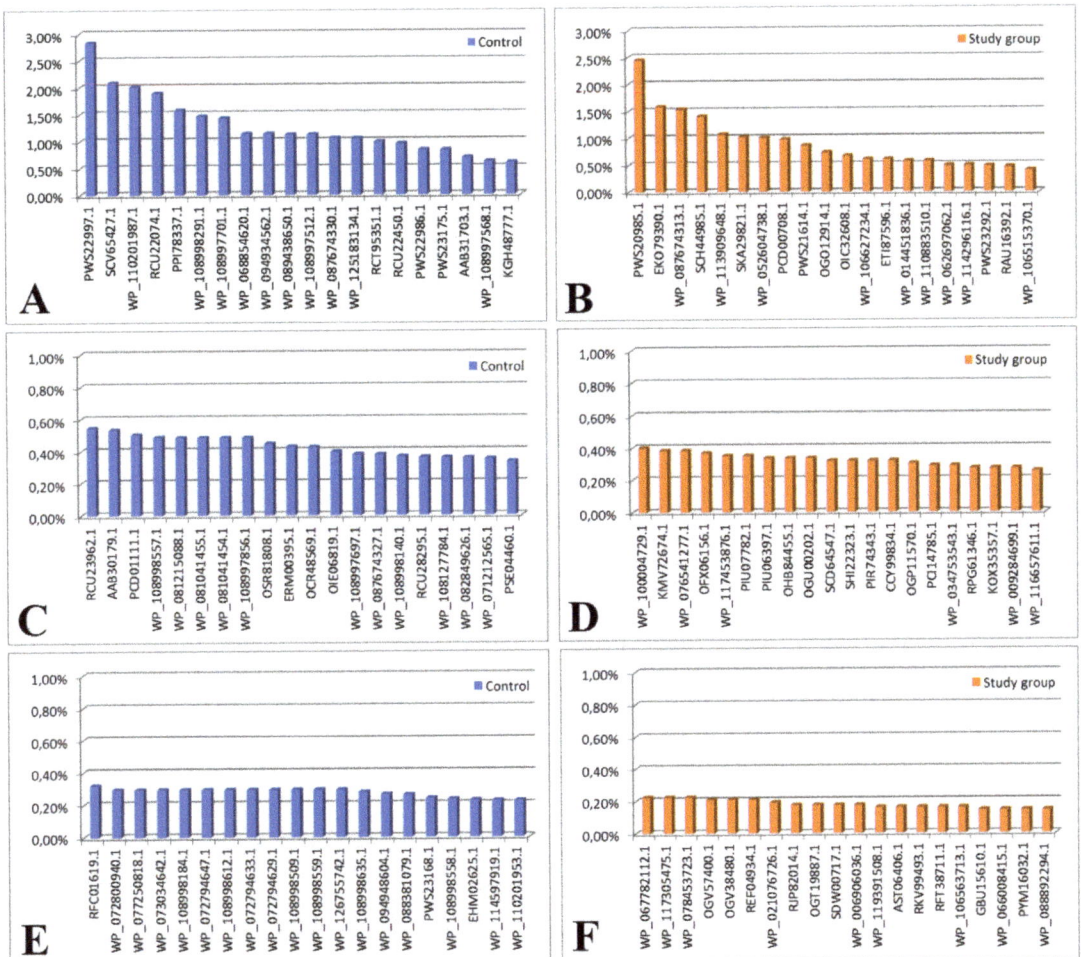

Figure 3. Bar graphs showing the content of proteins present only in the material from the study group or control. Graph showing the content of proteins (in order of decreasing emPAI value) found only in the material from the control group: proteins 1–20 (**A**); proteins 21–40 (**C**); proteins 41–60 (**E**) or tested: proteins 1–20 (**B**); proteins 21–40 (**D**); proteins 41–60 (**F**). Expressions from Figure 3 are explained in Table 3.

In addition, bacteria that may be pathological were identified in the study group (although data insignificantly higher): *Splinomonas* sp., *Pseudoalteromonas*, *Stenoprophomonas maltophila*, *Pseudomonas cichorii*, *Enterococcus faecium*, *Deltaproteobacteria bacterium*, *Acinetobacter baumannii*, *Firmicutes bacterium*, *Microbacterium*, *Archangium gephora*, *Veillonella magna*, *Hyphomonas* sp., *Enterococcus faecium* and *Lactobacillus harbinensis*.

In turn, in the control group, statistically more often, based on proteomic data, the following were found: *Flavobacterial bacterium*, *Aureimonas* sp., *Bacillus cereus* and *Klebsiella* were on the verge of statistical significance, as well as *Pneumoniae*, *Enterococcus faecium* and *E. coli*.

Table 4. Proteins for which emPAI was significantly higher in the study group compared to the control group.

Bacteria Species	Domain	Phylum	Class	Order/Genus	Access Number
Actinopolyspora erythraea	Bacteria	Actinomycetota	Actinomycetia	Actinosporaceae	WP_043569372.1
Listeria costaricensis	Firmicutes	Listeria	Bacilli	Listeriacea	WP_0999222156.1
Escherichia colli	proteobacteria	Pseudomonadot	Gammaproteobacteria	Enterobacteriacea	AQU017941.1
Methylobacterium sp. ap11	Bacteria	Methylobacterium	Aphaproteobacteria	Methylobacteriaceae	WP_091753941.1
Acidobacteria bacterium	Bacteria	Acidobacteriota	Acidobacteria	Acidobacteriales	RMG44463.1
candidate entotheonella factor	Bacteria	Tetomicrobia		entotheonella	ETW97925.1
Bacteroidet bacterium	Bacteria	Bacteroid	Saprospira	Bacteroides	PIQ27132.1
Paenisporasarcina sp. TG20	Bacteria	Paenisporosarcin	Bacilli	Planococcaceae	WP_019414340.1
candidate Thiodiazotropha endoloripes	Nomenclatural status: not validly published				WP_0690002724.1
Clostridiales bacterium	Bacteria	Eubacteriales	Clostrid	Clostridaceae	PWM01737.1

Table 5. Proteins for which emPAI was significantly higher in the control group compared to the study group.

Bacteria Species	Domain	Phylum	Class	Order/Genus	Access Number
Flavobacteriales bacterium 33_180_T64	Bacteria	Bacteroides	Flavobacteria	Flavobacteriales	OUS03466.1
Aureimonas sp. AU12	Bacteria	Pseudomonadot	Alphaproteo bacteria	Hyphomicrobiales	WP_062208650.1
Bacillus cerus	Bacteria	Bacillot	Bacilli	Bacillales	WP_000124192.1

3. Discussion

Advances in molecular methodology reveal the details of the human-microbial relationship, allowing for increased identification of microbiota composition and function. Recently, the maternal microbiome has been shown to prepare the newborn for host–microbial symbiosis, driving postnatal innate immune development [28]. However, the viability of placental bacteria cannot be determined due to discrepancies with the culture results [24]. On the other hand, some of these microorganisms may not be easily cultured, but they can be detected by DNA analysis.

The results of a review evaluating the microbiological composition of the placenta in a healthy pregnant woman and the potential relationship between the placental microbiome and the oral microbiome have shown the existence of a low biomass placental microflora in pregnant women with a normal course of pregnancy [29].

In turn, animal studies have shown that despite differences in gut physiology and morphology, both humans and cattle require a functional microbiome early in life (pre-implantation and organogenesis) and throughout pregnancy [25]. Studies indicate that both species acquire intestinal microbes before birth, possibly from the mother, which would indicate the existence of similar mechanisms and timing of fetal intestinal colonization.

Other studies have shown that gut microbiota dysbiosis is an important etiology of pre-eclampsia (PE) [30,31]. The intestinal microbiota and its active metabolites have great potential in the treatment and diagnosis of PE. The results of the cited work enrich the theory of the enteroplacental axis and contribute to the development of microecological products for preeclampsia. PE and FGR are placental-mediated disorders, and metabolomic studies of maternal-fetal pairings may aid in understanding their pathogenesis. Microbiome profiles from 37 overweight and obese pregnant women enrolled in the SPRING cohort were examined by 16SrRNA sequencing [32,33]. Consistent with our findings, four main bacterial phyla (*Firmicutes*, *Bacteroidetes*, *Actinobacteria* and *Proteobacteria*) were identified in all microbiomes. The possible origin of the placental microbiome was both the maternal oral and gut.

FGR is a complex obstetric complication with various causes and a wide spectrum of complications, especially for the fetus, as it is associated with an increased risk of perinatal mortality and morbidity. As highlighted above, the pathogenesis of FGR is unclear, which limits its effective treatment. It has been found that the dysbiosis of the intestinal microflora plays an important role in the pathogenesis of various diseases. However, its role in the development of FGR remains unclear and requires clarification.

In our study, significantly higher in the study group were bacteria: *Actinopolyspora erythraea*, *Listeria costaricensis*, *E. coli*, Methylobacterium, *Acidobacteria bacterium*, *Bacteroidetes bacterium*, *Paenisporsarcina* sp., *Thiodiazotropha endoloripes* and *Clostridiales bacterium*. On the other hand, in the control group, statistically more frequently, based on proteomic data, the following were found: *Flavobacterial bacterium*, *Aureimonas* sp. and *Bacillus cereus*.

Correlations between, e.g., *Helicobacteria pylori*, and the development of FGR in a group of 600 women were demonstrated by den Hollender et al. [34]. In turn, the important factor, which is the intestinal microbiome of infants, is indicated by the results of research by Groer et al. and Yang et al. [35]. Yang's research has shown correlations between an infant's physical development and fecal cysteine concentrations [36]. It also turned out that *Oscillospira* and *Coprococcus* are involved in the synthesis of butyrate, which is a source of energy for intestinal epithelial cells. Consistent with our results, a study by Tu et al., evaluating the feces of infants with FGR, showed significant differences in the growth of *Bacteroides*, *Faecalibacterium* and *Lachnospira* in patients with growth restriction [37].

In a pilot study by Hu et al., the relationship of FGR with the reproductive microbiome has been studied [38]. The reproductive microbiome was studied by 16sRNA sequencing (20-IUGR, 20-controls). Microbiological screening of the placenta showed a diverse flora as in our results, mainly *Proteobacteria*, *Fusobacteria*, *Firmicutes* and *Bacteroidetes*. The study group with FGR was characterized by a higher incidence of β-hemolytic bacteria *Neisseriaceae* and an increase in the number of anaerobic bacteria *Desulfovibrio* reflective of placental hypoxia. Further analysis of the reproductive microbiome of the FGR samples revealed lower levels of H_2O_2-producing *Bifidobacterium* and *Lactobacillus* that go from respiration to fermentation, a less energetic metabolic process as oxygen levels drop. Source tracing analysis showed that placental microbial content was predominantly from an oral source, compared to an intestinal or vaginal source. The cited results suggest that reproductive microbiome profiles may be potential biomarkers for fetal health during pregnancy in the future, while *Neisseriaceae* may represent promising therapeutic targets for the treatment of IUGR.

The *Actinopolyspora erythraea* protein identified in our FGR placentas catalyzes the circularization of gamma-N-acetyl-alpha, gamma—diaminobutyric acid (ADABA) to ectoine (1,4,5,6-tetrahydro-2-methyl-4-pyrimidine carboxylic acid), an effective osmoprotectant [39]. This prokaryote occupies an "extreme or inhabitable environment" [40]. These bacteria (extremophiles) have evolved to harsh pH, temperature, salinity and pressure by biosynthesizing unique compounds, such as new enzymes. *Acidobacteria* appear to be able to resist numerous pollutants, such as PCBs and petroleum compounds, linear alkylbenzene sulfate, p-nitrophenol, and heavy metals, under low pH circumstances [41]. A high number of acidobacterial genes code for transporters belonging to the drug/metabolite transporter superfamily. Unfortunately, no data supporting real actions linked to pollution degradation have been documented. The role of these bacteria in the pathophysiology of FGR is unknown.

Methylobacterium was also identified in FGR placentas; it is an emerging opportunistic premise plumbing pathogen (OPPsP) [42]. It possesses chlorine resistance, biofilm development, desiccation tolerance, and resilience to temperatures above 50 degrees Celsius. *Methylobacterium extorquens*, like other OPPPs, was isolated from amoebae in drinking water systems, making it an amoeba-resistant bacteria.

The sophisticated methods used in our research are based on the identification of proteins using LC-ESI-MS/MS by pooling material from 18 FGR and 18 control placentas. To distinguish between placental samples and contamination introduced during DNA extraction, purification and amplification, unsupervised ordination methods showed a separate clustering between pooled negative control and placental samples like in studies performed by others [32]. These methods do not distinguish between live, dead or ruptured bacterial fragments. Differences in relation to the data of other researchers may be statistically significant because the statistical analysis does not concern individual cases but material from the studied population, which seems to be more convincing in terms of the population.

The clinical implication of our research could be a careful consideration in the rational prescription and use of antibiotics to avoid infections while at the same time protecting the fetus from the adverse effects of pharmacotherapy.

A limitation of our study would be that we did not perform any bacterial culture of the tested bearings due to the presence of potentially viable bacteria. The material for the study was collected during cesarean section in sterile conditions. However, other researchers have confirmed that this method is devoid of the possibility of contamination [43]. Moreover, none of the taxa of bacteria mentioned in other studies were found to have different abundance between vaginally delivered and cesarean placentas [32].

Another limitation of our work is that we did not collect reference material for microbiome analysis from other parts of the body of pregnant women, such as saliva, vaginal secretions or feces. Our main goal was to determine the occurrence of individual bacteria traces, not their origin. However, it is known that the placental core microbiome shares phylotypes with the maternal oral and gut microbiome [32].

4. Materials and Methods

Patients hospitalized at the Department of Obstetrics and Pathology of Pregnancy at the Medical University of Lublin between 2019 and 2021 and between 32 and 36 weeks' gestation with a singleton pregnancy and late-onset FGR were selected for the research. Multiple pregnancies, the presence of any antenatal infections, a positive TORCH test result, treatment with antibiotics during pregnancy, any form of hypertension in pregnancy, pre-pregnancy and gestational diabetes, nephropathy, thyroid dysfunction and any other general diseases before pregnancy, the use of any drugs or stimulants, cigarette smoking, and fetuses with birth defects and chromosomal abnormalities were excluded from the study.

Thirty-six pregnant Caucasian women participated in the study, comprising 18 women with physiological pregnancy and eutrophic fetus (EFW > 10th percentile) (control group) and 18 women with late FGR identified after 32 weeks of pregnancy, according to Delphi consensus (study group) [3]. Placenta samples were successfully obtained from all eligible participants. Hadlock et al. devised a regression equation using the biparietal diameter, the length of the femur, and the head and belly circumferences to estimate the fetal weight during an ultrasound examination [44]. During one week before the birth, Doppler measurements of the umbilical artery free loop were taken using a Voluson E9 with RA4B 3D 4–8 MHz curvilinear probe (GE Healthcare, Hatfield, UK). Then, the pulsatility index (PI), resistance index (RI) and cerebroplacental ratio (CPR) were computed. PI = $(S - D)/A$ and RI = $(S - D)/S$, where S represents the systolic peak, D represents the end-diastolic flow, and A represents the temporal average frequency. In contrast, the CPR is the ratio between the PI of the middle cerebral artery (MCA) and the umbilical artery (UA) (PI MCA/PI UA) and reflects the distribution of cardiac output in favor of cerebral blood flow. It is one of the criteria with the highest predictive accuracy for perinatal outcomes [45]. In response to intrauterine hypoxia, fetal blood flow is redistributed to the brain, and the value of CPR reduces by 1. In cases of late-onset FGR, hypoxia tolerance is lower than in cases of early-onset FGR [46].

Using standardized medical records and patient interviews, smoking, age, weight, and body mass index (BMI) at the beginning of the first trimester, pregnancy weight increase, and TORCH were determined for the mothers. The BMI was computed by dividing body weight (kg) by height (m^2). Moreover, data including information on infants: gestational age at delivery, gender and birth weight of the newborn, placental weight, body length, head circumference, and neonatal problems. The gestational age was calculated using the latest menstrual period and the first-trimester ultrasonography (based on crown–rump length (CRL)). Immediately after birth, placenta weight and the neonate birth weight, body length, and head circumference were measured using the proper measuring instruments.

Material for proteomic investigation consisted of pieces of normal placentas serving as controls and fragments of placentas obtained from mothers with FGR. Following the process, trained employees collected all samples. During the cesarean section, soon after childbirth, the placenta was put in sterile containers containing ice under aseptic circumstances. Those responsible for collecting specimens wore a sterile protective apron, face masks and sterile gloves to guarantee sterility throughout the sampling procedure. The placentae were collected and weighed. Four placenta samples measuring $1.0 \times 1.0 \times 1.5$ cm were taken from each placenta (overall number of samples: 144), around 3 to 4 cm from the umbilical cord attachment point, from four separate quadrants of the placenta. To reduce the possibility of infection after cesarean delivery, only portions from the inner placenta were obtained for evaluation (risk of contamination). Each placenta sample was put in a sterile, labeled cryovial, frozen in liquid nitrogen, and kept at -80 degrees Celsius for future study.

4.1. Identification of Proteins Using LC-ESI-MS/MS

Liquid chromatography–mass spectrometry (LC-MS/MS) is an exceedingly sensitive and specific analytical technique that can precisely determine the identities and concentration of compounds within samples [47]. Because it identifies the proteins that are present in a sample and quantifies the abundance levels of the discovered proteins, it is utilized in proteomic research.

4.1.1. Protein Extraction

One hundred milligram sections were taken from the collected clinical material. Eighteen sections from normal placentas (control group) and eighteen FGR placentas (study group) were pooled and proteins were isolated. Clinical material in both samples was homogenized in liquid nitrogen (by mechanical homogenization in liquid nitrogen) and then suspended in a solution of 0.2 M $(NH_4)_2SO_4$ and left on ice for 30 min. After this time, the samples were centrifuged ($10,000 \times g$) for 39 min to remove cell debris. Proteins were isolated from the supernatant according to the procedure described by Diffley [48]. The quality of the preparations was assessed using 1-D gel electrophoresis separation [49].

4.1.2. Mass Spectrometry Examination

In the Laboratory of Mass Spectrometry, Institute of Biochemistry and Biophysics, Polish Academy of Sciences, Warsaw, Poland, proteins were examined by liquid chromatography linked to a mass spectrometer. Using two technical replicates, tryptic peptide mixtures were evaluated by LC-ESI-MS/MS employing nanoflow HPLC and an LTQ-Orbitrap XL (Thermo Fisher Scientific, Waltham, MA, USA) as the mass analyzer. Trypsin was used to break down the proteins. The synthesized peptides were concentrated, desalted on an RP-C18 precolumn (LC Packings, Coventry, UK), and then separated by UltiMate nano-HPLC (LC Packings, San Diego, CA, USA) with a linear acetonitrile gradient (from 10 to 30%) over 50 min. The column was linked directly to a nanospray ion source working in a data-dependent MS to MS/MS mode transition. Proteins were identified by tandem mass spectrometry (MS/MS) by acquiring fragmentation spectra of multiple-charged peptides in a manner dependent on information.

4.1.3. Identification Method for Proteins

MASCOT 2.4.1 (Matrix Science, London, UK) was used to search the Uniprot 2019_02 (561356 sequences; 201858328 residues) database with bacterial sequences and a filter to examine the spectrum data. These were the search criteria for mascots: With variable carbamidomethyl (C) and oxidation (M) modifications, peptide mass tolerance of 50 ppm and fragment mass tolerance of 0.8 Da. Acceptable protein identification required the identification of at least two peptide fragments per protein.

4.1.4. Quantitative Evaluation

The Exponentially Modified Protein Abundance Index (emPAI) was utilized to perform a non-label quantitative comparison of proteins between studied samples [50]. The protein abundance index (PAI) is the quantity of peptides per protein normalized by the theoretical number of peptides. The exponential version of PAI minus one (emPAI = 10PAI 1) is used to calculate protein abundance from nano-LC–MS/MS investigations. The value of emPAI is proportional to the abundance of proteins in a protein mixture. In Excel files, the resulting protein and peptide lists were preserved.

4.2. Statistical Analysis

The statistical analysis of the data collected in the spreadsheet was carried out using the Statistica program (v. 13 PL, TIBCO Software Inc. Palo Alto, CA, USA). The content (expressed by percentages calculated based on the emPAI value) of individual bacterial proteins in the test material (derived from the study group or control) was compared using the *Chi*-squared test with Yates' correction. All reported *p*-values are two-sided (or two-tailed). Since the analysis was based on multiple comparisons, Bonferroni correction was applied. Thus, only results with $p < 0.001$ were considered statistically significant.

4.3. Ethics

Written informed consent was obtained from all subjects included, and the study was performed in accordance with the principles of the Helsinki Declaration. The research was issued by the Bioethics Committee at the Medical University of Lublin (Approval No. KE-0254/87/2020). Derived data supporting the findings of this study are available from the corresponding author on request.

5. Conclusions

To sum up, the presence of numerous bacterial proteins present in the control material, which are absent in the material taken from the study group, may indicate their protective role. Similarly, the presence of bacterial proteins found only in the material obtained from people from the study group may indicate their potentially pathogenic nature.

However, we must remember that the proteome does not necessarily correspond to the content of the bacteria themselves, due to the variable expression of many proteins depending on their type and needs.

Supplementary Materials: The following supporting information can be downloaded at: https://www.mdpi.com/article/10.3390/ijms24086922/s1.

Author Contributions: Conceptualization, A.S., A.K. and A.G.-J.; Methodology, R.M., R.N. and A.G.-J.; Software, T.G.; Validation, P.P.; Formal analysis, R.M. and R.N.; Investigation, A.S., T.G., R.M. and A.G.-J.; Resources, P.P. and R.N.; Data curation, A.S., T.G. and W.K.; Writing—original draft, A.S. and A.G.-J.; Writing—review & editing, T.G., A.K. and R.M.; Visualization, R.M.; Supervision, A.K. and W.K.; Project administration, W.K.; Funding acquisition, A.K. All authors have read and agreed to the published version of the manuscript.

Funding: This research was funded by Medical University of Lublin grant number DS 128.

Institutional Review Board Statement: Not applicable.

Informed Consent Statement: Informed consent was obtained from all subjects involved in the study.

Data Availability Statement: The data presented in this study are available on request from the corresponding author.

Conflicts of Interest: The authors declare no conflict of interest.

Abbreviations

ADABA	circularization of gamma-N-acetyl-alpha: gamma-diaminobutyric acid
APGAR	appearance, pulse, grimace, activity, respiration score
BMI	body mass index
CRL	crown–rump length
CPR	cerebroplacental ratio
EFW	estimated fetal weight
emPAI	Exponentially Modified Protein Abundance Index
FGR	fetal growth restriction
HMP	Human Microbiome Project
NGS	next-generation sequencing
OPPsP	opportunistic premise plumbing pathogen
PE	preeclampsia
PI	pulsation index
RI	resistance index
TNF	tumor necrosis factor
TORCH	toxoplasmosis, other, rubella, cytomegalic and herpes infection

References

1. Romo, A.; Carceller, R.; Tobajas, J. Intrauterine growth retardation (IUGR): Epidemiology and etiology. *Pediatr. Endocrinol. Rev.* **2009**, *6* (Suppl. 3), 332–336.
2. Nardozza, L.M.; Caetano, A.C.; Zamarian, A.C.; Mazzola, J.B.; Silva, C.P.; Marçal, V.M.G.; Lobo, T.F.; Peixoto, A.B.; Júnior, E.A. Fetal growth restriction: Current knowledge. *Arch. Gynecol. Obstet.* **2017**, *295*, 1061–1077. [CrossRef]
3. Gordijn, S.J.; Beune, I.M.; Thilaganathan, B.; Papageorghiou, A.; Baschat, A.A.; Baker, P.N.; Silver, R.M.; Wynia, K.; Ganzevoort, W. Consensus definition of fetal growth restriction: A Delphi procedure. *Ultrasound Obs. Gynecol.* **2016**, *48*, 333–339. [CrossRef] [PubMed]
4. Kamphof, H.D.; Posthuma, S.; Gordijn, S.J.; Wessel, G. Fetal Growth Restriction: Mechanisms, Epidemiology, and Management. *Matern.-Fetal Med.* **2022**, *4*, 186–196. [CrossRef]
5. Chew, L.C.; Verma, R.P. Fetal Growth Restriction. In *StatPearls [Internet]*; StatPearls Publishing: Treasure Island, FL, USA, 2022. Available online: https://www.ncbi.nlm.nih.gov/books/NBK562268/ (accessed on 5 March 2023).
6. Melamed, N.; Baschat, A.; Yinon, Y.; Athanasiadis, A.; Mecacci, F.; Figueras, F.; Berghella, V.; Nazareth, A.; Tahlak, M.; McIntyre, H.D.; et al. FIGO (international Federation of Gynecology and obstetrics) initiative on fetal growth: Best practice advice for screening, diagnosis, and management of fetal growth restriction. *Int. J. Gynaecol. Obstet.* **2021**, *152* (Suppl. 1), 3–57. [CrossRef]
7. Maulik, D. Fetal Growth Restriction: The Etiology. *Clin. Obstet. Gynecol.* **2006**, *49*, 228–235. [CrossRef] [PubMed]
8. Longo, S.; Borghesi, A.; Tzialla, C.; Stroti, M. IUGR and infections. *Early Hum. Dev.* **2014**, *90* (Suppl. 1), S42–S44. [CrossRef]
9. Germain, M.; Krohn, M.A.; Hillier, S.L.; Eschenbach, D.A. Genital flora in pregnancy and its association with intrauterine growth retardation. *J. Clin. Microbiol.* **1994**, *32*, 2162–2168. [CrossRef] [PubMed]
10. Fernandez-Gonzalez, S.; Ortiz-Arrabal, O.; Torrecillas, A.; Pérez-Cruz, M.; Chueca, N.; Gómez-Roig, M.D.; Gómez-Llorente, C. Study of the Fetal and Maternal Microbiota in Pregnant Women with Intrauterine Growth Restriction and Its Relationship with Inflammatory Biomarkers: A Case-Control Study Protocol (SPIRIT Compliant). *Medicine* **2020**, *99*, e22722. [CrossRef]

11. Fujimura, K.E.; Sitarik, A.R.; Havstad, S.; Lin, D.L.; Levan, S.; Fadrosh, D.; Panzer, A.R.; LaMere, B.; Rackaityte, E.; Lukacs, N.W.; et al. Neonatal gut microbiota associates with childhood multisensitized atopy and T cell differentiation. *Nat. Med.* **2016**, *22*, 1187–1191. [CrossRef]
12. Ruohtula, T.; de Goffau, M.C.; Nieminen, J.K.; Honkanen, J.; Siljander, H.; Hämäläinen, A.; Peet, A.; Tillmann, V.; Ilonen, J.; Niemelä, O.; et al. Maturation of Gut Microbiota and Circulating Regulatory T Cells and Development of IgE Sensitization in Early Life. *Front. Immunol.* **2019**, *10*, 2494. [CrossRef]
13. Soderborg, T.K.; Clark, S.E.; Mulligan, C.E.; Janssen, R.C.; Babcock, L.; Ir, D.; Young, B.; Krebs, N.; Lemas, D.J.; Johnson, L.K.; et al. The gut microbiota in infants of obese mothers increases inflammation and susceptibility to NAFLD. *Nat. Commun.* **2018**, *9*, 4462, Erratum in *Nat. Commun.* **2019**, *10*, 2965. [CrossRef]
14. Available online: https://www.nature.com/subjects/microbiome (accessed on 30 March 2023).
15. Whipps, J.M.; Lewis, K.; Cooke, R.C. Mycoparasitism and plant disease control. In *Fungi in Biological Control Systems, ed 2001*; Manchester University Press: Manchester, NH, USA, 1988; pp. 161–187.
16. Bolte, E.E.; Moorshead, D.; Aagaard, K.M. Maternal and early life exposures and their potential to influence development of the microbiome. *Genome Med.* **2022**, *14*, 4. [CrossRef] [PubMed]
17. Bull, M.J.; Plummer, N.T. Part 1: The Human Gut Microbiome in Health and Disease. *Integr. Med.* **2014**, *13*, 17–22.
18. Shreiner, A.B.; Kao, J.Y.; Young, V.B. The gut microbiome in health and in disease. *Curr. Opin. Gastroenterol.* **2015**, *31*, 69–75. [CrossRef] [PubMed]
19. Cani, P.D. Human gut microbiome: Hopes, threats and promises. *Gut* **2018**, *67*, 1716–1725. [CrossRef] [PubMed]
20. Available online: http://www.commonfund.nih.gov/hmp (accessed on 30 March 2023).
21. Sirota, I.; Zarek, S.M.; Segars, J.H. Potential influence of the microbiome on infertility and assisted reproductive technology. *Semin. Reprod. Med.* **2014**, *32*, 35–42. [CrossRef]
22. Lamont, R.F.; Sobel, J.D.; Akins, R.A.; Hassan, S.S.; Chaiworapongsa, T.; Kusanovic, J.P.; Romero, R. The vaginal microbiome: New information about genital tract flora using molecular based techniques. *BJOG Int. J. Obstet. Gynaecol.* **2011**, *118*, 533–549. [CrossRef]
23. Verstraelen, H.; Vieira-Baptista, P.; De Seta, F.; Ventolini, G.; Lonnee-Hoffmann, R.; Lev-Sagie, A. The Vaginal Microbiome: I. Research Development, Lexicon, Defining "Normal" and the Dynamics Throughout Women's Lives. *J. Low. Genit. Tract Dis.* **2022**, *26*, 73–78. [CrossRef]
24. Cariño, R., 3rd; Takayasu, L.; Suda, W.; Masuoka, H.; Hirayama, K.; Konishi, S.; Umezaki, M. The search for aliens within us: A review of evidence and theory regarding the fetal microbiome. *Crit. Rev. Microbiol.* **2022**, *48*, 611–623. [CrossRef]
25. Hummel, G.L.; Austin, K.; Cunningham-Hollinger, H.C. Comparing the maternal-fetal microbiome of humans and cattle: A translational assessment of the reproductive, placental, and fetal gut microbiomes. *Biol. Reprod.* **2022**, *107*, 371–381. [CrossRef]
26. Hayward, C.E.; Jones, R.L.; Sibley, C.P. Mechanisms of transfer across the human placenta. In *Fetal and Neonatal Physiology*, 5th ed.; Polin, R.A., Abman, S.H., Rowitch, D.H., Benitz, W.E., Fox, W.W., Eds.; Elsevier: Philadelphia, PA, USA, 2017; pp. 121–133.
27. Gęca, T.; Stupak, A.; Nawrot, R.; Goździcka-Józefiak, A.; Kwaśniewska, A.; Kwaśniewski, W. Placental proteome in late-onset of fetal growth restriction. *Mol. Med. Rep.* **2022**, *26*, 356. [CrossRef]
28. Gomez de Agüero, M.; Ganal-Vonarburg, S.C.; Fuhrer, T.; Rupp, S.; Uchimura, Y.; Li, H.; Steinert, A.; Heikenwalder, M.; Hapfelmeier, S.; Sauer, U.; et al. The maternal microbiota drives early postnatal innate immune development. *Science* **2016**, *351*, 1296–1302. [CrossRef] [PubMed]
29. Zakis, D.R.; Paulissen, E.; Kornete, L.; Kaan, A.; Nicu, E.A.; Zaura, E. The evidence for placental microbiome and its composition in healthy pregnancies: A systematic review. *J. Reprod. Immunol.* **2022**, *149*, 103455. [CrossRef] [PubMed]
30. Altemani, F.; Barrett, H.L.; Gomez-Arango, L.; Josh, P.; McIntyre, H.D.; Callaway, L.K.; Morrison, M.; Tyson, G.W.; Nitert, M.D. Pregnant Women Who Develop Preeclampsia Have Lower Abundance of the Butyrate-Producer Coprococcus in Their Gut Microbiota. *Pregnancy Hypertens.* **2021**, *23*, 211–219. [CrossRef] [PubMed]
31. Jin, J.; Gao, L.; Zou, X.; Zhang, Y.; Zheng, Z.; Zhang, X.; Li, J.; Tian, Z.; Wang, X.; Gu, J.; et al. Gut Dysbiosis Promotes Preeclampsia by Regulating Macrophages and Trophoblasts. *Circ. Res.* **2022**, *131*, 492–506. [CrossRef] [PubMed]
32. Gomez-Arango, L.F.; Barrett, H.L.; McIntyre, H.D.; Callaway, L.K.; Morrison, M.; Nitert, M.D. Contributions of the maternal oral and gut microbiome to placental microbial colonization in overweight and obese pregnant women. *Sci. Rep.* **2017**, *7*, 2860. [CrossRef]
33. Nitert, M.D.; Barrett, H.L.; Foxcroft, K.; Tremellen, A.; Wilkinson, S.; Lingwood, B.; Tobin, J.M.; McSweeney, C.; O'Rourke, P.; McIntyre, H.; et al. SPRING: An RCT study of probiotics in the prevention of gestational diabetes mellitus in overweight and obese women. *BMC Pregnancy Childbirth* **2013**, *13*, 50. [CrossRef]
34. Den Hollander, W.J.; Schalekamp-Timmermans, S.; Holster, I.L.; Jaddoe, V.W.; Hofman, A.; Moll, H.A.; Perez-Perez, G.I.; Blaser, M.J.; Steegers, E.A.P.; Kuipers, E.J. Helicobacter Pylori Colonization and Pregnancies Complicated by Preeclampsia, Spontaneous Prematurity, and Small for Gestational Age Birth. *Helicobacter* **2017**, *22*, e12364. [CrossRef]
35. Groer, M.W.; Luciano, A.A.; Dishaw, L.J.; Ashmeade, T.L.; Miller, E.; Gilbert, J.A. Development of the Preterm Infant Gut Microbiome: A Research Priority. *Microbiome* **2014**, *2*, 38. [CrossRef]
36. Yang, J.; Hou, L.; Wang, J.; Xiao, L.; Zhang, J.; Yin, N.; Yao, S.; Cheng, K.; Zhang, W.; Shi, Z.; et al. Unfavourable Intrauterine Environment Contributes to Abnormal Gut Microbiome and Metabolome in Twins. *Gut* **2022**, *71*, 2451–2462. [CrossRef] [PubMed]

37. Tu, X.; Duan, C.; Lin, B.; Li, K.; Gao, J.; Yan, H.; Wang, K.; Zhao, Z. Characteristics of the Gut Microbiota in Pregnant Women with Fetal Growth Restriction. *BMC Pregnancy Childbirth* **2022**, *22*, 297. [CrossRef] [PubMed]
38. Hu, J.; Benny, P.; Wang, M.; Ma, Y.; Lambertini, L.; Peter, I.; Xu, Y.; Lee, M.J. Intrauterine Growth Restriction Is Associated with Unique Features of the Reproductive Microbiome. *Reprod. Sci.* **2021**, *28*, 828–837. [CrossRef] [PubMed]
39. Available online: https://www.uniprot.org/uniprotkb/A0A099D2A0/entry (accessed on 30 March 2023).
40. Zhao, L.-X.; Huang, S.-X.; Tang, S.-K.; Jiang, C.-L.; Duan, Y.; Beutler, J.A.; Henrich, C.J.; McMahon, J.B.; Schmid, T.; Blees, J.S.; et al. Actinopolysporins AC and tubercidin as a Pdcd4 stabilizer from the halophilic actinomycetes *Actinopolyspora erythraea* YIM 90600. *J. Nat. Prod.* **2011**, *74*, 1990–1995. [CrossRef]
41. Kielak, A.M.; Barreto, C.C.; Kowalchuk, G.A.; Van Veen, J.A.; Kuramae, E.E. The Ecology of Acidobacteria: Moving beyond Genes and Genomes. *Front. Microbiol.* **2016**, *7*, 744. [CrossRef]
42. Szwetkowski, K.J.; Falkinham, J.O., III. *Methylobacterium* spp. as Emerging Opportunistic Premise Plumbing Pathogens. *Pathogens* **2020**, *9*, 149. [CrossRef]
43. Gschwind, R.; Fournier, T.; Kennedy, S.; Tsatsaris, V.; Cordier, A.G.; Barbut, F.; Butel, M.J.; Wydawu-Dematteis, S. Evidence for contamination as the origin for bacteria found in human placenta rather than a microbiota. *PLoS ONE* **2020**, *15*, e0237232. [CrossRef]
44. Hadlock, F.P.; Harrist, R.B.; Sharman, R.S.; Deter, R.L.; Park, S.K. Estimation of fetal weight with the use of head, body, and femur measurements—A prospective study. *Am. J. Obstet. Gynecol.* **1985**, *151*, 333–337. [CrossRef]
45. Ebbing, C.; Rasmussen, S.; Kiserud, T. Middle cerebral artery blood flow velocities and pulsatility index and the cerebroplacental pulsatility ratio: Longitudinal reference ranges and terms for serial measurements. *Ultrasound Obs. Gynecol.* **2007**, *30*, 287–296. [CrossRef]
46. Jugović, D.; Tumbri, J.; Medić, M.; Jukić, M.K.; Kurjak, A.; Arbeille, P.; Salihagić-Kadić, A. New Doppler index for prediction of perinatal brain damage in growth-restricted and hypoxic fetuses. *Ultrasound Obs. Gynecol.* **2007**, *30*, 303–311. [CrossRef]
47. Karpievitch, Y.V.; Polpitiya, A.D.; Anderson, G.A.; Smith, R.D.; Dabney, A.R. Liquid Chromatography Mass Spectrometry-Based Proteomics: Biological and Technological Aspects. *Ann. Appl. Stat.* **2010**, *4*, 1797–1823. [CrossRef] [PubMed]
48. Diffley, J.F.; BStillman, B. Similarity between the transcriptional silencer binding proteins ABF1 and RAP1. *Science* **1998**, *246*, 1034–1038. [CrossRef] [PubMed]
49. Nawrot, R.; Kalinowski, A.; Goździcka-Józefiak, A. Proteomic analysis of Chelidonium majus milky sap using two-dimensial gel electrophoresis and tandem mass spectrometry. *Phyochemistry* **2007**, *68*, 1612–1622. [CrossRef] [PubMed]
50. Ishihama, Y.; Oda, Y.; Tabata, T.; Sato, T.; Nagasu, T.; Rappsilber, J.; Mann, M. Exponentially modified protein abundance index (emPAI) for estimation of absolute protein amount in proteomics by the number of sequenced peptides per protein. *Mol. Cell. Proteom.* **2005**, *4*, 1265–1272. [CrossRef]

Disclaimer/Publisher's Note: The statements, opinions and data contained in all publications are solely those of the individual author(s) and contributor(s) and not of MDPI and/or the editor(s). MDPI and/or the editor(s) disclaim responsibility for any injury to people or property resulting from any ideas, methods, instructions or products referred to in the content.

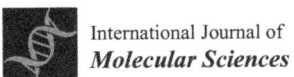

Review

What the Gut Tells the Brain—Is There a Link between Microbiota and Huntington's Disease?

Dorota Wronka [1,†], Anna Karlik [1,†], Julia O. Misiorek [2] and Lukasz Przybyl [1,*]

1. Laboratory of Mammalian Model Organisms, Institute of Bioorganic Chemistry Polish Academy of Sciences, Noskowskiego 12/14, 61-704 Poznan, Poland
2. Department of Molecular Neurooncology, Institute of Bioorganic Chemistry Polish Academy of Sciences, Noskowskiego 12/14, 61-704 Poznan, Poland
* Correspondence: lukasz.przybyl@ibch.poznan.pl
† These authors contributed equally to this work.

Abstract: The human intestinal microbiota is a diverse and dynamic microenvironment that forms a complex, bi-directional relationship with the host. The microbiome takes part in the digestion of food and the generation of crucial nutrients such as short chain fatty acids (SCFA), but is also impacts the host's metabolism, immune system, and even brain functions. Due to its indispensable role, microbiota has been implicated in both the maintenance of health and the pathogenesis of many diseases. Dysbiosis in the gut microbiota has already been implicated in many neurodegenerative diseases such as Parkinson's disease (PD) and Alzheimer's disease (AD). However, not much is known about the microbiome composition and its interactions in Huntington's disease (HD). This dominantly heritable, incurable neurodegenerative disease is caused by the expansion of CAG trinucleotide repeats in the huntingtin gene (*HTT*). As a result, toxic RNA and mutant protein (mHTT), rich in polyglutamine (polyQ), accumulate particularly in the brain, leading to its impaired functions. Interestingly, recent studies indicated that mHTT is also widely expressed in the intestines and could possibly interact with the microbiota, affecting the progression of HD. Several studies have aimed so far to screen the microbiota composition in mouse models of HD and find out whether observed microbiome dysbiosis could affect the functions of the HD brain. This review summarizes ongoing research in the HD field and highlights the essential role of the intestine-brain axis in HD pathogenesis and progression. The review also puts a strong emphasis on indicating microbiome composition as a future target in the urgently needed therapy for this still incurable disease.

Keywords: Huntington's disease; neurodegeneration; gastrointestinal microbiome; gut-brain axis; dysbiosis; immune

1. Introduction

1.1. Intestinal Microbiome

The intestinal microbiome is the largest and most active group of microorganisms in the human body. It plays an essential role in health and disease, but due to its complexity, it is challenging to elucidate the specific interactions between the bacterial species and the impact on host metabolism. The large intestine (colon) is the main place inhabited by microbiota. It is built up by several tissue types, including lumen-facing colonocytes that form the inner epithelial layer. A healthy microbiome is advantageous to the host due to its ability to digest various large molecules, like long plant-derived polysaccharides, into smaller nutrients, like short chain fatty acids (SCFA), that can be absorbed and utilized by the host. It also produces various other molecules, such as amino acids, vitamins, and neurotransmitters, that contribute to the host's health [1,2]. Over 1000 different bacterial species colonize the human gut, the vast majority of which have yet to be functionally characterized. The microbiota composition is dynamic and influenced by a variety of environmental factors such as diet, physical activity, host genetics, age, and antibiotic treatment, all of which contribute to the great diversity observed in healthy individuals. It is thus a challenge to accurately characterize a healthy microbiome [3]. We took a closer look at several large-scale studies that point to the genera *Bacteroides* and *Clostridium* as being the most prevalent, with *Clostridium* being less abundant than *Bacteroides* in the human intestine. Several genera, including *Bifidobacterium, Eubacterium, Lactobacillus, Streptococcus,* and *Escherichia*, were also present but in much lower abundance [3]. Determining a clear definition of a "healthy" microbiome is challenging, and many various factors need to be considered. The microbiome composition is dependent on a multitude of factors that may seem insignificant at first glance. In 2010, studies conducted by the MetaHIT consortium made an attempt to quantify microbiome diversity. According to the obtained results, there are 3.3 million non-redundant genes in the human gut microbiome [4], however, it had been known until early 2000s that the human genome consists of about 22,000 genes [5]. Further research confirms that the diversity of the microbiome is enormous between individuals and can differ by up to 90% in terms of microbiome localization (e.g., those found on the hands vs. those present in the gut) [6,7]. These findings drive scientists and physicians towards developing a highly personalized treatment plan. The profile and microbiota composition changes with the host's lifespan, starting from embryos which were thought to be sterile till now. The microbiota colonizes newborns' intestines, but studies have also revealed the microbiome's presence in semen, placenta, amniotic fluid, umbilical cord blood, and meconium [8]. Moreover, factors such as delivery and feeding methods are essential for microbiota composition in infants and adults. Further, when children start to ingest solid food, their intestinal microbiome becomes more diversified, and during puberty, the release of sex hormones also contributes to microbiome maturation [9]. Next, diversification of the microbiome occurs naturally with the physiological development of the organism, i.e., the increase in length and volume of the intestines provides the microbiome with appropriate niches. Numerous studies indicate that there is a correlation between aging and microbiome composition. In 2011, a pioneering study was conducted to compare the composition of the microbiome in fecal samples from people aged 64 to 102 (study group) and young adults with an average age of 36 (control group). The results showed that the "core" microbiome—defined as the specific species found in the microbiome of at least 50% of study participants—was significantly different between the groups [10,11]. So far, the main function of the intestinal microbiome has been identified as maintaining body homeostasis. Researchers emphasize that despite the fact that technological progress is at a high level, the individual composition of the microbiome, functional characteristics, or interactions between the host and microbes have not yet been established [12]. Data collected by the Human Microbiome Project [13,14] and MetaHIT [4,15] report that 2776 species of prokaryotic microorganisms isolated from human feces have been identified (data for 2019) [16]. They have been classified into 11 different phyla, including *Proteobacteria, Firmicutes, Actinobacteria,* and *Bacteroidetes*, which make up over 90% of the microbiome, [15,17,18], while *Fusobacteria* and *Verrucomicrobia* are present in trace amounts [19]. As mentioned earlier, microbiota are essential for the proper function and homeostasis of the intestines. Interactions between gut colonocytes, immune cells, and microbiota are heavily involved in shaping the immune response throughout the body [20]. In support of this, gut microbiota transplants from healthy individuals have been found to alleviate symptoms and reduce inflammation in disorders like ulcerative colitis, irritable bowel syndrome (IBS), and hepatic encephalopathy [21,22].

1.2. Short Chain Fatty Acid Production and Their Importance

Key end products of microbial fermentation in the large intestine are short chain fatty acids. They are saturated carboxylic acids containing less than six carbons in their chain structure. The main sources of SCFAs are dietary macromolecules, especially fiber-rich plant-derived polysaccharides that are indigestible to humans due to the lack of enzymes required for breaking the glycosidic bonds. Thus, they are available to microbes in the intestinal lumen, which ferment them and make them available to the host. SCFAs are transported into the colonic epithelial cells by solute transporters or by simple diffusion across the membranes [23]. 95% of the total SCFAs in the human gut are acetate, propionate, and butyrate, and their levels are largely dependent on the diet and the amount of fiber, which affect the microbiota composition. The main species involved in the production of acetate are *Akkermansia muciniphila*, *Bacteroidetes* spp., and *Prevetolla* spp. Propionate is mostly produced by *Bacteroidetes* and *Firmicutes*, with the latter also producing butyrate. SCFAs are an important energy source for colonocytes and hepatocytes, but they also enter the systemic circulation and act as signaling molecules to exert a variety of regulatory functions. The presence of SCFAs is closely linked to gut integrity, not only through increased expression of tight junction (TJ) proteins but also through modulation of the host immune system. They act as ligands for G-protein-coupled receptors (GPR), their main targets being GPR43 and GPR41, also called free fatty acid receptor-2 (FFAR2) and free fatty acid receptor-3 (FFAR3), respectively. It has also been reported that butyrate can interact with GPR109/HCA2 (hydroxycarboxylic acid receptor 2). These receptors are involved in the glucose metabolism, lipid regulation, and gut homeostasis, as well as being expressed on immune cells, where they can influence the inflammation. Indeed, acetate has been implicated in resolving enteritis through GPR43 signaling [24]. Propionate, butyrate, and valerate can influence gene transcription by inhibiting histone deacetylase (HDAC) and thus making chromatin more accessible to transcription factors. Butyrate has been shown to be a potent suppressor of $CD4^+$ T cell activation, acting through GPR43 and HDAC inhibition to decrease proliferation and production of proinflammatory cytokines (IFN-γ, IL-17) [25,26]. Studies show that butyrate-mediated inhibition of class II HDAC in the gut $CD4^+$ T cells epigenetically induces the transcription of genes responsible for regulatory T cell (Treg) function [27]. There are many examples of the anti-inflammatory roles of SCFAs, but some studies report a dual effect, inducing both Treg and cytotoxic effector T cells, which points out the need for further studies [23].

Importantly, SCFAs can also cross the blood-brain barrier and affect the brain, which renders them as a potential target in neuroinflammatory diseases [20]. Supplementation of sodium butyrate has been tested on the R6/2 mouse model of HD, yielding positive results. When compared to untreated controls, the supplemented group showed improved motor performance, increased brain weight, and decreased striatal neuronal atrophy. However, sodium butyrate supplementation had no effect on the formation of mutant huntingtin (mHTT) aggregates or weight loss [28]. The study conducted on the YAC128 mouse HD model has also shown a beneficial effect of sodium butyrate supplementation, as the treated group displayed improved learning and motor skills, as well as improved cortical energy levels and increased histone 3 acetylation, suggesting that butyrate acting as an HDAC inhibitor can improve mitochondrial and transcriptional dysfunctions present in HD [29].

1.3. Tryptophan Metabolism

Tryptophan is an essential amino acid, since in mammals it is mainly derived from diet and used for protein synthesis or converted through two main pathways: serotonin or kynurenine. In the body, there are two pools of serotonin: the brain and the gut. In the brain, serotonin is synthesized in the midbrain by neurons of the raphe nucleus, although the vast majority of serotonin is produced in the gut and can impact the brain through the stimulation of the vagus nerve. Other microbial metabolites, such as butyrate, can also impact serotonin production by stimulating the activity of the tryptophan hydroxylase 1 (TPH1) enzyme. The serotonin pathway can also lead to the synthesis of melatonin, which regulates the biological rhythm and can have antioxidant and anti-inflammatory effects [30].

The kynurenine pathway utilizes the vast majority of available tryptophan and leads to the synthesis of NAD^+, which is essential for the proper functioning of the cells. There are two enzymes responsible for the conversion of tryptophan into kynurenine: IDO1 and IDO2. The IDO1 enzyme has been implicated as a key molecule regulating the host-microbiome symbiotic relationship and immune responses. L-kynurenine acts as a ligand for the aryl hydrocarbon receptor (AhR), which is expressed in lymphoid tissues and has been linked to promoting Treg development in the periphery, thus stimulating homeostasis and immune tolerance. AhR signaling is also responsible for promoting IL-22 expression in gut-resident type 3 innate lymphoid cells (ILC3) [31]. There are two major metabolites synthesized along this pathway that have neuroactive properties: kynurenic acid (KYNA) and quinolinic acid (QUIN). KYNA has a neuroprotective function and is mainly produced by astrocytes, while QUIN has neurotoxic effects and is synthesized by microglia. The presence of IFN-γ and a proinflammatory environment has been found to promote QUIN production and skew the balance towards neurotoxicity.

Additionally, the gut microbiome can metabolize tryptophan along the indole pathway. *Escherichia coli*, *Clostridium* spp., and *Bacteroides* spp. are known to utilize this pathway. About 5% of ingested tryptophan is used by microbes for a variety of physiological processes, like biofilm formation, drug resistance, virulence, and others, which are required for the maintenance of a variable microbial community, but indole and its derivatives also influence the host [30,32]. Similar to kynurenine, several indole derivatives can act as ligands for AhR and have been linked to promoting IL-22 expression. A study has shown that regulation of gut IL-22 expression by indole-3-aldehyde allows for the survival of a varied microbial community while providing resistance to opportunistic fungi (*C. albicans*) infection [31].

1.4. Gut-Brain Axis

The gut-brain axis is the main link between the digestive tract and the central nervous system (CNS). It is a specific two-way communication system consisting of neural pathways such as the enteric nervous system (ENS), the sympathetic and spinal vagus nerves, and the humoral pathways involving cytokines, hormones, and neuropeptides [33]. The factors regulating the work of the axis include cortisol, SCFAs, neurotransmitters, neuromodulators, and the intestinal microbiota, which has been recognized relatively recently and is still gaining popularity. For a long time, the gut-brain axis has been known to play a role in maintaining homeostasis in the body. Disturbances of the brain-gut axis are believed to lead to systemic disorders, such as dysregulation of the intestinal system and CNS disorders, e.g., depression [34,35]. The direct impact of the microbiome on the CNS is still poorly understood. The gut microbiome is known to produce neurotransmitters such as gamma-aminobutyric acid (GABA), histamine, dopamine, norepinephrine, and serotonin, as well as most likely other neuroactive molecules [16]. The ENS is the internal nervous system of the gastrointestinal tract, where neurons organized in microarrays enable modulation of gastrointestinal function independently from the CNS, although the systems are interconnected and interact with each other [36]. This combination is also believed to allow the neurodegenerative diseases to progress. In 80% of individuals affected by Parkinson's disease, the symptoms of neurodegeneration were preceded by digestive system symptoms. It has been suggested that alpha-synucleopathy of the gastrointestinal nervous system is an early indicator of Parkinson's disease. The regular expression of the *APP* gene in the ENS indicates that it is also involved in the pathogenesis of Alzheimer's disease [37,38].

2. Neurodegenerative Disease Characterization and Link to Microbiome

2.1. Parkinson's Disease and Alzheimer's Disease

Two of the most prevalent neurodegenerative diseases are Parkinson's disease (PD) and Alzheimer's disease (AD), with the latter being more common. They are both progressive and associated with advanced age, but their exact causes are not fully understood, although it is believed that a combination of both genetic and environmental factors play a role in their development and progression. AD is mostly associated with memory loss, disorientation, and behavioral issues. In the brain, there is a progressive loss of neurons and the formation of amyloid plaques and neurofibrillary tangles originating from the amyloid-beta (Aβ) precursor protein (APP). PD is characterized by abnormal accumulation and aggregation of alpha-synuclein in the form of Lewy bodies and loss of dopaminergic neurons in the substantia nigra, which causes dopamine deficiency. The most common motor symptoms are tremors, stiffness, bradykinesia, and loss of coordination, with accompanying cognitive disorders such as depression, anxiety, and apathy [39,40].

The composition of the intestinal microbiota is not only important for maintaining the proper health of the body but can also affect the physiological, behavioral, and cognitive functions of the brain. There is ample evidence for differences in the microbiome between healthy individuals and PD patients. Patients suffering from PD were characterized by a reduced presence of *Prevotellaceae* bacteria and an increased number of *Enterobacteriaceae* bacteria. Currently, it is difficult to clearly define the role of SCFAs in the pathogenesis of neurodegenerative diseases. However, the vast majority of publications indicate pathological SCFA activity in PD patients. Studies in mice overexpressing alpha-synuclein demonstrate the effect of a microbial-free environment on the elimination of the PD phenotype, and oral feeding of SCFAs to the same mice restores the neuropathology associated with PD. Counterintuitively, SCFA administration to patients increases motor dysfunction and inflammation [41–43]. According to a study published in 2019, bacteria from the *Prevotellaceae* family have been found to provide high levels of health-promoting neuroactive SCFAs, which in turn contribute to a healthy environment in the gut [44]. Decreased *Prevotella* abundance has also been linked to multiple sclerosis (MS), type 1 diabetes, and autism spectrum disorders. Furthermore, the presence of *Prevotella* is significantly influenced by a plant-based diet. Increased abundance of *Lactobacillus* has been associated with type 2 diabetes and constipation, suggesting that the prognostic value of *Lactobacillus* is not specific to PD. Multiple bacterial taxa have been reported to be altered in individuals with PD. Potential interactions between them indicate that the effects of altered gut microbiota in PD may be the result of many complex cascades of events within the entire gut microbiota as well as relationships with the host [45].

Recent results suggest a strong link between the pathogenesis of AD and intestinal microbiota dysfunctions. Studies conducted on the ADLPAPT mouse model of AD show that changes in the composition of the intestinal microflora led to a loss of intestinal epithelial integrity, which in turn caused systemic inflammation. Intestinal abnormalities coincided with Aβ deposition, Tau protein pathology, progressive gliosis, and cognitive impairment in the animals. It was also noted that the transplantation of microbiota from healthy animals into animals suffering from AD significantly attenuated the progression of AD pathogenesis [46]. A number of studies indicate significant changes in the composition of the gut microbiota during the course of AD. There was an increase in *Firmicutes/Bacteroidetes* and a decrease in *Actinobacteria* and SCFA-producing bacteria in AD mice [47,48]. A large body of research supports the idea that the gut microbiome in mouse models of AD is less diverse than in wild type (WT) mice [48–52]. Some association has also been noted between the presence of butyrate- and lactate-producing bacteria. Furthermore, a decrease in the number of butyrate-producing *Faecalibacterium* and an increase in the number of lactate-producing bacteria of the *Bifidobacterium* family were found using the sequencing of 16S rRNA from stool samples [50]. Metagenomic studies have proven the relationship between *Lachnospiraceae* and type 2 diabetes. The aforementioned family of bacteria contributes to the development of diabetes, which, along with insulin resistance, is one of the risk factors for AD [53–55]. Functional studies show that *Pseudomonas aeruginosa* infection can increase endothelial Tau phosphorylation and permeability, a common pathophysiological mechanism in the genesis of Alzheimer's disease [56,57]. To date, little has been established about the interactions between pathogenic and non-pathogenic *Pseudomonas* strains in the bodies of patients with AD. Future research should focus on further understanding the role of specific bacterial clusters in the gut microbiome in the pathogenesis of AD [58]. A study where the young WT mice received a gut microbiota transplant from old AD mice has shown that this intervention significantly impaired the recovery from a traumatic brain injury. The study has also shown increased activation of microglia and macrophages and reduced motor recovery. In addition, there was a higher relative count of *Muribaculum* bacteria and a decrease in *Lactobacillus johnsonii* in WT mice transplanted with a microbiome derived from old AD mice. Another study confirms that the microflora derived from AD mice has a significant effect on the deterioration of the neurological response [59].

2.2. Microbiome in Huntington's Disease

2.2.1. Trinucleotide Repeat Expansion Disorders

The expansion of microsatellite repeats is the cause of several neurodegenerative diseases. They are usually caused by replication errors such as polymerase dissociation or arrest, or sliding of the 5′ and or 3′ ends of the Okazaki fragment, which results in the formation of a hairpin structure [60,61]. Neurodegenerative diseases that are classified as trinucleotide repeat expansion disorders (TREDs) are caused by the repetition of the CNG sequence (where N is one of the 4 nucleotides) in certain genes. These disorders can further be subclassified as PolyQ (where the repeated sequence CAG encodes glutamine), like Huntington's disease (HD), and Spinocerebellar Ataxia types 1, 2, 3, 6, 7, 12, 17, and non-PolyQ (where other triplets are repeated), like myotonic dystrophy (DM) or Friedreich's ataxia (FRDA) [62,63].

2.2.2. Huntington's Disease Etiology

Huntington's disease is a rare disorder of the CNS. It affects 5–10 in 100,000 people [64]. It is the most common disorder in Europe and USA, and the least in Asia [65–67].

HD symptoms include uncontrolled body movements, weight loss, facial grimaces, psychological disorders, personality changes, and apathy. First non-specific symptoms can start 10 years before full manifestation of HD, which usually occurs between 35 and 40 years of age. The disease can also affect juveniles, but it is extremely rare in patients under the age of 10 and over the age of 70. The life expectancy after first symptoms is 15–20 years, with the most common causes of death being aspiration pneumonia, heart disease, and suicide [68–70]. The mutation that causes HD is located in the first exon of the *HTT* gene and is inherited in an autosomal dominant manner. In healthy individuals, the first exon contains between 10 and 35 CAG repeats, and the disease severity varies depending on the number of repeats: 27–35 repeats do not cause the disease but increase the probability of HD manifestation in progeny; 36–38 repeats cause the disease with incomplete penetrance; and more than 39 repeats cause the disease with complete penetrance, where the first symptoms occur in patients at the age of 40–55. More than 60 repeats cause the juvenile form, where the first symptoms occur before the age of 21 [71]. This specific mutation in *HTT* leads to the expression of mutant HTT (mHTT) protein, which tends to form intracellular insoluble aggregates that are the pathologic hallmark of HD [72]. The longer the polyQ repeats, the more aggregates it forms. In the brain, the disease pathology is linked to neuronal loss in the striatum, which is responsible for control of motor functions and the reward center. Medium spiny neurons make up the structure of the striatum, and these cells are mainly affected by pathogenic mHTT aggregates, which lead to neuronal loss and secondary gliosis. The other hallmarks of HD pathology are weight loss, gastritis, esophagitis, and nutritional deficiencies, all of which point to a strong link with dysfunction of the digestive tract. mHTT has been found to be expressed in the majority of tissues, including the gastrointestinal tract. Interestingly, studies performed on mouse models have shown that mHTT forms aggregates in the enteric nervous system even before neurological and motoric symptoms appear. It has also been reported that HD affects the functions of the gastrointestinal (GI) system through impaired gut motility, diarrhea, and malabsorption of food, and even influences the gut anatomy by reducing mucosal thickness and villus length, as well as the loss of various neuropeptides that stimulate or inhibit gut motility [73]. There are also pathological changes in gene transcription—mHTT aggregates have been found to interact with several proteins involved in various transcriptional pathways. They have been found to interact with specificity protein 1 (SP1), CREB-binding protein (CBP), peroxisome proliferator-activated receptor-γ coactivator 1α (PGC1α), Nuclear factor κ light-chain-enhancer of activated B cells (NF-κB), and Repressor element 1 (RE1)-silencing transcription factor (REST) [74]. Altered transcription in HD is also linked to mitochondrial dysfunction. Diminished transcription of PGC1α negatively impacts energy metabolism and mitochondrial biogenesis. The mHTT has also been found to have a strong association with the translocase of mitochondrial inner membrane 23 (TIM23) complex, which impairs protein import and disrupts mitochondrial function [74–76].

2.2.3. Immunoprofiling of Huntington's Disease

Chronic inflammation is a hallmark of HD. Inflammatory responses predate motor and psychiatric symptoms, suggesting that chronic inflammation contributes to disease progression. mHTT is highly expressed in immune cells, and its aggregates have been found to have a proinflammatory effect [77]. Even in premanifest patients, peripheral inflammation is characterized by elevated plasma levels of IL-6, and IL-8, IL-4, IL-10, and TNF-α levels rise as the disease progresses. The increase of both IL-6 and IL-8 in the early stages suggests, that it is the innate immunity that drives the initial immunopathology in HD. Indeed, monocytes, macrophages, and microglia isolated from HD patients were found to be hyperreactive to stimulation [78]. The mHTT has been found to drive up the release of IL-6 by upregulating the NF-κB pathway in mice [79]. Interestingly, a study has shown that the presence of mHTT does not directly impact the function of T cells, as their frequencies and functions did not differ from healthy controls [80].

Central inflammation in HD is characterized by chronic activation of microglia and astrocytes. Microglia are the primary mediators of neuroinflammation and in their activated state they release proinflammatory cytokines, such as IL-6, IL-1β, and TNF-α, as well as cytotoxic factors, such as reactive oxygen species (ROS), nitric oxide (NO) and QUIN. Prolonged microglial activation can lead to chronic neuroinflammation and tissue damage [81]. The number of activated microglial cells has been shown to positively correlate with the degree of neuronal loss in the striatum and cortex [82]. It has also been found that activation of microglia is present in very early stages of disease prior to the onset of symptoms [83]. Unlike microglia, the activation of astrocytes occurs in later stages of disease, when neurodegeneration is already present [81]. Reactive astrocytes can contribute to the proinflammatory environment through the production of pro-inflammatory cytokines, such as IL-12 and TNF-α; however, they can also contribute to neuroprotection by expressing anti-inflammatory cytokines, such as IL-10 and TGF-β [84].

Several studies have found a link between T helper 17 (Th17) cells and immunopathology in HD. In premanifest gene expansion carriers, it has been found that Th17.1 cells are activated while the number of Tregs is diminished. IL-17 is a proinflammatory cytokine that plays a role in communication between immune cells and tissue. In animal models, it has been shown to interact with endothelial cells, which induces the breakdown of the blood-brain barrier. The presence of IL-17 in cerebrospinal fluid (CSF) activates microglia, astrocytes, and oligodendrocytes, causing neuroinflammation. Early therapeutic intervention targeting Th17 cells might be beneficial and delay the onset of symptoms [85].

2.2.4. Microbiome in Huntington's Disease

HD—mouse model studies

There are several commercially available mouse models of HD. They differ in the genetic background, the structure of the transgene, and the disease phenotype. The most commonly used lines are R6/1 and R6/2, which are characterized by early symptoms and rapid progression of the disease, compared to the BACHD line. The BACHD mouse model shows the first symptoms of the disease between 2 and 6 months of age, but their severity appears after about a year. The BACHD line shows somatic stability in embryos [86].

Studying the microbiome is an increasingly emerging trend in HD research. One study showed an impact of the transplantation of a microbiome derived from WT mice into a mouse model of HD on its phenotype. The results show that especially the females responded positively to this procedure, as improvements in cognitive function have been observed in animals suffering from HD. The same study proved the ineffectiveness of this approach in males. Researchers speculated that the possible reasons for that phenomenon might be more extensive changes in structure, instability in the gut microbiome and the imbalance in acetate immune profiles [87]. In order to characterize the gut microbiome in a mouse model of HD, 16S RNA sequencing was performed. The research was carried out on R6/1 mice. Sequencing results revealed significant differences in the composition of the microbiome. Furthermore, the amount of water in the feces of HD mice at 12 weeks of age was significantly changed. Most notably, there was an increase in *Bacteroidetes* and a proportional decrease in *Firmicutes*. Interestingly, an increase in microbiome diversity was also observed in HD males compared to WT control mice, but these differences were not observed in females. The changes coincided with an increased food intake and a simultaneous decrease in body weight [88]. It has been proven that PD is characterized by a decrease in the expression of TJ proteins, which under physiological conditions maintain the integrity of the intestinal barrier [89]. Björkqvist and coauthors evaluated whether the same mechanism is responsible for the pathologies occurring in another mouse model of HD (R6/2). The results showed a significant decrease in body weight and body length in these mice. They were also accompanied by a decrease in colon length compared to WT mice, but TJ protein levels showed no statistically significant changes between groups. Moreover, along with the observed changes, differences in the composition of the gut microbiota were also found in the R6/2 mice. Increased amounts of *Bacteroidetes* and *Proteobacteria* and decreased amounts of *Firmicutes*, relative to levels maintained in the control group were demonstrated [90]. A very interesting and detailed study was performed by Gubert et al. They focused on comparing the study group (R6/1 mouse line), which consisted of 3 subgroups: animals with standard living conditions, mice with additional environmental enrichment, and groups of animals with increased physical activity, with WT mice as controls. The results indicated a possible modulation of the gut microbiome by the environment. Therapeutic effects on psychomotor symptoms and the brain have been reported in groups of animals with an enriched environment and greater activity compared to the control group. Changes in the composition of the microbiome at the level of orders such as *Bacteroidales*, *Lachnospirales*, and *Oscillospirales* have also been demonstrated. The results obtained in this experiment show higher alpha diversity for all HD mice compared to WT mice. There was no difference in food intake, but there was a previously expected decrease in body weight in the HD mice compared to the control group. Increased water intake by animals from the test groups was shown, which was associated with the increase in alpha diversity. With the aging of the HD animals, increased fecal excretion was noted. Post-mortem analysis showed a statistically significant decrease in the brain weight of HD mice. There were also significant differences between males and females. The brain weight of females was lower in the group of mice with standard living conditions. Based on the study of the concentration of SCFAs and branched chain fatty acids (BCFAs) in the feces, an attempt was made to check what role these metabolites may play in living condition changes. Male mice from the group with increased physical activity were characterized by a decrease in the concentration of butyrate and valerate. There was no correlation between the concentration of substances, such as acetate and propionate, and the living conditions, genotype, or gender. Statistically significant differences were found between HD and WT mice in the alpha diversity index. The test groups showed increased alpha diversity indices in contrast to the control group. The results of the beta diversity analysis showed differences between the sexes of the animals. Certain orders of microbial bacteria have been identified as those that play the greatest role in microbiome changes under different animal housing conditions. These include the orders *Bacteroidales*, *Lachnospirales*, and *Oscillospirales* [91].

Early pathological features associated with HD are molecular deficits in myelination and progressive neurodegeneration. Experiments conducted on germ-free (GF) animals suggested that there is a two-way communication between the microbiome, gut, and brain [11,92]. Research conducted on the BACHD mouse model was intended to answer the question of what impact the microbiome has on myelin plasticity and oligodendrocyte dynamics. The experiment compared GF, specific pathogen-free (SPF), and WT mice. Animals of both sexes were used in the experiment. Analysis of myelin in the corpus callosum revealed changes in myelin thickness in BACHD GF mice compared to SPF mice, while no intergroup changes were observed in WT mice. However, significant differences in myelin density were noted in all groups compared to WT SPF mice. In the GF conditions, a reduced level of myelin-associated proteins, such as myelin basic protein (MBP), proteolipid protein (PLP), and Ermin (Ermn), and a lower number of mature oligodendrocytes in the prefrontal cortex were observed compared to the SPF conditions, regardless of the mouse genotype. Slight differences in family and genus were also observed in the commensal bacteria of the gut microbiome in the BACHD and WT groups maintained under SPF conditions. However, the differences were not statistically significant. Researchers concluded that the *HTT* mutation in BACHD mice does not cause profound disturbances in the intestinal microflora, and thus plasticity defects are not associated with disturbances in the structure of the microbiome. Analysis of the brain structures of GF animals showed that then environment had a greater effect on the myelination caliber of callosum axons in BACHD animals compared to WT controls, while a possible distribution of myelin plaques was observed in both genotypes. The axons of mice maintained under GF conditions were characterized by a reduced diameter and a lower g-ratios, which could suggest thicker myelin. Examination of the myelin membranes, however, showed that the observed features may have been due to the decompaction of the laminae and not an increase in their number. A similar trend of increased periodicity, suggesting decompaction, was also observed in BACHD mice under SPF conditions compared to WT, prompting the conclusion that the *HTT* mutation in BACHD animals causes this pathology. Supportive is the observation of a trend towards lower levels of the cortical myelin-associated proteins MBP and PLP, which play a key role in myelin compaction. The researchers did not observe significant changes in the gut bacterial community. Slight disparities were observed in BACHD mice at 3 and 6 months of age compared to WT mice, with reduced numbers of *Prevotella* and *Bacteroides* at the genus level and part of the *Bacteroidetes* type [93]. More reports indicate the importance of the intestinal microbiome in the communication between the digestive system and the brain and its impact on the pathologies of neurodegenerative diseases. Subsequent studies involved shotgun sequencing of the gut microbiome from R6/1 mice, aged 4–12 weeks (from early adolescent to adult stages). Metabolomic analyses, in addition to those performed on fecal samples, were also performed on blood plasma collected from 12-week-old animals. The results showed an upregulation of bacterial gene expression, which may indicate potential early effects of the HTT protein mutation in the gut. In addition, mice at 12 weeks of age were found to have disturbed gut microbiome function. In particular, the researchers' attention was drawn to the increase in the butanoate metabolic pathway, which leads to increased production of SCFA playing a protective role. This increase was not observed when analyzing plasma from 12-week-old mice. Statistical analysis of the results obtained in metagenomic and metabolomic studies allowed for the observation of a negative correlation of several species of *Bacteroides* with ATP and pipecolic acid in plasma. During the experiment, feces were collected at five different time points. No statistically significant differences in the composition of the microbiome were observed when comparing the mice from the study group and the control WT group. The dominance of two phyla, *Bacteroidetes* and *Firmicutes*, was observed, followed by the *Proteobacteria*, *Actinobacteria*, and *Verrucomicrobia* phyla. It was determined that at the family level, the most numerous group was *Lachnospiraceae*, followed by similar numbers in the groups of *Bacteroidaceae*, *Porphyromonadaceae*, *Prevotellaceae*, and *Clostridiaceae*. No statistically significant differences were found between bacterial families at any timepoint when comparing WT mice. At 12 weeks of age, which corresponds to the timepoint before the onset of overt motor symptoms in HD mice, differences in 30 bacterial species were observed between HD and WT mice. These included *Clostridium mt 5, Treponema phagedenis, Clostridium leptum CAG: 27, Desulfatirhabdium butyrativorans, Plasmodium chabaudi, Defulfuribacillus alkaliarsenatis, Plasmodium yoelii,* and *Chlamydia abortus.* No differences in the abundance of butyrate producers such as *Roseburia intestinalis*, *Clostridium symbiosum*, and *Eubacterium rectale* were found when comparing samples from HD and WT mice [94].

HD—human studies

Studies were also performed on a diverse group of people suffering from HD. Participants were clinically characterized using a battery of cognitive tests, and 16S RNA sequencing was performed on stool samples. The study involved healthy individuals (control group; n = 36) and carriers of the expanded mutated gene (n = 42). Nineteen of them were previously diagnosed with HD, and the rest were pre-symptomatic. The groups were matched by gender and age. Microbiome evaluation showed differences between the control group and the study group in the composition of the microbial community (beta diversity) as well as significantly lower species richness (alpha diversity). The results of the sequencing analysis show statistically significant differences at the phylum level (differences apply only to the group of men) in *Euryarchaeota*, *Firmicutes*, and *Verrucomicrobia*. Further changes were also observed at the family level, including: *Acidaminococcaceae*, *Akkermansiaceae*, *Bacteroidaceae*, *Bifidobacteriaceae*, *Christensenellaceae*, *Clostridiaceae*, *Coriobacteriaceae*, *Eggerthellaceae*, *Enterobacteriaceae*, *Erysipelotrichaceae*, *Flavobacteriaceae*, *Lachnospiraceae*, *Methanobacteriaceae*, *Peptococcaceae*, *Peptostreptococcaceae*, and *Rikenellaceae*, concerned only men. No significant changes at the phylum and family levels were observed in women. The obtained results confirmed the researchers' assumptions and showed changes in the composition of the microbiome between the test and control groups. In addition, the observations made provide evidence that the composition of the intestinal microbiome affects the cognitive abilities of patients. However, the results obtained in this study should be interpreted with caution. According to the authors, the study and control groups were too small to make adequate statistical analyses. Nevertheless, the information provided is essential for further research [95]. Another study conducted on patients suffering from HD indicates a correlation between changes in the composition of the gut microbiome and the immune response. The study included 33 HD patients and 33 healthy individuals; the groups were matched in terms of sex and age. In addition to assessing the fecal microflora in terms of microbial richness, structure, and diversity of abundance of individual taxa, IFN-γ, IL-1β, IL-2, IL-4, IL-6, IL-8, IL-10, IL-12p70, IL-13, and TNF-α concentrations in patients' plasma were measured. The results obtained in both experiments were correlated with each other to find connotations between them. It was shown that HD patients were distinguished by increased richness and altered microbiome structure. The analysis showed that the higher number of *Intestinimonas* bacteria is positively correlated with the Total Functional Capacity score (measured in HD patients to evaluate disease progression). It is also positively correlated with the level of the anti-inflammatory cytokine IL-4. The study also showed that the genus *Bilophila* is negatively correlated with pro-inflammatory IL-6 levels. In addition, negative correlations between *Oscillibacter*, *Gemmier*, and IL-6; *Clostridium XVIII*, TNF-α and IL-8; and positive correlations between *Porphyromonas* and IL-4, IL-10, and IL-13 were also noted. The results obtained in these experiments clearly indicate the relationship between the composition of the intestinal microbiome and the immune response in HD patients [96].

All results described in the paragraph are summarized in Table 1.

Table 1. Summarized results of microbiome studies performed in HD mouse models and HD patients. The table shows bacterial species changed in HD, ↑ signifies increase, ↓ signifies decrease. C – Class, O – Order, F – Family, G – Genus.

Host	Phylum	Class/Order	Family/Genus	Alpha Diversity	Beta Diversity	Source
Mouse R6/1	*Bacteroidetes* ↑ *Firmicutes* ↓			males↑	ns	[88]
Mouse R6/2	*Bacteroidetes* ↑ *Proteobacteria* ↑ *Firmicutes* ↓		G *Bacteroides* ↑ G *Parabacteroides* ↑ G *Lactobacillus* ↑ G *Coprobacillus* ↑ G *Enterobacteriaceae* ↑	ns		[90]
Mouse R6/1		O *Bacteroidales* O *Lachnospirales* O *Oscillospirales*		↑	differed	[91]
Mouse BACHD 3 months old	*Bacteroidetes* ↓ *Firmicutes* ↑		F *Bacteroidaceae* ↓ F *Anaeroplasmataceae* ↓ G *Prevotella* ↓ G *Bacteroides* ↓ G *Oscillospira* ↑ G *Adlercreutzia* ↑	ns		[93]
Mouse BACHD 6 months old	*Bacteroidetes* ↑ *Firmicutes* ↓		F *Mogibacteriaceae* ↓	ns		[93]
Human Males	*Firmicutes* ↓ *Euryarchaeota* *Verrucomicrobia*		F *Lachnospiraceae* ↓ F *Akkermansiaceae* ↓ F *Acidaminococcaceae* F *Akkermansiaceae* F *Bacteroidaceae* F *Bifidobacteriaceae* F *Christensenellaceae* F *Clostridiaceae* F *Coriobacteriaceae* F *Eggerthellaceae* F *Enterobacteriaceae* F *Erysipelotrichaceae* F *Flavobacteriaceae* F *Lachnospiraceae* F *Methanobacteriaceae* F *Peptococcaceae* F *Peptostreptococcaceae* F *Rikenellaceae*	↓	differed	[95]
Human	*Actinobacteria* ↑	C *Deltaproteobacteria* ↑ C *Actinobacteria* ↑ O *Desulfovibrionales* ↑	F *Oxalobacteraceae* ↑ F *Lactobacillaceae* ↑ F *Desulfovibrionaceae* ↑ G *Clostridium XVIII* ↓ G *Intestinimonas* ↑ G *Bilophila* ↑ G *Lactobacillus* ↑ G *Oscillibacter* ↑ G *Gemmiger* ↑ G *Dialister* ↑	↑	differed	[96]

3. Discussion and Future Prospects

Increasing advancement in research on neurodegenerative diseases indicates that these pathologies are very complex processes with often forgotten microbiome- and immune-related components. The publications and studies mentioned in this review present evidence for the relationship between neurodegenerative diseases, mainly HD, and the intestinal microbiome. So far, the focus has been on understanding the pathology of the disease based on molecular biomarkers, which hopefully could effectively contribute to the development of future therapies [97]. Recent studies on the effect of the intestinal microbiome and its metabolites also pave the way for new branches in the field of HD. Microbial metabolites have the potential to modulate the pathogenesis of HD. SCFAs can influence the immune system and ameliorate inflammation, both in the CNS and the peripheral nerves. Studies on mouse models that were supplemented with sodium butyrate showed a beneficial effect on their motor skills, mitochondrial and transcriptional dysfunction [28,29]. This suggests that therapeutic interventions promoting butyrate production by patients' microbiota have the potential to ameliorate disease symptoms. However, there are still many open questions regarding the bacteria inhabiting healthy and diseased digestive systems. The results of research involving microbiota carried out so far are still not entirely conclusive due to microbiome complexity and numerous contributing factors. Therefore, there is still a long way to go to fully understand the communication in the gut—brain axis, including in pathological conditions like HD.

Moreover, the microbiome results are not always consistent. The large amount of data generated in experiments is hard to compile, and one needs to be attentive when analyzing and drawing conclusions based on it. Insufficiently known taxonomies of species inhabiting the intestines and inaccurate and non-standardized terminology related to the subject of the microbiome are often misleading and generate mistakes when classifying individual bacteria into appropriate classes, groups, or families. Furthermore, the choice of mouse model, its strain, sex, or age is essential in the studies concerning the microbiome. For example, two studies in a mouse model of HD confirm an increase in *Bacteriodetes* and a decrease in *Firmicutes* [88,90]. The first one was carried out on the R6/1 line, and the second on the R6/2 mouse model. Additionally, the study conducted on another HD model contradicts these results. At 3 months of age, BACHD mice exhibit the opposite trend of increased *Firmicutes* and decreased *Bacteriodetes*. Interestingly, re-analysis on 6-month-old mice showed the opposite, which rather confirms the results of the previous two studies [93]. The presented results display certain consistency, despite the use of different models, but only when using older mice from the BACHD line. It can be assumed that the microbiome diversity changes in the same fashion as organisms mature. It is also worth noting that some of the results show statistical significance only in the group of males, both in animal and human studies [88,95]. On the other hand, only female mice showed a positive reaction to the transplant of a healthy microbiome [87]. These findings also indicate the effect of female hormones on microbiome composition. In the study conducted by the Hannan group, the body weight of WT and HD mice differed significantly, as HD mice lost weight with age. This could be due to differences in the composition of the microbiome and the level of food absorption, which is inversely proportional to body weight [98]. Increased thirst was also noted, possibly due to xerostomia, which both patients and HD mice suffer from, or hypothalamic degeneration, which is associated with increased thirst [99]. Interestingly, increased water intake by the animals did not change the water content of the feces. The reason could be the microbiological environment in the intestines. This result may suggest a very precise regulation of water absorption [100]. Some of the cited studies indicate an increased level of alpha diversity compared to other groups [88,91,96]. A higher level of this index is believed to indicate a healthier and more resilient microbial environment [101]. Studies in other models of neurodegenerative diseases, such as AD and PD, have also linked movement deficits with lower levels of alpha diversity in patients compared to controls [102–104]. Human HD studies have shown lower [95] and higher [96] values of alpha diversity in CAG repeat overexpressors compared to healthy controls. Recent extensive meta-analyses have found no associations between alpha diversity and neurological disorders, particularly in PD and MS [105]. Interestingly, there are also studies that prove that increased diversity does not always correlate with better patient conditions [106,107]. According to Coyte et al., a decrease in the stability of the microbiome environment may also result in higher alpha diversity [108]. Research also shows that the alpha level of diversity may also be related to diet, body weight, and gastrointestinal physiology [109].

Another essential factor that should be considered when conducting experiments related to the microbiome and neurodegeneration in humans is the environment. Each of the mentioned experiments was performed under slightly different conditions, especially in humans. Environmental changes are noticeable among the participants of a project, despite the fact that the control group was chosen from the close family members of the patients [96]. The composition of the gut microbiome is also influenced by various factors, such as physical activity [110,111]. The difference in this respect between healthy and disease-affected individuals certainly existed during the project. This proves how difficult it is to compose appropriate groups in experiments assuming the study of the microbiome. In addition to differences in physical activity, each person has different nutritional preferences, which certainly influence the composition of the microbiome and are a burden for bioinformaticians to be leveled in statistical analyses [112,113]. In addition, the quoted research was performed on distinct continents, which results in diametrically different environmental conditions such as climate or local food accessibility that affect diet [114]. Sampling for testing is an extremely important point in the whole experiment. Typically, the collected samples are snap frozen to eliminate the adverse effect of air on aerophobic bacteria in the samples. In both of these experiments [95,96], the samples were obtained in a different way, and the patients were responsible for collecting and delivering the samples to the laboratory, which might have affected the composition of the microbiome in the samples. Conducting research on mouse models can be better standardized and reproducible by applying a specific sampling and storage protocol. Collection should be as quick as possible, with a caution not to contaminate the sample with other DNA or with bacteria residing on fur.

Animal experiments also have the advantage of breeding in more standardized conditions, typically SPF, though the microbiome may vary slightly. On the other hand, the place of origin of the animal, lineage, strain, age, disease model, maintenance method, or even environmental enrichment in the cages are all aspects that should be considered when studying the microbiome. Mice are also known to be coprophages to reabsorb essential nutrients such as vitamins; thus, when housing a few mice in the same cage, one should consider the natural microbiome transfer between them and dodge the "cage effect" [91]. Additionally, all existing mouse models of HD differ from each other by the dynamics of disease progression or the degree of interference in the animal's genome [115,116]. At this point, it is worth considering at what age and on what model such tests should be carried out. The studies we quoted were based on various models and were carried out on animals of different ages. As with human studies, comparing results obtained in mouse experiments is equally problematic, although the experiments were more standardized.

Animal models of HD provide us with tools to study the mammalian microbiome and its possible implications for disease progression in a highly controlled environment. Most studies presented in this review used R6/1 or R6/2 models, which are well established for HD; however, they are characterized by early onset, rapid disease progression, and premature death. As previously mentioned, in humans, the symptoms of HD occur well into adulthood, at 35–40 years of age, with continuous progression for the next 10–15 years, which points to a need for other models with slower disease progression, such as YAC128, Hu128/21, or BACHD. Aging is also closely linked to changes in microbiome composition, so these models might be more applicable for long term studies of changes in microbiome composition and possible dietary or therapeutic interventions that might better translate to humans. There was only one study utilizing the BACHD model that showed pronounced differences in microbiota composition at different ages [93]. Long-term studies on both pre- and post-symptomatic animals are important for a better understanding of the microbiome and HD pathology, but they also have the unique ability to find the most suitable timepoints for therapeutic interventions. Using these models might also be relevant in fecal microbiota transfer studies, as the R6/2 model used by Gubert and colleagues has shown that the engraftment was unsuccessful in male mice [87]. Using models with slower disease progression might provide the researchers with a variety of timepoints and disease phenotypes to choose from, which might impact the success of the microbiota transplant.

There is also a fruit fly model of HD (FL-HD) that exhibits similar symptoms such as motor deficits, mHTT aggregates, disrupted gene expression, and dysbiosis in the gut. The *Drosophila* microbiome is, however, much less complex than the mammalian microbiome, which can help in analyzing single species and their impact on dysbiosis. A study conducted on female fruit flies has found that gut colonization by *E. coli* worsened the HD symptoms, as there was an increase in aggregate buildup and earlier death. A therapy using crocin was used in *Drosophila* with beneficial effects. This therapy ameliorated motor deficits and extended the lifespan, but what is more interesting is that it provided resistance to *E. coli* colonization and had positive effects on the microbiome [117]. Crocin is a carotenoid exhibiting anti-inflammatory, antioxidant, and neuroprotective properties. Crocin, or its major byproduct, crocetin, has been suggested to act in the gut and modulate the gut microbiome. Another study has shown that oral administration of crocin was beneficial for cerebral ischemic/reperfusion (I/R) injuries in rats, while the intravenous route of administration was not. It suggests that the therapeutic effects are mediated through the gut microbiota [118]. As such, crocin might provide beneficial effects in HD, ameliorating inflammation, oxidative stress, and gut dysbiosis, which makes it a promising target for further studies.

Interestingly, a few studies have found that prion infection can also lead to dysbiosis and significant changes in microbial metabolites. The microbial richness (alpha diversity) was higher in healthy controls, and the microbiome structure was significantly different between healthy and infected groups. Prion diseases are linked to neuroinflammation, and while the mechanism underlying the gut dysbiosis in this type of disease is not well understood, it is nonetheless an interesting topic to further examine the relationship between the gut and the brain [119,120].

According to the latest research, taking pro- and pre-biotics can help with nervous system diseases. So far, the effect of taking these substances on the progression of HD has not been proven, but it has been studied in other neurodegenerative diseases. There are several studies confirming the psychophysiological effect of prebiotics on the body. Chitosan oligosaccharide (COS) has been shown to have a positive effect on cognitive deficits in a rat model of AD by reducing oxidative stress and neuroinflammatory responses [121]. In studies on amyotrophic lateral sclerosis, it was proven that the use of galactooligosaccharides (GOS) reduced the activation of microglia and astrocytes and caused less death of motor neurons [122]. Other studies conducted in a mouse model of PD showed that long-term intake of probiotics resulted in a neuroprotective effect on dopaminergic neurons, effectively counteracting motor disorders in animals [123]. Unfortunately, few similar studies have been conducted in humans so far. The examples of research cited above prove that the use of products containing both pro- and prebiotic bacterial strains could act as an effective supporting therapy in the treatment of neurodegenerative diseases. Perhaps in the future, effective and personalized drugs based solely on these compounds will be developed.

Author Contributions: Conceptualization, L.P.; writing—original draft preparation, L.P., A.K., D.W. and J.O.M.; writing—review and editing, L.P., A.K., D.W. and J.O.M.; visualization, A.K.; supervision, L.P.; funding acquisition, L.P. All authors have read and agreed to the published version of the manuscript.

Funding: This research received no external funding.

Institutional Review Board Statement: Not applicable.

Informed Consent Statement: Not applicable.

Data Availability Statement: Not applicable.

Acknowledgments: We would like to thank Anna Zimniewicz for her support in gathering material for this review article.

Conflicts of Interest: The authors declare no conflict of interest.

References

1. Magnúsdóttir, S.; Thiele, I. Modeling Metabolism of the Human Gut Microbiome. *Curr. Opin. Biotechnol.* **2018**, *51*, 90–96. [CrossRef]
2. Sochocka, M.; Donskow-Łysoniewska, K.; Diniz, B.S.; Kurpas, D.; Brzozowska, E.; Leszek, J. The Gut Microbiome Alterations and Inflammation-Driven Pathogenesis of Alzheimer's Disease—A Critical Review. *Mol. Neurobiol.* **2019**, *56*, 1841–1851. [CrossRef]
3. Lloyd-Price, J.; Abu-Ali, G.; Huttenhower, C. The Healthy Human Microbiome. *Genome Med.* **2016**, *8*, 51. [CrossRef] [PubMed]
4. Qin, J.; Li, R.; Raes, J.; Arumugam, M.; Burgdorf, K.S.; Manichanh, C.; Nielsen, T.; Pons, N.; Levenez, F.; Yamada, T.; et al. A Human Gut Microbial Gene Catalogue Established by Metagenomic Sequencing. *Nature* **2010**, *464*, 59–65. [CrossRef] [PubMed]
5. International Human Genome Sequencing Consortium Finishing the Euchromatic Sequence of the Human Genome. *Nature* **2004**, *431*, 931–945. [CrossRef] [PubMed]
6. Fierer, N.; Hamady, M.; Lauber, C.L.; Knight, R. The Influence of Sex, Handedness, and Washing on the Diversity of Hand Surface Bacteria. *Proc. Natl. Acad. Sci. USA* **2008**, *105*, 17994–17999. [CrossRef]
7. Turnbaugh, P.J.; Hamady, M.; Yatsunenko, T.; Cantarel, B.L.; Duncan, A.; Ley, R.E.; Sogin, M.L.; Jones, W.J.; Roe, B.A.; Affourtit, J.P.; et al. A Core Gut Microbiome in Obese and Lean Twins. *Nature* **2009**, *457*, 480–484. [CrossRef]
8. Collado, M.C.; Rautava, S.; Aakko, J.; Isolauri, E.; Salminen, S. Human Gut Colonisation May Be Initiated in Utero by Distinct Microbial Communities in the Placenta and Amniotic Fluid. *Sci. Rep.* **2016**, *6*, 23129. [CrossRef]
9. Koenig, J.E.; Spor, A.; Scalfone, N.; Fricker, A.D.; Stombaugh, J.; Knight, R.; Angenent, L.T.; Ley, R.E. Succession of Microbial Consortia in the Developing Infant Gut Microbiome. *Proc. Natl. Acad. Sci. USA* **2011**, *108*, 4578–4585. [CrossRef]
10. Claesson, M.J.; Jeffery, I.B.; Conde, S.; Power, S.E.; O'Connor, E.M.; Cusack, S.; Harris, H.M.B.; Coakley, M.; Lakshminarayanan, B.; O'Sullivan, O.; et al. Gut Microbiota Composition Correlates with Diet and Health in the Elderly. *Nature* **2012**, *488*, 178–184. [CrossRef]
11. Kundu, P.; Blacher, E.; Elinav, E.; Pettersson, S. Our Gut Microbiome: The Evolving Inner Self. *Cell* **2017**, *171*, 1481–1493. [CrossRef] [PubMed]
12. Ruan, W.; Engevik, M.A.; Spinler, J.K.; Versalovic, J. Healthy Human Gastrointestinal Microbiome: Composition and Function After a Decade of Exploration. *Dig. Dis. Sci.* **2020**, *65*, 695–705. [CrossRef] [PubMed]
13. Human Microbiome Jumpstart Reference Strains Consortium; Nelson, K.E.; Weinstock, G.M.; Highlander, S.K.; Worley, K.C.; Creasy, H.H.; Wortman, J.R.; Rusch, D.B.; Mitreva, M.; Sodergren, E.; et al. A Catalog of Reference Genomes from the Human Microbiome. *Science* **2010**, *328*, 994–999. [CrossRef] [PubMed]
14. Huttenhower, C.; Gevers, D.; Knight, R.; Abubucker, S.; Badger, J.H.; Chinwalla, A.T.; Creasy, H.H.; Earl, A.M.; FitzGerald, M.G.; Fulton, R.S.; et al. Structure, Function and Diversity of the Healthy Human Microbiome. *Nature* **2012**, *486*, 207–214. [CrossRef]
15. Li, J.; Jia, H.; Cai, X.; Zhong, H.; Feng, Q.; Sunagawa, S.; Arumugam, M.; Kultima, J.R.; Prifti, E.; Nielsen, T.; et al. An Integrated Catalog of Reference Genes in the Human Gut Microbiome. *Nat. Biotechnol.* **2014**, *32*, 834–841. [CrossRef]
16. Cryan, J.F.; O'Riordan, K.J.; Cowan, C.S.M.; Sandhu, K.V.; Bastiaanssen, T.F.S.; Boehme, M.; Codagnone, M.G.; Cussotto, S.; Fulling, C.; Golubeva, A.V.; et al. The Microbiota-Gut-Brain Axis. *Physiol. Rev.* **2019**, *99*, 1877–2013. [CrossRef]
17. Bilen, M.; Dufour, J.-C.; Lagier, J.-C.; Cadoret, F.; Daoud, Z.; Dubourg, G.; Raoult, D. The Contribution of Culturomics to the Repertoire of Isolated Human Bacterial and Archaeal Species. *Microbiome* **2018**, *6*, 94. [CrossRef]
18. Hugon, P.; Dufour, J.-C.; Colson, P.; Fournier, P.-E.; Sallah, K.; Raoult, D. A Comprehensive Repertoire of Prokaryotic Species Identified in Human Beings. *Lancet Infect. Dis.* **2015**, *15*, 1211–1219. [CrossRef]
19. Eckburg, P.B.; Bik, E.M.; Bernstein, C.N.; Purdom, E.; Dethlefsen, L.; Sargent, M.; Gill, S.R.; Nelson, K.E.; Relman, D.A. Diversity of the Human Intestinal Microbial Flora. *Science* **2005**, *308*, 1635–1638. [CrossRef]
20. Rebeaud, J.; Peter, B.; Pot, C. How Microbiota-Derived Metabolites Link the Gut to the Brain during Neuroinflammation. *Int. J. Mol. Sci.* **2022**, *23*, 10128. [CrossRef]
21. Costello, S.P.; Hughes, P.A.; Waters, O.; Bryant, R.V.; Vincent, A.D.; Blatchford, P.; Katsikeros, R.; Makanyanga, J.; Campaniello, M.A.; Mavrangelos, C.; et al. Effect of Fecal Microbiota Transplantation on 8-Week Remission in Patients with Ulcerative Colitis: A Randomized Clinical Trial. *JAMA* **2019**, *321*, 156. [CrossRef]
22. Ooijevaar, R.E.; Terveer, E.M.; Verspaget, H.W.; Kuijper, E.J.; Keller, J.J. Clinical Application and Potential of Fecal Microbiota Transplantation. *Annu. Rev. Med.* **2019**, *70*, 335–351. [CrossRef]
23. Park, J.; Kim, M.; Kang, S.G.; Jannasch, A.H.; Cooper, B.; Patterson, J.; Kim, C.H. Short-Chain Fatty Acids Induce Both Effector and Regulatory T Cells by Suppression of Histone Deacetylases and Regulation of the MTOR–S6K Pathway. *Mucosal Immunol.* **2015**, *8*, 80–93. [CrossRef]
24. Maslowski, K.M.; Vieira, A.T.; Ng, A.; Kranich, J.; Sierro, F.; Yu, D.; Schilter, H.C.; Rolph, M.S.; Mackay, F.; Artis, D.; et al. Regulation of Inflammatory Responses by Gut Microbiota and Chemoattractant Receptor GPR43. *Nature* **2009**, *461*, 1282–1286. [CrossRef]

25. Rekha, K.; Venkidasamy, B.; Samynathan, R.; Nagella, P.; Rebezov, M.; Khayrullin, M.; Ponomarev, E.; Bouyahya, A.; Sarkar, T.; Shariati, M.A.; et al. Short-Chain Fatty Acid: An Updated Review on Signaling, Metabolism, and Therapeutic Effects. *Crit. Rev. Food Sci. Nutr.* **2022**, *62*, 1–29. [CrossRef]
26. Kibbie, J.J.; Dillon, S.M.; Thompson, T.A.; Purba, C.M.; McCarter, M.D.; Wilson, C.C. Butyrate Directly Decreases Human Gut Lamina Propria CD4 T Cell Function through Histone Deacetylase (HDAC) Inhibition and GPR43 Signaling. *Immunobiology* **2021**, *226*, 152126. [CrossRef] [PubMed]
27. Furusawa, Y.; Obata, Y.; Fukuda, S.; Endo, T.A.; Nakato, G.; Takahashi, D.; Nakanishi, Y.; Uetake, C.; Kato, K.; Kato, T.; et al. Commensal Microbe-Derived Butyrate Induces the Differentiation of Colonic Regulatory T Cells. *Nature* **2013**, *504*, 446–450. [CrossRef] [PubMed]
28. Ferrante, R.J.; Kubilus, J.K.; Lee, J.; Ryu, H.; Beesen, A.; Zucker, B.; Smith, K.; Kowall, N.W.; Ratan, R.R.; Luthi-Carter, R.; et al. Histone Deacetylase Inhibition by Sodium Butyrate Chemotherapy Ameliorates the Neurodegenerative Phenotype in Huntington's Disease Mice. *J. Neurosci.* **2003**, *23*, 9418–9427. [CrossRef] [PubMed]
29. Naia, L.; Cunha-Oliveira, T.; Rodrigues, J.; Rosenstock, T.R.; Oliveira, A.; Ribeiro, M.; Carmo, C.; Oliveira-Sousa, S.I.; Duarte, A.I.; Hayden, M.R.; et al. Histone Deacetylase Inhibitors Protect Against Pyruvate Dehydrogenase Dysfunction in Huntington's Disease. *J. Neurosci.* **2017**, *37*, 2776–2794. [CrossRef]
30. Lukić, I.; Ivković, S.; Mitić, M.; Adžić, M. Tryptophan Metabolites in Depression: Modulation by Gut Microbiota. *Front. Behav. Neurosci.* **2022**, *16*, 987697. [CrossRef]
31. Zelante, T.; Iannitti, R.G.; Cunha, C.; De Luca, A.; Giovannini, G.; Pieraccini, G.; Zecchi, R.; D'Angelo, C.; Massi-Benedetti, C.; Fallarino, F.; et al. Tryptophan Catabolites from Microbiota Engage Aryl Hydrocarbon Receptor and Balance Mucosal Reactivity via Interleukin-22. *Immunity* **2013**, *39*, 372–385. [CrossRef] [PubMed]
32. Lee, J.-H.; Lee, J. Indole as an Intercellular Signal in Microbial Communities. *FEMS Microbiol. Rev.* **2010**, *34*, 426–444. [CrossRef] [PubMed]
33. Bercik, P.; Collins, S.M.; Verdu, E.F. Microbes and the Gut-Brain Axis: Microbiota-Gut-Brain Axis. *Neurogastroenterol. Motil.* **2012**, *24*, 405–413. [CrossRef]
34. Liang, S.; Wu, X.; Jin, F. Gut-Brain Psychology: Rethinking Psychology from the Microbiota–Gut–Brain Axis. *Front. Integr. Neurosci.* **2018**, *12*, 33. [CrossRef] [PubMed]
35. Margolis, K.G.; Cryan, J.F.; Mayer, E.A. The Microbiota-Gut-Brain Axis: From Motility to Mood. *Gastroenterology* **2021**, *160*, 1486–1501. [CrossRef] [PubMed]
36. Spencer, N.J.; Hu, H. Enteric Nervous System: Sensory Transduction, Neural Circuits and Gastrointestinal Motility. *Nat. Rev. Gastroenterol. Hepatol.* **2020**, *17*, 338–351. [CrossRef] [PubMed]
37. Kowalski, K.; Mulak, A. Brain-Gut-Microbiota Axis in Alzheimer's Disease. *J. Neurogastroenterol. Motil.* **2019**, *25*, 48–60. [CrossRef]
38. Mulak, A.; Koszewicz, M.; Panek-Jeziorna, M.; Koziorowska-Gawron, E.; Budrewicz, S. Fecal Calprotectin as a Marker of the Gut Immune System Activation Is Elevated in Parkinson's Disease. *Front. Neurosci.* **2019**, *13*, 992. [CrossRef]
39. Antony, P.M.A.; Diederich, N.J.; Krüger, R.; Balling, R. The Hallmarks of Parkinson's Disease. *FEBS J.* **2013**, *280*, 5981–5993. [CrossRef]
40. Lane, C.A.; Hardy, J.; Schott, J.M. Alzheimer's Disease. *Eur. J. Neurol.* **2018**, *25*, 59–70. [CrossRef]
41. Chen, S.-J.; Chen, C.-C.; Liao, H.-Y.; Lin, Y.-T.; Wu, Y.-W.; Liou, J.-M.; Wu, M.-S.; Kuo, C.-H.; Lin, C.-H. Association of Fecal and Plasma Levels of Short-Chain Fatty Acids with Gut Microbiota and Clinical Severity in Patients with Parkinson Disease. *Neurology* **2022**, *98*, e848–e858. [CrossRef]
42. Bedarf, J.R.; Hildebrand, F.; Coelho, L.P.; Sunagawa, S.; Bahram, M.; Goeser, F.; Bork, P.; Wüllner, U. Functional Implications of Microbial and Viral Gut Metagenome Changes in Early Stage L-DOPA-Naïve Parkinson's Disease Patients. *Genome Med.* **2017**, *9*, 39. [CrossRef] [PubMed]
43. Sampson, T.R.; Debelius, J.W.; Thron, T.; Janssen, S.; Shastri, G.G.; Ilhan, Z.E.; Challis, C.; Schretter, C.E.; Rocha, S.; Gradinaru, V.; et al. Gut Microbiota Regulate Motor Deficits and Neuroinflammation in a Model of Parkinson's Disease. *Cell* **2016**, *167*, 1469–1480.e12. [CrossRef] [PubMed]
44. Uyar, G.Ö.; Yildiran, H. A Nutritional Approach to Microbiota in Parkinson's Disease. *Biosci. Microbiota Food Health* **2019**, *38*, 115–127. [CrossRef]
45. Bullich, C.; Keshavarzian, A.; Garssen, J.; Kraneveld, A.; Perez-Pardo, P. Gut Vibes in Parkinson's Disease: The Microbiota-Gut-Brain Axis. *Mov. Disord. Clin. Pract.* **2019**, *6*, 639–651. [CrossRef] [PubMed]
46. Kim, M.-S.; Kim, Y.; Choi, H.; Kim, W.; Park, S.; Lee, D.; Kim, D.K.; Kim, H.J.; Choi, H.; Hyun, D.-W.; et al. Transfer of a Healthy Microbiota Reduces Amyloid and Tau Pathology in an Alzheimer's Disease Animal Model. *Gut* **2020**, *69*, 283–294. [CrossRef]
47. Yan, Y.; Gao, Y.; Fang, Q.; Zhang, N.; Kumar, G.; Yan, H.; Song, L.; Li, J.; Zhang, Y.; Sun, J.; et al. Inhibition of Rho Kinase by Fasudil Ameliorates Cognition Impairment in APP/PS1 Transgenic Mice via Modulation of Gut Microbiota and Metabolites. *Front. Aging Neurosci.* **2021**, *13*, 755164. [CrossRef]
48. Gu, X.; Zhou, J.; Zhou, Y.; Wang, H.; Si, N.; Ren, W.; Zhao, W.; Fan, X.; Gao, W.; Wei, X.; et al. Huanglian Jiedu Decoction Remodels the Periphery Microenvironment to Inhibit Alzheimer's Disease Progression Based on the "Brain-Gut" Axis through Multiple Integrated Omics. *Alzheimers Res. Ther.* **2021**, *13*, 44. [CrossRef]

49. Liu, P.; Wu, L.; Peng, G.; Han, Y.; Tang, R.; Ge, J.; Zhang, L.; Jia, L.; Yue, S.; Zhou, K.; et al. Altered Microbiomes Distinguish Alzheimer's Disease from Amnestic Mild Cognitive Impairment and Health in a Chinese Cohort. *Brain Behav. Immun.* **2019**, *80*, 633–643. [CrossRef]
50. Ling, Z.; Zhu, M.; Yan, X.; Cheng, Y.; Shao, L.; Liu, X.; Jiang, R.; Wu, S. Structural and Functional Dysbiosis of Fecal Microbiota in Chinese Patients with Alzheimer's Disease. *Front. Cell Dev. Biol.* **2021**, *8*, 634069. [CrossRef]
51. Zhang, X.; Wang, Y.; Liu, W.; Wang, T.; Wang, L.; Hao, L.; Ju, M.; Xiao, R. Diet Quality, Gut Microbiota, and MicroRNAs Associated with Mild Cognitive Impairment in Middle-Aged and Elderly Chinese Population. *Am. J. Clin. Nutr.* **2021**, *114*, 429–440. [CrossRef]
52. Li, B.; He, Y.; Ma, J.; Huang, P.; Du, J.; Cao, L.; Wang, Y.; Xiao, Q.; Tang, H.; Chen, S. Mild Cognitive Impairment Has Similar Alterations as Alzheimer's Disease in Gut Microbiota. *Alzheimers Dement.* **2019**, *15*, 1357–1366. [CrossRef] [PubMed]
53. Rawlings, A.M.; Sharrett, A.R.; Schneider, A.L.C.; Coresh, J.; Albert, M.; Couper, D.; Griswold, M.; Gottesman, R.F.; Wagenknecht, L.E.; Windham, B.G.; et al. Diabetes in Midlife and Cognitive Change over 20 Years: A Cohort Study. *Ann. Intern. Med.* **2014**, *161*, 785. [CrossRef]
54. Ott, A.; Stolk, R.P.; van Harskamp, F.; Pols, H.A.P.; Hofman, A.; Breteler, M.M.B. Diabetes Mellitus and the Risk of Dementia: The Rotterdam Study. *Neurology* **1999**, *53*, 1937. [CrossRef] [PubMed]
55. De la Monte, S.M.; Wands, J.R. Review of Insulin and Insulin-like Growth Factor Expression, Signaling, and Malfunction in the Central Nervous System: Relevance to Alzheimer's Disease. *J. Alzheimers Dis.* **2005**, *7*, 45–61. [CrossRef] [PubMed]
56. Yahr, T.L.; Vallis, A.J.; Hancock, M.K.; Barbieri, J.T.; Frank, D.W. ExoY, an Adenylate Cyclase Secreted by the *Pseudomonas Aeruginosa* Type III System. *Proc. Natl. Acad. Sci. USA* **1998**, *95*, 13899–13904. [CrossRef] [PubMed]
57. Ochoa, C.D.; Alexeyev, M.; Pastukh, V.; Balczon, R.; Stevens, T. Pseudomonas Aeruginosa Exotoxin Y Is a Promiscuous Cyclase That Increases Endothelial Tau Phosphorylation and Permeability. *J. Biol. Chem.* **2012**, *287*, 25407–25418. [CrossRef]
58. Xi, J.; Ding, D.; Zhu, H.; Wang, R.; Su, F.; Wu, W.; Xiao, Z.; Liang, X.; Zhao, Q.; Hong, Z.; et al. Disturbed Microbial Ecology in Alzheimer's Disease: Evidence from the Gut Microbiota and Fecal Metabolome. *BMC Microbiol.* **2021**, *21*, 226. [CrossRef] [PubMed]
59. Soriano, S.; Curry, K.; Wang, Q.; Chow, E.; Treangen, T.J.; Villapol, S. Fecal Microbiota Transplantation Derived from Alzheimer's Disease Mice Worsens Brain Trauma Outcomes in Wild-Type Controls. *Int. J. Mol. Sci.* **2022**, *23*, 4476. [CrossRef]
60. Paulson, H. Repeat Expansion Diseases. In *Handbook of Clinical Neurology*; Elsevier: Amsterdam, The Netherlands, 2018; Volume 147, pp. 105–123; ISBN 978-0-444-63233-3.
61. Stoyas, C.A.; La Spada, A.R. The CAG–Polyglutamine Repeat Diseases: A Clinical, Molecular, Genetic, and Pathophysiologic Nosology. In *Handbook of Clinical Neurology*; Elsevier: Amsterdam, The Netherlands, 2018; Volume 147, pp. 143–170; ISBN 978-0-444-63233-3.
62. Orr, H.T.; Zoghbi, H.Y. Trinucleotide Repeat Disorders. *Annu. Rev. Neurosci.* **2007**, *30*, 575–621. [CrossRef]
63. Cohen-Carmon, D.; Meshorer, E. Polyglutamine (PolyQ) Disorders: The Chromatin Connection. *Nucleus* **2012**, *3*, 433–441. [CrossRef] [PubMed]
64. Ghosh, R.; Tabrizi, S.J. Huntington Disease. In *Handbook of Clinical Neurology*; Elsevier: Amsterdam, The Netherlands, 2018; Volume 147, pp. 255–278; ISBN 978-0-444-63233-3.
65. Baine, F.K.; Kay, C.; Ketelaar, M.E.; Collins, J.A.; Semaka, A.; Doty, C.N.; Krause, A.; Jacquie Greenberg, L.; Hayden, M.R. Huntington Disease in the South African Population Occurs on Diverse and Ethnically Distinct Genetic Haplotypes. *Eur. J. Hum. Genet.* **2013**, *21*, 1120–1127. [CrossRef] [PubMed]
66. Kay, C.; Tirado-Hurtado, I.; Cornejo-Olivas, M.; Collins, J.A.; Wright, G.; Inca-Martinez, M.; Veliz-Otani, D.; Ketelaar, M.E.; Slama, R.A.; Ross, C.J.; et al. The Targetable A1 Huntington Disease Haplotype Has Distinct Amerindian and European Origins in Latin America. *Eur. J. Hum. Genet.* **2017**, *25*, 332–340. [CrossRef] [PubMed]
67. Warby, S.C.; Visscher, H.; Collins, J.A.; Doty, C.N.; Carter, C.; Butland, S.L.; Hayden, A.R.; Kanazawa, I.; Ross, C.J.; Hayden, M.R. HTT Haplotypes Contribute to Differences in Huntington Disease Prevalence between Europe and East Asia. *Eur. J. Hum. Genet.* **2011**, *19*, 561–566. [CrossRef]
68. Paulsen, J.S.; Langbehn, D.R.; Stout, J.C.; Aylward, E.; Ross, C.A.; Nance, M.; Guttman, M.; Johnson, S.; MacDonald, M.; Beglinger, L.J.; et al. Detection of Huntington's Disease Decades before Diagnosis: The Predict-HD Study. *J. Neurol. Neurosurg. Psychiatry* **2008**, *79*, 874–880. [CrossRef]
69. Tabrizi, S.J.; Scahill, R.I.; Durr, A.; Roos, R.A.; Leavitt, B.R.; Jones, R.; Landwehrmeyer, G.B.; Fox, N.C.; Johnson, H.; Hicks, S.L.; et al. Biological and Clinical Changes in Premanifest and Early Stage Huntington's Disease in the TRACK-HD Study: The 12-Month Longitudinal Analysis. *Lancet Neurol.* **2011**, *10*, 31–42. [CrossRef]
70. Tabrizi, S.J.; Scahill, R.I.; Owen, G.; Durr, A.; Leavitt, B.R.; Roos, R.A.; Borowsky, B.; Landwehrmeyer, B.; Frost, C.; Johnson, H.; et al. Predictors of Phenotypic Progression and Disease Onset in Premanifest and Early-Stage Huntington's Disease in the TRACK-HD Study: Analysis of 36-Month Observational Data. *Lancet Neurol.* **2013**, *12*, 637–649. [CrossRef]
71. Quigley, J. Juvenile Huntington's Disease: Diagnostic and Treatment Considerations for the Psychiatrist. *Curr. Psychiatry Rep.* **2017**, *19*, 9. [CrossRef]
72. Sassone, J.; Colciago, C.; Cislaghi, G.; Silani, V.; Ciammola, A. Huntington's Disease: The Current State of Research with Peripheral Tissues. *Exp. Neurol.* **2009**, *219*, 385–397. [CrossRef]

73. Van der Burg, J.M.M.; Winqvist, A.; Aziz, N.A.; Maat-Schieman, M.L.C.; Roos, R.A.C.; Bates, G.P.; Brundin, P.; Björkqvist, M.; Wierup, N. Gastrointestinal Dysfunction Contributes to Weight Loss in Huntington's Disease Mice. *Neurobiol. Dis.* **2011**, *44*, 9478630. [CrossRef]
74. Jurcau, A. Molecular Pathophysiological Mechanisms in Huntington's Disease. *Biomedicines* **2022**, *10*, 1432. [CrossRef] [PubMed]
75. Jesse, S.; Bayer, H.; Alupei, M.C.; Zügel, M.; Mulaw, M.; Tuorto, F.; Malmsheimer, S.; Singh, K.; Steinacker, J.; Schumann, U.; et al. Ribosomal Transcription Is Regulated by PGC-1alpha and Disturbed in Huntington's Disease. *Sci. Rep.* **2017**, *7*, 8513. [CrossRef] [PubMed]
76. Yablonska, S.; Ganesan, V.; Ferrando, L.M.; Kim, J.; Pyzel, A.; Baranova, O.V.; Khattar, N.K.; Larkin, T.M.; Baranov, S.V.; Chen, N.; et al. Mutant Huntingtin Disrupts Mitochondrial Proteostasis by Interacting with TIM23. *Proc. Natl. Acad. Sci. USA* **2019**, *116*, 16593–16602. [CrossRef] [PubMed]
77. Valadão, P.A.C.; Santos, K.B.S.; e Vieira, T.H.F.; e Cordeiro, T.M.; Teixeira, A.L.; Guatimosim, C.; de Miranda, A.S. Inflammation in Huntington's Disease: A Few New Twists on an Old Tale. *J. Neuroimmunol.* **2020**, *348*, 577380. [CrossRef] [PubMed]
78. Björkqvist, M.; Wild, E.J.; Thiele, J.; Silvestroni, A.; Andre, R.; Lahiri, N.; Raibon, E.; Lee, R.V.; Benn, C.L.; Soulet, D.; et al. A Novel Pathogenic Pathway of Immune Activation Detectable before Clinical Onset in Huntington's Disease. *J. Exp. Med.* **2008**, *205*, 1869–1877. [CrossRef] [PubMed]
79. Khoshnan, A.; Ko, J.; Watkin, E.E.; Paige, L.A.; Reinhart, P.H.; Patterson, P.H. Activation of the IκB Kinase Complex and Nuclear Factor-KB Contributes to Mutant Huntingtin Neurotoxicity. *J. Neurosci.* **2004**, *24*, 7999–8008. [CrossRef]
80. Miller, J.R.C.; Träger, U.; Andre, R.; Tabrizi, S.J. Mutant Huntingtin Does Not Affect the Intrinsic Phenotype of Human Huntington's Disease T Lymphocytes. *PLoS ONE* **2015**, *10*, e0141793. [CrossRef]
81. Palpagama, T.H.; Waldvogel, H.J.; Faull, R.L.M.; Kwakowsky, A. The Role of Microglia and Astrocytes in Huntington's Disease. *Front. Mol. Neurosci.* **2019**, *12*, 258. [CrossRef]
82. Sapp, E.; Kegel, K.B.; Aronin, N.; Hashikawa, T.; Uchiyama, Y.; Tohyama, K.; Bhide, P.G.; Vonsattel, J.P.; Difiglia, M. Early and Progressive Accumulation of Reactive Microglia in the Huntington Disease Brain. *J. Neuropathol. Exp. Neurol.* **2001**, *60*, 161–172. [CrossRef]
83. Politis, M.; Lahiri, N.; Niccolini, F.; Su, P.; Wu, K.; Giannetti, P.; Scahill, R.I.; Turkheimer, F.E.; Tabrizi, S.J.; Piccini, P. Increased Central Microglial Activation Associated with Peripheral Cytokine Levels in Premanifest Huntington's Disease Gene Carriers. *Neurobiol. Dis.* **2015**, *83*, 115–121. [CrossRef]
84. Cekanaviciute, E.; Buckwalter, M.S. Astrocytes: Integrative Regulators of Neuroinflammation in Stroke and Other Neurological Diseases. *Neurotherapeutics* **2016**, *13*, 685–701. [CrossRef] [PubMed]
85. Von Essen, M.R.; Hellem, M.N.N.; Vinther-Jensen, T.; Ammitzbøll, C.; Hansen, R.H.; Hjermind, L.E.; Nielsen, T.T.; Nielsen, J.E.; Sellebjerg, F. Early Intrathecal T Helper 17.1 Cell Activity in Huntington Disease. *Ann. Neurol.* **2020**, *87*, 246–255. [CrossRef]
86. Farshim, P.P.; Bates, G.P. Mouse Models of Huntington's Disease. In *Huntington's Disease*; Precious, S.V., Rosser, A.E., Dunnett, S.B., Eds.; Methods in Molecular Biology; Springer: New York, NY, USA, 2018; Volume 1780, pp. 97–120; ISBN 978-1-4939-7824-3.
87. Gubert, C.; Choo, J.M.; Love, C.J.; Kodikara, S.; Masson, B.A.; Liew, J.J.M.; Wang, Y.; Kong, G.; Narayana, V.K.; Renoir, T.; et al. Faecal Microbiota Transplant Ameliorates Gut Dysbiosis and Cognitive Deficits in Huntington's Disease Mice. *Brain Commun.* **2022**, *4*, fcac205. [CrossRef] [PubMed]
88. Kong, G.; Cao, K.-A.L.; Judd, L.M.; Li, S.; Renoir, T.; Hannan, A.J. Microbiome Profiling Reveals Gut Dysbiosis in a Transgenic Mouse Model of Huntington's Disease. *Neurobiol. Dis.* **2020**, *135*, 104268. [CrossRef] [PubMed]
89. Clairembault, T.; Leclair-Visonneau, L.; Coron, E.; Bourreille, A.; Le Dily, S.; Vavasseur, F.; Heymann, M.-F.; Neunlist, M.; Derkinderen, P. Structural Alterations of the Intestinal Epithelial Barrier in Parkinson's Disease. *Acta Neuropathol. Commun.* **2015**, *3*, 12. [CrossRef]
90. Stan, T.L.; Soylu-Kucharz, R.; Burleigh, S.; Prykhodko, O.; Cao, L.; Franke, N.; Sjögren, M.; Haikal, C.; Hållenius, F.; Björkqvist, M. Increased Intestinal Permeability and Gut Dysbiosis in the R6/2 Mouse Model of Huntington's Disease. *Sci. Rep.* **2020**, *10*, 18270. [CrossRef]
91. Gubert, C.; Love, C.J.; Kodikara, S.; Mei Liew, J.J.; Renoir, T.; Lê Cao, K.-A.; Hannan, A.J. Gene-Environment-Gut Interactions in Huntington's Disease Mice Are Associated with Environmental Modulation of the Gut Microbiome. *iScience* **2022**, *25*, 103687. [CrossRef]
92. Hoban, A.E.; Stilling, R.M.; Ryan, F.J.; Shanahan, F.; Dinan, T.G.; Claesson, M.J.; Clarke, G.; Cryan, J.F. Regulation of Prefrontal Cortex Myelination by the Microbiota. *Transl. Psychiatry* **2016**, *6*, e774. [CrossRef]
93. Radulescu, C.I.; Garcia-Miralles, M.; Sidik, H.; Bardile, C.F.; Yusof, N.A.B.M.; Lee, H.U.; Ho, E.X.P.; Chu, C.W.; Layton, E.; Low, D.; et al. Manipulation of Microbiota Reveals Altered Callosal Myelination and White Matter Plasticity in a Model of Huntington Disease. *Neurobiol. Dis.* **2019**, *127*, 65–75. [CrossRef]
94. Kong, G.; Ellul, S.; Narayana, V.K.; Kanojia, K.; Ha, H.T.T.; Li, S.; Renoir, T.; Cao, K.-A.L.; Hannan, A.J. An Integrated Metagenomics and Metabolomics Approach Implicates the Microbiota-Gut-Brain Axis in the Pathogenesis of Huntington's Disease. *Neurobiol. Dis.* **2021**, *148*, 105199. [CrossRef]
95. Wasser, C.I.; Mercieca, E.-C.; Kong, G.; Hannan, A.J.; McKeown, S.J.; Glikmann-Johnston, Y.; Stout, J.C. Gut Dysbiosis in Huntington's Disease: Associations among Gut Microbiota, Cognitive Performance and Clinical Outcomes. *Brain Commun.* **2020**, *2*, fcaa110. [CrossRef]

96. Du, G.; Dong, W.; Yang, Q.; Yu, X.; Ma, J.; Gu, W.; Huang, Y. Altered Gut Microbiota Related to Inflammatory Responses in Patients With Huntington's Disease. *Front. Immunol.* **2021**, *11*, 603594. [CrossRef] [PubMed]
97. Przybyl, L.; Wozna-Wysocka, M.; Kozlowska, E.; Fiszer, A. What, When and How to Measure—Peripheral Biomarkers in Therapy of Huntington's Disease. *Int. J. Mol. Sci.* **2021**, *22*, 1561. [CrossRef] [PubMed]
98. Liot, G.; Valette, J.; Pépin, J.; Flament, J.; Brouillet, E. Energy Defects in Huntington's Disease: Why "in Vivo" Evidence Matters. *Biochem. Biophys. Res. Commun.* **2017**, *483*, 1084–1095. [CrossRef] [PubMed]
99. Wood, N.I.; Goodman, A.O.G.; van der Burg, J.M.M.; Gazeau, V.; Brundin, P.; Björkqvist, M.; Petersén, Å.; Tabrizi, S.J.; Barker, R.A.; Jennifer Morton, A. Increased Thirst and Drinking in Huntington's Disease and the R6/2 Mouse. *Brain Res. Bull.* **2008**, *76*, 70–79. [CrossRef]
100. Vandeputte, D.; Falony, G.; Vieira-Silva, S.; Tito, R.Y.; Joossens, M.; Raes, J. Stool Consistency Is Strongly Associated with Gut Microbiota Richness and Composition, Enterotypes and Bacterial Growth Rates. *Gut* **2016**, *65*, 57–62. [CrossRef]
101. Lozupone, C.A.; Stombaugh, J.I.; Gordon, J.I.; Jansson, J.K.; Knight, R. Diversity, Stability and Resilience of the Human Gut Microbiota. *Nature* **2012**, *489*, 220–230. [CrossRef]
102. Keshavarzian, A.; Green, S.J.; Engen, P.A.; Voigt, R.M.; Naqib, A.; Forsyth, C.B.; Mutlu, E.; Shannon, K.M. Colonic Bacterial Composition in Parkinson's Disease. *Mov. Disord.* **2015**, *30*, 1351–1360. [CrossRef]
103. Rowin, J.; Xia, Y.; Jung, B.; Sun, J. Gut Inflammation and Dysbiosis in Human Motor Neuron Disease. *Physiol. Rep.* **2017**, *5*, e13443. [CrossRef]
104. Vogt, N.M.; Kerby, R.L.; Dill-McFarland, K.A.; Harding, S.J.; Merluzzi, A.P.; Johnson, S.C.; Carlsson, C.M.; Asthana, S.; Zetterberg, H.; Blennow, K.; et al. Gut Microbiome Alterations in Alzheimer's Disease. *Sci. Rep.* **2017**, *7*, 13537. [CrossRef]
105. Plassais, J.; Gbikpi-Benissan, G.; Figarol, M.; Scheperjans, F.; Gorochov, G.; Derkinderen, P.; Cervino, A.C.L. Gut Microbiome Alpha-Diversity Is Not a Marker of Parkinson's Disease and Multiple Sclerosis. *Brain Commun.* **2021**, *3*, fcab113. [CrossRef] [PubMed]
106. Cardinale, B.J.; Srivastava, D.S.; Emmett Duffy, J.; Wright, J.P.; Downing, A.L.; Sankaran, M.; Jouseau, C. Effects of Biodiversity on the Functioning of Trophic Groups and Ecosystems. *Nature* **2006**, *443*, 989–992. [CrossRef] [PubMed]
107. Shade, A. Diversity Is the Question, Not the Answer. *ISME J.* **2017**, *11*, 1118–1129. [CrossRef] [PubMed]
108. Coyte, K.Z.; Schluter, J.; Foster, K.R. The Ecology of the Microbiome: Networks, Competition, and Stability. *Science* **2015**, *350*, 663–666. [CrossRef] [PubMed]
109. Reese, A.T.; Dunn, R.R. Drivers of Microbiome Biodiversity: A Review of General Rules, Feces, and Ignorance. *mBio* **2018**, *9*, e01294-18. [CrossRef] [PubMed]
110. Magzal, F.; Shochat, T.; Haimov, I.; Tamir, S.; Asraf, K.; Tuchner-Arieli, M.; Even, C.; Agmon, M. Increased Physical Activity Improves Gut Microbiota Composition and Reduces Short-Chain Fatty Acid Concentrations in Older Adults with Insomnia. *Sci. Rep.* **2022**, *12*, 2265. [CrossRef] [PubMed]
111. Wegierska, A.E.; Charitos, I.A.; Topi, S.; Potenza, M.A.; Montagnani, M.; Santacroce, L. The Connection Between Physical Exercise and Gut Microbiota: Implications for Competitive Sports Athletes. *Sport. Med.* **2022**, *52*, 2355–2369. [CrossRef]
112. Horn, J.; Mayer, D.E.; Chen, S.; Mayer, E.A. Role of Diet and Its Effects on the Gut Microbiome in the Pathophysiology of Mental Disorders. *Transl. Psychiatry* **2022**, *12*, 164. [CrossRef]
113. Yeşilyurt, N.; Yılmaz, B.; Ağagündüz, D.; Capasso, R. Microbiome-Based Personalized Nutrition as a Result of the 4.0 Technological Revolution: A Mini Literature Review. *Process. Biochem.* **2022**, *121*, 257–262. [CrossRef]
114. Huang, G.; Qu, Q.; Wang, M.; Huang, M.; Zhou, W.; Wei, F. Global Landscape of Gut Microbiome Diversity and Antibiotic Resistomes across Vertebrates. *Sci. Total Environ.* **2022**, *838*, 156178. [CrossRef]
115. Brooks, S.P.; Jones, L.; Dunnett, S.B. Comparative Analysis of Pathology and Behavioural Phenotypes in Mouse Models of Huntington's Disease. *Brain Res. Bull.* **2012**, *88*, 81–93. [CrossRef] [PubMed]
116. Brooks, S.P.; Dunnett, S.B. Mouse Models of Huntington's Disease. In *Behavioral Neurobiology of Huntington's Disease and Parkinson's Disease*; Nguyen, H.H.P., Cenci, M.A., Eds.; Current Topics in Behavioral Neurosciences; Springer: Berlin/Heidelberg, Germany, 2015; pp. 101–133; ISBN 978-3-662-46344-4.
117. Chongtham, A.; Yoo, J.H.; Chin, T.M.; Akingbesote, N.D.; Huda, A.; Marsh, J.L.; Khoshnan, A. Gut Bacteria Regulate the Pathogenesis of Huntington's Disease in Drosophila Model. *Front. Neurosci.* **2022**, *16*, 830.
118. Zhang, Y.; Geng, J.; Hong, Y.; Jiao, L.; Li, S.; Sun, R.; Xie, Y.; Yan, C.; Aa, J.; Wang, G. Orally Administered Crocin Protects Against Cerebral Ischemia/Reperfusion Injury through the Metabolic Transformation of Crocetin by Gut Microbiota. *Front. Pharmacol.* **2019**, *10*, 440. [CrossRef] [PubMed]
119. Trichka, J.; Zou, W.-Q. Modulation of Neuroinflammation by the Gut Microbiota in Prion and Prion-like Diseases. *Pathogens* **2021**, *10*, 887. [CrossRef]
120. Yang, D.; Zhao, D.; Shah, S.Z.A.; Wu, W.; Lai, M.; Zhang, X.; Li, J.; Guan, Z.; Zhao, H.; Li, W.; et al. Implications of Gut Microbiota Dysbiosis and Metabolic Changes in Prion Disease. *Neurobiol. Dis.* **2020**, *135*, 104704. [CrossRef] [PubMed]
121. Jia, S.; Lu, Z.; Gao, Z.; An, J.; Wu, X.; Li, X.; Dai, X.; Zheng, Q.; Sun, Y. Chitosan Oligosaccharides Alleviate Cognitive Deficits in an Amyloid-B1-42-Induced Rat Model of Alzheimer's Disease. *Int. J. Biol. Macromol.* **2016**, *83*, 416–425. [CrossRef]

122. Schmidt, K.; Cowen, P.J.; Harmer, C.J.; Tzortzis, G.; Errington, S.; Burnet, P.W.J. Prebiotic Intake Reduces the Waking Cortisol Response and Alters Emotional Bias in Healthy Volunteers. *Psychopharmacology* **2015**, *232*, 1793–1801. [CrossRef]
123. Hsieh, T.-H.; Kuo, C.-W.; Hsieh, K.-H.; Shieh, M.-J.; Peng, C.-W.; Chen, Y.-C.; Chang, Y.-L.; Huang, Y.-Z.; Chen, C.-C.; Chang, P.-K.; et al. Probiotics Alleviate the Progressive Deterioration of Motor Functions in a Mouse Model of Parkinson's Disease. *Brain Sci.* **2020**, *10*, 206. [CrossRef]

Disclaimer/Publisher's Note: The statements, opinions and data contained in all publications are solely those of the individual author(s) and contributor(s) and not of MDPI and/or the editor(s). MDPI and/or the editor(s) disclaim responsibility for any injury to people or property resulting from any ideas, methods, instructions or products referred to in the content.

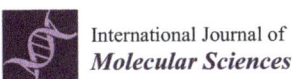

Review

The Impact of Non-Pathogenic Bacteria on the Spread of Virulence and Resistance Genes

Francisco Dionisio [1,*], Célia P. F. Domingues [1,2], João S. Rebelo [1], Francisca Monteiro [1] and Teresa Nogueira [1,2]

[1] cE3c—Centre for Ecology, Evolution and Environmental Changes & CHANGE, Global Change and Sustainability Institute, Faculdade de Ciências, Universidade de Lisboa, 1749-016 Lisboa, Portugal
[2] INIAV—National Institute for Agrarian and Veterinary Research, 2780-157 Oeiras, Portugal
* Correspondence: dionisio@fc.ul.pt

Abstract: This review discusses the fate of antimicrobial resistance and virulence genes frequently present among microbiomes. A central concept in epidemiology is the mean number of hosts colonized by one infected host in a population of susceptible hosts: R_0. It characterizes the disease's epidemic potential because the pathogen continues its propagation through susceptible hosts if it is above one. R_0 is proportional to the average duration of infections, but non-pathogenic microorganisms do not cause host death, and hosts do not need to be rid of them. Therefore, commensal bacteria may colonize hosts for prolonged periods, including those harboring drug resistance or even a few virulence genes. Thus, their R_0 is likely to be (much) greater than one, with peculiar consequences for the spread of virulence and resistance genes. For example, computer models that simulate the spread of these genes have shown that their diversities should correlate positively throughout microbiomes. Bioinformatics analysis with real data corroborates this expectation. Those simulations also anticipate that, contrary to the common wisdom, human's microbiomes with a higher diversity of both gene types are the ones that took antibiotics longer ago rather than recently. Here, we discuss the mechanisms and robustness behind these predictions and other public health consequences.

Keywords: antibiotic resistance; virulence; microbiome; metagenomics; human gut; antibiotic consumption

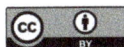

1. Introduction

"What is essential is invisible to the eye".
Antoine de Saint-Exupéry.
"The Little Prince" (1943) [1].

Antibiotic-resistant bacteria caused 1.27 million human deaths worldwide in 2019 [2]. This estimation indicates, once more, that antimicrobial resistance is a severe world health problem [3,4]. Bacterial pathogens are, by definition, the etiological agents of bacterial diseases. However, one must consider commensal bacteria in the list of public health concerns because they are also reservoirs of genes encoding adaptive traits (non-housekeeping genes), e.g., virulence, heavy-metal resistance, and antibiotic-resistance genes that can transfer to pathogenic bacteria [5–11]. For example, a recent work involving bacteria of the *Neisseria* genus has shown that the phenotypic resistance profile of four commensal *Neisseria* species was higher than that of four pathogenic *Neisseria gonorrhoeae* strains [12].

Gene transfer occurs through three major mechanisms. Bacteria can directly uptake DNA from the environment or with the connivance of vectors such as conjugative plasmids, conjugative integrative elements, or bacteriophages [13,14]. For example, in a study of the donor ability of a naturally isolated conjugative plasmid conferring resistance to six antibiotics between 14 enterobacteria, the best plasmid donor was a commensal *Escherichia coli* [7].

These DNA transfer events may occur between different bacteria within microbiomes. Human microbiomes–the collection of all microorganisms (and their genomes) living in human tissues–are complex [15], comprising more than 10^{13} bacterial cells belonging to hundreds of species [16]. In the human body, microorganisms are especially numerous and diverse in the skin, mucosa, and gastrointestinal tract, possibly comprising both pathogenic and non-pathogenic bacteria [17]. The metagenome refers to the set of all genes in a microbiome, including chromosomal genes and extra-chromosomal genetic elements, e.g., bacteriophages, transposons, plasmids, and other mobile genetic elements. Several microbiomes can also be very complex, namely that of other animals, soil, plant roots, sewage, etc.

Generally, in human and veterinary medicine, the onset of a symptomatic infectious disease leads to the prescription of antibiotics. However, we argue here that this does not necessarily mean that bacterial pathogenicity is directly associated with antibiotic resistance (see next sections).

Consider the following arguments:

(i) People that have not used antibiotics for a long time have a lower diversity of drug-resistance genes in their microbiomes;
(ii) The diversity of resistance genes in a person's microbiome increases when that person takes an antibiotic;
(iii) Antibiotic overuse increases the diversity of resistance genes in human microbiomes;
(iv) The co-location of virulence and resistance genes in bacterial genomes explains the positive correlation between the resistance and virulence genes' diversities in microbiomes observed over human microbiomes.

Readers that feel some of these arguments are accurate should keep reading this paper. The vast majority of microorganisms in human microbiomes are non-pathogenic, and we will see how they might play critical roles in the spread of virulence and resistance genes. Paraphrasing Antoine de Saint-Exupéry [1], what is essential, is often unnoticed.

2. The Fate of Commensal Bacteria

2.1. Brief Review of the R_0, the Basic Reproductive Number

A central concept in the epidemiology of infectious disease transmission is the basic reproductive number: also called the basic reproduction number or basic reproduction ratio. It is the expected number of infected individuals by a single infected individual in a susceptible population. Denoted as R_0, this number is a measure of the pathogen's fitness but is also a threshold that characterizes the epidemic potential of the disease because: if $R_0 > 1$, the pathogen continues its propagation through susceptible hosts, with the number of infected hosts increasing exponentially; if $R_0 < 1$, the number of infected hosts decreases exponentially, and the pathogen is extinct. The number of infected hosts is stable in the unlikely case where R_0 equals one [18,19].

R_0 is a dimensionless number defined as $R_0 = \beta \cdot c \cdot d$, where β is the probability of infection if an infected individual contacts a susceptible one, c is the number of contacts between infected and susceptible individuals per time unit, and d is the duration of the infectious period. Its mathematical formula shows that R_0 is proportional to the mean duration of infections d. This period decreases when the intrinsic mortality (i.e., mortality not caused by the pathogen) increases, the pathogen-induced mortality increases, and the rate at which the host recovers (e.g., through immunity) increases. When the colonizing agents are pathogens, typically, either the hosts die or manage to clear the pathogen. If the host's death or recovery is quick, the R_0 of the pathogen is lower than if the pathogen remains a long time in the host. Therefore, there is something peculiar about non-pathogenic microorganisms with public-health consequences.

Non-pathogenic agents do not cause host death, and the hosts do not need to eliminate them. Consequently, commensal or mutualistic bacteria, including those harboring drug resistance or even a few virulence genes, may colonize their hosts for longer, so their R_0 is prone to be larger than one. This conclusion may impact public health because an R_0 larger than one implies that the microorganism may spread through the host population, and as mentioned above, non-pathogenic bacteria may harbor non-housekeeping genes and mobile genetic elements such as virulence and resistance genes.

Even if newly arrived non-pathogenic bacterial cells cannot persist in a microbiome for more than a few days, its mobile genetic elements can have several opportunities to transfer to one of the other established cells in that microbiome [20–22], and may thus remain there for a long time. This is possible due to the presence of hundreds of bacterial species in many microbiomes, including the human gut, and because bacteria can receive foreign DNA through three primary mechanisms: (i) transformation, where bacteria directly uptakes DNA from the surroundings [23]; (ii) transduction, where bacteriophages bring DNA from their previous hosts [24]; and (iii) bacterial conjugation, where bacteria receive conjugative plasmids or integrative conjugative elements from neighboring cells [25]. A bacterial cell can uptake DNA from phylogenetically distant bacteria cells, and conjugative plasmids can transfer between cells belonging to different bacterial species [26]. Therefore, both pathogenic and non-pathogenic bacteria can share a gene pool that includes virulence and resistance genes.

Moreover, some bacterial populations containing neither mobile genetic elements nor virulence or resistance genes can become great "amplifiers" of these genes after receiving some plasmids. Some bacterial strains are excellent donors of conjugative plasmids and are able to "amplify" it among them while quickly transmitting the plasmid to other cells in a microbiome [7,27]. These amplifiers are present among strains of *Escherichia coli* and other enterobacterial species [7], among soil bacteria [27], and most probably in the majority of microbiomes.

2.2. The Human Network of Physical Contacts

2.2.1. Brief Review of Small-World Networks

People establish many networks involving physical contact with each other through family relationships, friendships, sexual relationships, and many others. Networks have nodes (or vertices) and edges (connections). For example, consider the "handshaking" network in which each node is a person, and two persons are connected in this network if they had at least a handshaking, e.g., last year.

In a typical network established by people, each person connects to a tiny subset of another person included in that network. Therefore, most people have no direct connections (each one of us gave a handshake to just a few people last year).

In some networks involving people, if a given person connects to two others, these two persons are likely connected to each other, but each person can reach most people (through the network's connections) by a small number of connections. The last sentence sounds somewhat contradictory, but it is not–strikingly, many networks established by people are similar to this–the so-called small-world networks–and we will discuss how that is relevant to understanding microorganisms' spread.

We first consider a regular network (Figure 1, left panel) and then change it to make it a small-world network (Figure 1, middle panel). Consider, for example, the network of friendships. For clarification, let us assume that individuals in a population are organized in alphabetic order: A, B, C, ..., Y, Z, AA, AB, ... and that all individuals have precisely four friends. Frequently, if individual C is a friend of two individuals on his/her right, A and B, and the two individuals on his/her left, D and E, then probably B and D are friends of each other, and A and B or D and E.

Meanwhile, D is a friend of B, C (right), E, and F (left), so B and C are friends to each other, as well as E and F, and so on. Therefore, the clustering of these networks' nodes (people) is high. If all friendships were similar to this, the friendships' network would be regular. In such a network, if, for example, individual G has an exciting gossip, it takes nine steps to reach, say, individual X. These nine steps are the following: G first informs I, which would transmit the story to K, then M, O, Q, S, U, V, X.

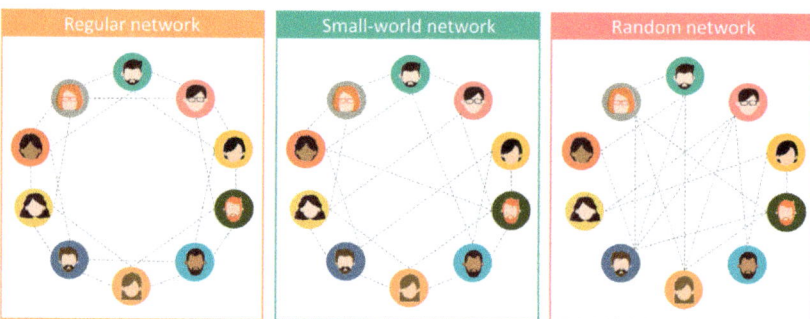

Figure 1. Regular, small-world, and random networks.

Of course, some exceptions to the regular network of friendships may substantially impact information spread. For example, according to the rule described above, individual K may be a friend of I, J, and L. Nevertheless, in this new network version, the fourth K's friend is Z, not M. With this exception, the network is no longer a regular one. In this case, a gossip would take just four steps to progress from G to X (G => I => K => Z => X). With a few more changes in other individuals, such as the one we introduced in K, the network becomes a "small-world" network.

In small-world networks, the clustering of nodes (people) is high, but the path of friendships between any human being is short. Rumors may spread in regular networks, but the speed would be much higher in small-world networks [28].

What makes small-world networks so relevant to epidemiology? As mentioned above, if people organize themselves in small-world networks, the spread of information is fast because, although most people do not have direct contact with each other, most can be reached in a few steps. Suppose physical proximity or even contact is involved in these networks. In that case, microorganisms may quickly spread because the typical distance between two randomly chosen people (the network nodes) grows proportionally to its logarithm [28] instead of the number of people in the network as in regular networks. This difference is relevant because the logarithm function grows much slower than a linear function (Figure 2A). For example, when a given variable X increases from one to a billion (i.e., from 1 to 10^9), $Log_{10}X$ goes from zero to nine only. Therefore, in small-world networks, the path between two random persons is low, even if the network contains millions or billions of people.

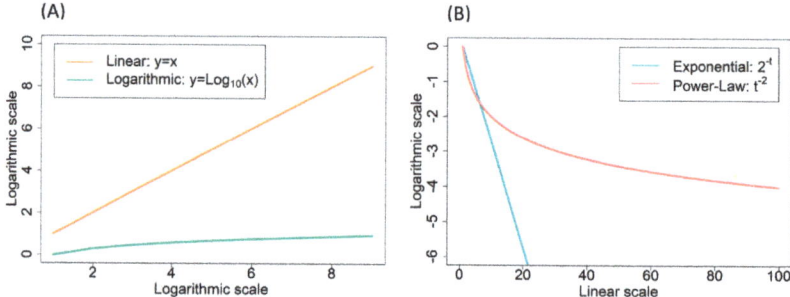

Figure 2. (A): Linear and logarithmic functions. Suppose that x increases from 1 to 10^9, close to the world population size. Then, y increases from 1 to 10^9 in the case of the $y = x$ linear function, whereas the $y = Log_{10}(x)$ function increases from zero to nine only. Note that both axes are at the logarithmic scale (base 10). **(B)**: Exponential and power-law decay. The exponential function 2^{-t} decreases much faster than the power-law function t^{-2}. Note that the vertical axis is at the logarithmic scale (base 10) but not the horizontal axis.

Of course, people spontaneously build other contact networks. For example, people in our working place are not necessarily our friends, but we contact them daily. These networks, which usually involve physical proximity or sharing a working environment, may be relevant concerning the microorganisms' evolution or spread. For example, previous studies have shown that the shorter path lengths in small-world networks increase the effectiveness of natural selection while maintaining the fittest clones in bacterial populations because the probability of encounters between individuals is higher than in regular networks [29,30].

Liljeros et al. studied the web of human sexual connections among 2810 adult Swedish people and found that those connections defined a scale-free network [31,32]. In scale-free networks, the distribution of links in each node follows a power law [33]. In the case of the network of sexual contacts, $p(k)$ describes the proportion of people with k sexual contacts in the previous year, $p(k) \approx c \cdot k^{-\alpha}$, where c and α are positive parameters. Therefore, all people in that Swedish database had at least one sexual partner in the previous year, but a lower fraction had two partners; an even lower fraction, some people had three sexual partners, and so on. Power-law distributions characteristically decreased slowly, so some individuals had 20 partners in the previous year. These few individuals are "hubs" of this network, which is relevant, for example, for sexually transmitted diseases [32]. In this study, the exponent α is slightly above three. The exponent α for women is higher than that for men, which means that the proportion of women with k sexual partners is lower than that of men; however, the statistical error of these estimations is higher than their difference [31,32,34]. The same authors have also shown that the cumulative distribution $P(k)$ similarly follows a decreasing power-law distribution, $P(\geq k) \approx c \cdot k^{-\rho}$, where $\rho = \alpha - 1$. The word "cumulative" in the previous sentence means that $P(\geq k)$ quantifies the fraction of people with k or more contacts [31].

2.2.2. Power-Laws and Scale-Free Networks

Power-laws are mathematical functions such as x^q, where x is the independent variable and q is a negative or positive constant. They are common in physical laws; for example, the gravitational force between two bodies decreases with distance d according to a power law proportional to d^{-2}. Similarly, the electric force between two charged bodies falls with d^{-2}.

In microbiology, we also find power laws. For example, the mutation rate per replication per nucleotide of DNA-based microorganisms decreases with the genome size according to $\mu \approx c \cdot G^{-\beta}$. Because $\beta \approx -1$, this equation means that the mutation rate per replication per nucleotide is inversely proportional to the genome size ($\mu \cdot G \approx c$) so that the mutation rate per replication per genome is a constant ($c \approx 0.003$): Drake's rule [35–37]. Another example concerns the death rate of persister bacterial populations in the presence of a bactericidal antibiotic. Some authors have argued that the death rate of persister populations of some strains follows a power law with an exponent close to -2 [38,39]. A power-law decay is slower than an exponential decay, which means that bacterial cells under antibiotic exposure decay according to a power law can persist alive for longer, sometimes causing health problems and persistent food contamination (Figure 2B).

Concerning the spread of microorganisms through human-contact networks (i.e., with people as nodes), it is relevant to know if the networks are scale-free, that is, if the proportion of people with a k connection follows a power-law distribution. That would mean that a non-negligible proportion of people have many connections, as we have seen with the web of sexual contacts [31]. However, there are more examples of scale-free networks relevant to epidemiology.

In 2006, Brockmann et al. found something striking concerning the dispersal of banknotes in the USA. They studied banknote dispersion as a proxy of people traveling. As intuitively expected, most banknotes travel less than 10 km in four days; also, according to our intuition, the number of banknotes detected further away decreases when the distance increases. Gaussian or Exponential distributions would mostly predict that none or very few banknotes travel more than a few hundred kilometers. However, contrary to common intuition, many banknotes travel thousands of kilometers in those four days. Banknote traveling follows a decreasing power law [40]. The transactions of these banknotes may be twofold in their relevance to epidemiological studies: (i) banknotes move between physically close people, enabling cross-contagion with microorganisms; (ii) banknotes may carry microorganisms, so a person may contaminate another one without being physically close.

Tracking the position of 100,000 mobile phones for six months provides a similar distribution [41]. Most mobile phones only travel a few kilometers, and the proportion of phones traveling decays when the distance increases. A non-negligible number of cell phones traveled hundreds of kilometers. As we have seen for banknotes, the overall traveling of mobile phones follows a decreasing power law. These long-distance traveling people (measured through their banknotes and mobile phones) may constitute relevant microorganism spreaders.

As we have seen, networks where the proportion of people with k connections decreases according to $p(k) \approx k^{-\alpha}$, where α is a positive fixed number are epidemiologically relevant. However, concerning the diseases' spread, some are even more relevant such as those power laws where the parameter α is between two and three. We have seen above that a suitable parameter commonly discussed in epidemiological studies is that of R_0, which informs us how many people a single infected person will transmit the infection to on average in a fully susceptible population. Strikingly, there is no such threshold in networks whose connections between people follow a decreasing power-law distribution with $2 < \alpha < 3$. Therefore, an epidemic spread may occur even with low rates of disease transmission between the hosts [42,43]. Networks with $\alpha < 3$ have very high standard deviations in terms of the number of connections to each node. Therefore, in the context of the equation $R_0 = \beta \cdot c \cdot d$, the number of contacts between infected and susceptible individuals per time unit, c, may also be extremely high.

If the human population network structure (small word, sometimes following a power-law distribution) somewhat facilitates microorganism spread, why do novel pathogens not almost instantly infect humans worldwide? In the case of scale-free networks, the α parameter mentioned above is sometimes lower than two or above three. For example, we have seen above that, in the case of sexual partners in the previous year, that α is slightly higher than three [31,32]. With the α parameter outside that interval, the network is still a small world, but there is an epidemic transition value [34]. Moreover, real-life scale-free networks are finite (i.e., have a limited number of people), which implies that, even if the α parameter falls between two and three, there is a non-null epidemic threshold.

Moreover, humans do not become infectious immediately after contagion, which may take a few days, depending on the disease. Furthermore, people are not permanently in contact with each other, particularly if they feel ill. Additionally, people, medical doctors, and the government commonly implement measures to halt disease spread. Even so, we have seen that with, for example, the COVID-19 pandemic, and despite arduous efforts employed by the governments of several countries, two and a half months (between December 2019 and the first days of March 2020) were sufficient to spread the SARS-CoV-2 virus to most countries worldwide. Governments employed compulsory confinements and other demanding measures because COVID-19 would kill many people and cause morbidity to many others [44].

2.3. Selection and Weak Counter-Selection of Virulence and Resistance Genes

Proteins encoded by virulence genes—e.g., toxins and cell surface proteins that enable bacterial attachment to host tissues, among others—can help bacteria colonize hosts [45]. Therefore, newly acquired virulence genes may not affect fitness or confer immediate advantages to bacteria, while recently acquired resistance determinants often impose a fitness cost on the bacterial cell. Therefore, these gene types may have different effects on their new hosts when newly acquired. However, the claim that resistant determinants are costly is somewhat complex.

The fitness costs of drug resistance determinants may evolve towards lower values or even become zero. For example, compensatory mutations often arise and diminish or even eliminate the deleterious effects of resistance mutations [46–56]. Moreover, resistance determinants (mutations or plasmids) can decrease the fitness cost of other resistant determinants, e.g., through epistatic interactions [57–59]. Furthermore, plasmid–plasmid interactions may facilitate plasmid transfer [60–62], sometimes compensating for plasmid costs [63,64].

Sometimes compensatory mutations arise in the resistance-encoding mobile genetic element, not the bacterial chromosome. In this case, when moving into another bacterial host, this genetic element carries both the resistance gene and the compensatory mutations, therefore imposing no cost on its new host [52,65].

A recent study involved 9275 patients during hospital stays over two years at the Ramon y Cajal University Hospital (Madrid, Spain). Alonso-del Valle et al. measured the cost of *pOXA-48_K8*: a naturally isolated plasmid. This plasmid was the most successful *pOXA-48*-like plasmid in an extensive collection of extended-spectrum ß-lactamase- and carbapenemase-producing enterobacteria isolated from the gut of 105 out of those 9275 patients (1.13%). The authors introduced this plasmid in 25 isolates of *Klebsiella pneumoniae* and 25 of *Escherichia coli* naïve to the *pOXA-48_K8* plasmid to determine the distribution of fitness effects on the plasmid in those 50 strains. These strains were isolated from patients coinciding on the hospital ward with others colonized with bacteria harboring *pOXA-48*-like plasmids [66].

As expected, the plasmid imposed a fitness cost to bacterial cells: a mean cost of 2.9%. Although small, this effect is statistically significant. However, individual values varied considerably. Most fitness effects were null, and the authors only observed a fitness cost in 14 strains (28%). Interestingly, the plasmid conferred a fitness advantage to the host in seven strains (14%) [66]. It is crucial to note that, even if the plasmid decreases bacterial fitness in 28% of the strains, the plasmid can succeed and "amplify" in the other 58% of the strains where the plasmid is neutral or among the 14% where the plasmid confers a fitness benefit [7,27,67].

Alonso-del Valle et al. measured the fitness of plasmid-bearing strains through competition assays. This method is appropriate because it mimics the real competition taking place between plasmid-bearing and plasmid-free cells in the gut microbiota. These competition assays were performed in agitated liquid media to avoid plasmid transfer into the competitor [66].

All the accumulated knowledge about the cost of resistant determinants points in the same direction: even if plasmid-encoded resistance determinants impose a fitness cost to naïve recipient cells, soon the cost diminishes or disappears. Therefore, resistant cells may avoid being outcompeted by sensitive cells after a critical adaptation period to a resistance-encoding gene.

One must remember that human tissues and the gut are structured media with minimal or no agitation. In such environments, plasmids can transfer to neighboring naïve cells. Possibly, the plasmid imposes a fitness cost to their neighbors, leaving resources to the donor cells. Therefore, even if plasmids are costly in the donor cells, these may succeed by imposing fitness costs on adjacent competitors, acting as harmful agents [68]. This harming behavior is advantageous to donor cells for the following reasons [68]: (i) donor cells have already adapted to the plasmid presence due, for example, to compensatory mutations [56]; (ii) the plasmid transfers to recipient cells (transconjugant cells); (iii) these cells are not adapted to the plasmid presence because they never harbored it; (iv) these non-adapted transconjugant cells replicate slower and use fewer resources than before the plasmid arrival; (v) donor cells may uptake the unused nutrients and replicate.

Furthermore, it is interesting to note that, just because they are transferable (and not due to the gain of additional genes), conjugative plasmids may have an adaptive value to their hosts, not only as harmful agents, as explained above [68], but also as promoters of bacterial biofilms, which confer protection against antimicrobials [63,69,70].

Therefore, epidemiological or evolutionary studies of antibiotic resistance must assume that resistance genes are widespread worldwide. For over eight decades, tons of antibiotics have been used and thrown into the environment [71]. The prolonged use of these drugs has promoted the clonal expansion of resistant cells and the worldwide spread of resistant clones and putative mobile genetic elements carrying resistance genes. Not surprisingly, nowadays, many metagenomes, including human and environmental ones, contain resistance genes; sometimes, this includes a diverse set of those genes as well as virulence genes [72].

2.4. The Diversity of Virulence and Resistance Genes across Microbiomes

We have argued above that non-housekeeping genes are somewhat free to spread within and between microbiomes (namely between people). Some people may use antibiotics, which select virulence genes that are present in resistant cells and resistance genes but counter-select other genes, including those that confer resistance to unrelated antibiotics and virulence genes encoded in bacterial cells susceptible to the used drug.

The use of antibiotics by sick people may select antibiotic-resistant pathogens, which, by definition, encode virulence genes. Perhaps this is why several studies have shown antibiotic and virulence genes co-occurrence in bacterial genomes [73–75]. In general, one could predict that the continuing use of tons of antibiotics through the decades would co-select virulence and resistance genes. However, it is also manifest that the administration of antibiotics hits several other bacteria, namely commensal and mutualistic bacteria, in the human microbiome [76–78]. Moreover, the use of antibiotics as growth promoters in livestock and agriculture or with prophylactic purposes may select resistant cells independently on whether or not they encode virulence genes [79].

Paradoxically, however, the diversity of resistance genes correlates positively with the diversity of virulence genes across human and environmental microbiomes [72]: microbiomes with a high diversity of one class of genes tend to have a high diversity of the other class. However, Darmancier et al. studied 16,632 bacterial genomes and concluded that no such positive correlation exists at the level of genomes, neither across chromosomes nor across plasmids [80]. The results of these two studies (references [72,80]) are compatible if, and only if, metagenomes with a high diversity of both gene types have those genes mostly located in different genomes. Why should there be a positive correlation at the level of metagenomes but not at the genome level?

In the previous two sections, we have also argued that virulence and resistance genes have conditions to remain in metagenomes for a long time. Each person receives diverse genes of both types during this period, accumulating them in their microbiomes, although not necessarily in the same bacterial cells. Meanwhile, pathogenic bacteria circulate through the human population. Some of those ill people take an antibiotic, which selects cells resistant to it but kills susceptible cells, including those resistant to other drugs. Therefore, a consequence of taking the antibiotic is a decrease in the diversity of drug-resistance genes [81]. Moreover, virulence genes are present in dead cells, decreasing their diversity. This process implies that people who took antibiotics recently are those with the lowest diversity of both resistant and virulence cells [82]. On the other hand, those that took antibiotics a long time ago have the highest diversity of both gene types [82]. The overall result is a positive correlation between the diversities of both gene types across human microbiomes [72,82].

What if there is a misuse (and overuse) of antibiotics, where some people use them even if they are not infected by a bacterial pathogen (or are randomly in contact with antibiotics from environmental contamination)? The process is very similar to the one described above, and the overall result is the same: a positive correlation of both genes' diversities. These are the predictions if the probability that a metagenome loses resistance determinants is lower than the transmission probability between people [82]. We have seen above how unlikely it is that metagenomes lose resistance determinants, so the transmission probability between people must prevail or even the contamination of people from the environment or, for example, non-cooked vegetables [83].

A computer model enabled the analysis and corroboration of the above predictions [82]. The model simulated the transfer of pathogenic bacteria and one hundred categories of resistance and virulence genes. Simulations ran with different network types (regular, small-world, and random), and the results were always similar (the only difference being that the simulations reached stable results much sooner in small-world and random networks than in the regular network as expected, and according to explanations given above). Control simulations included changing the number of interacting people, the number of virulence and resistance genes, the relative probabilities of losing genes and acquiring them through contacts, or even changing the initial number of people already containing virulence and resistant genes, providing similar results [82].

Until this point, we have shown why the arguments (i) to (iii) presented in the Introduction section are wrong. About the fourth one, our discussion above does not predict a co-location of virulence and resistance genes in bacterial genomes; moreover, the computer model did not need to postulate their co-location to explain the positive correlation between the resistance and virulence genes' diversities in microbiomes observed over human microbiomes. However, one must ask whether the last eighty years of intensive antibiotic use have put virulence and resistance genes together. As mentioned above, there is no correlation between resistance and virulence genes' diversities throughout genomes [80]. Nevertheless, there are indirect signs of the selection of antibiotic-resistant pathogens, given that some categories of resistance and virulence genes preferentially occur in the same genome [80]. For example, Darmancier et al. observed the co-occurrence between type VII secretion systems and fusidic acid resistance genes [80]: fusidic acid is used, e.g., to treat methicillin-resistant *S. aureus* infections, and is also active against tuberculosis [84,85].

3. Conclusions

We have known for decades that bacteria share some core genes (a common gene pool), so health professionals and microbiologists must consider the impact of commensal bacteria on pathogenesis and public health studies [5,7,9,10,86]. Moreover, non-pathogenic bacteria may contain virulence, drug resistance, and other non-housekeeping genes that are capable of increasing the pathogens' success during infection [6,11]. Furthermore, non-pathogenic cells that do not carry those genes may help pathogenic cells to receive those genes by amplifying their presence among microbiomes [7,27]. Finally, physical contact networks involving humans (see the above Sections 2.1 and 2.2) facilitate the pathogens' spread through our species. However, the vast majority of bacteria in human microbiomes, the non-pathogenic ones, must play critical roles in spreading virulence and resistance genes (Sections 2.3 and 2.4).

Author Contributions: F.D. and T.N. planned the paper. F.D. wrote the first draft of the manuscript, with contributions from all the other authors. All authors have read and agreed to the published version of the manuscript.

Funding: Célia P. F. Domingues, João S. Rebelo, and Francisca Monteiro acknowledge FCT-Fundação para a Ciência e a Tecnologia, IP for their fellowships (PhD grants UI/BD/153078/2022, SFRH/BD/04631/2021 and PostDoc grant SFRH/BPD/123504/2016, respectively). FCT also supports cE3c by contract UIDP/00329/2020.

Institutional Review Board Statement: Not applicable.

Informed Consent Statement: Not applicable.

Data Availability Statement: Not applicable.

Acknowledgments: The authors thank the work of the editor and two anonymous reviewers.

Conflicts of Interest: The authors declare that the research was conducted in the absence of any commercial or financial relationships that could be construed as a potential conflict of interest.

References

1. Saint-Exupery, A.D. *The Little Prince*; Farshore Picture Books: London, UK, 2017; ISBN 978-1-4052-8819-4.
2. Murray, C.J.; Ikuta, K.S.; Sharara, F.; Swetschinski, L.; Aguilar, G.R.; Gray, A.; Han, C.; Bisignano, C.; Rao, P.; Wool, E.; et al. Global burden of bacterial antimicrobial resistance in 2019: A systematic analysis. *Lancet* **2022**, *399*, 629–655. [CrossRef] [PubMed]
3. WHO. *Antimicrobial Resistance: Global Report on Surveillance*; WHO: Geneva, Switzerland, 2014.
4. WHO. *WHO Report on Surveillance of Antibiotic Consumption: 2016–2018 Early Implementation*; WHO: Geneva, Switzerland, 2018.
5. Salyers, A.A.; Gupta, A.; Wang, Y. Human intestinal bacteria as reservoirs for antibiotic resistance genes. *Trends Microbiol.* **2004**, *12*, 412–416. [CrossRef] [PubMed]
6. Rolain, J.-M. Food and human gut as reservoirs of transferable antibiotic resistance encoding genes. *Front. Microbiol.* **2013**, *4*, 173. [CrossRef] [PubMed]
7. Dionisio, F.; Matic, I.; Radman, M.; Rodrigues, O.R.; Taddei, F. Plasmids Spread Very Fast in Heterogeneous Bacterial Communities. *Genetics* **2002**, *162*, 1525–1532. [CrossRef] [PubMed]
8. Bailey, J.; Pinyon, J.; Anantham, S.; Hall, R.M. Commensal Escherichia coli of healthy humans: A reservoir for antibiotic-resistance determinants. *J. Med. Microbiol.* **2010**, *59*, 1331–1339. [CrossRef]
9. Sommer, M.O.A.; Dantas, G.; Church, G.M. Functional Characterization of the Antibiotic Resistance Reservoir in the Human Microflora. *Science* **2009**, *325*, 1128–1131. [CrossRef]
10. Smillie, C.S.; Smith, M.B.; Friedman, J.; Cordero, O.X.; David, L.A.; Alm, E.J. Ecology drives a global network of gene exchange connecting the human microbiome. *Nature* **2011**, *480*, 241–244. [CrossRef]
11. Balasubramanian, D.; López-Pérez, M.; Grant, T.-A.; Ogbunugafor, C.B.; Almagro-Moreno, S. Molecular mechanisms and drivers of pathogen emergence. *Trends Microbiol.* **2022**, *30*, 898–911. [CrossRef]
12. Goytia, M.; Thompson, S.; Jordan, S.; King, K. Antimicrobial Resistance Profiles of Human Commensal *Neisseria* Species. *Antibiotics* **2021**, *10*, 538. [CrossRef]
13. Arnold, B.J.; Huang, I.-T.; Hanage, W.P. Horizontal gene transfer and adaptive evolution in bacteria. *Nat. Rev. Genet.* **2021**, *20*, 206–218. [CrossRef]
14. Baquero, F.; Martínez, J.L.; Lanza, V.F.; Rodríguez-Beltrán, J.; Galán, J.C.; Millán, A.S.; Cantón, R.; Coque, T.M. Evolutionary Pathways and Trajectories in Antibiotic Resistance. *Clin. Microbiol. Rev.* **2021**, *34*, e0005019. [CrossRef] [PubMed]
15. Heintz-Buschart, A.; Wilmes, P. Human Gut Microbiome: Function Matters. *Trends Microbiol.* **2018**, *26*, 563–574. [CrossRef] [PubMed]
16. Sender, R.; Fuchs, S.; Milo, R. Revised Estimates for the Number of Human and Bacteria Cells in the Body. *PLoS Biol.* **2016**, *14*, e1002533. [CrossRef] [PubMed]
17. Ursell, L.K.; Metcalf, J.L.; Parfrey, L.W.; Knight, R. Defining the human microbiome. *Nutr. Rev.* **2012**, *70*, S38–S44. [CrossRef]
18. Anderson, R.M.; May, R.M. *Infectious Diseases of Humans: Dynamics and Control*; Oxford University Press: Oxford, UK; New York, NY, USA, 1992; ISBN 978-0-19-854040-3.
19. Frank, S.A. Models of Parasite Virulence. *Q. Rev. Biol.* **1996**, *71*, 37–78. [CrossRef]
20. Zeng, X.; Lin, J. Factors influencing horizontal gene transfer in the intestine. *Anim. Health Res. Rev.* **2017**, *18*, 153–159. [CrossRef]
21. McInnes, R.S.; McCallum, G.E.; Lamberte, L.E.; van Schaik, W. Horizontal transfer of antibiotic resistance genes in the human gut microbiome. *Curr. Opin. Microbiol.* **2020**, *53*, 35–43. [CrossRef]
22. Brito, I.L. Examining horizontal gene transfer in microbial communities. *Nat. Rev. Microbiol.* **2021**, *19*, 442–453. [CrossRef]
23. Johnston, C.; Martin, B.; Fichant, G.; Polard, P.; Claverys, J.-P. Bacterial transformation: Distribution, shared mechanisms and divergent control. *Nat. Rev. Microbiol.* **2014**, *12*, 181–196. [CrossRef]
24. Smillie, C.; Garcillán-Barcia, M.P.; Francia, M.V.; Rocha, E.P.C.; de la Cruz, F. Mobility of Plasmids. *Microbiol. Mol. Biol. Rev.* **2010**, *74*, 434–452. [CrossRef]
25. Sessions, S.K. Genome Size. In *Brenner's Encyclopedia of Genetics*, 2nd ed.; Maloy, S., Hughes, K., Eds.; Elsevier: London, UK, 2013; Volume 3, pp. 144–151. ISBN 978-0-08-096156-9.
26. McGowan, J.E.; Tenover, F.C. Confronting bacterial resistance in healthcare settings: A crucial role for microbiologists. *Nat. Rev. Genet.* **2004**, *2*, 251–258. [CrossRef] [PubMed]
27. Hall, J.P.J.; Wood, A.J.; Harrison, E.; Brockhurst, M.A. Source–sink plasmid transfer dynamics maintain gene mobility in soil bacterial communities. *Proc. Natl. Acad. Sci. USA* **2016**, *113*, 8260–8265. [CrossRef] [PubMed]
28. Watts, D.J.; Strogatz, S.H. Collective dynamics of 'small-world' networks. *Nature* **1998**, *393*, 440–442. [CrossRef] [PubMed]
29. Combadão, J.; Campos, P.R.A.; Dionisio, F.; Gordo, I. Small-world networks decrease the speed of Muller's ratchet. *Genet. Res.* **2007**, *89*, 7–18. [CrossRef]
30. Campos, P.R.A.; Combadão, J.; Dionisio, F.; Gordo, I. Muller's ratchet in random graphs and scale-free networks. *Phys. Rev. E* **2006**, *74*, 42901. [CrossRef]

31. Liljeros, F.; Edling, C.R.; Amaral, L.A.N.; Stanley, H.E.; Åberg, Y. The web of human sexual contacts. *Nature* **2001**, *411*, 907–908. [CrossRef]
32. Liljeros, F.; Edling, C.R.; Stanley, H.E.; Åberg, Y.; Amaral, L.A.N. Sexual contacts and epidemic thresholds. *Nature* **2003**, *423*, 606. [CrossRef]
33. Amaral, L.A.N.; Scala, A.; Barthélémy, M.; Stanley, H.E. Classes of small-world networks. *Proc. Natl. Acad. Sci. USA* **2000**, *97*, 11149–11152. [CrossRef]
34. Newman, M.E.J. Spread of epidemic disease on networks. *Phys. Rev. E* **2002**, *66*, 16128. [CrossRef]
35. Drake, J.W. A constant rate of spontaneous mutation in DNA-based microbes. *Proc. Natl. Acad. Sci. USA* **1991**, *88*, 7160–7164. [CrossRef]
36. Drake, J.W. The Distribution of Rates of Spontaneous Mutation over Viruses, Prokaryotes, and Eukaryotes. *Ann. N. Y. Acad. Sci.* **1999**, *870*, 100–107. [CrossRef] [PubMed]
37. Sung, W.; Ackerman, M.S.; Miller, S.F.; Doak, T.G.; Lynch, M. Drift-barrier hypothesis and mutation-rate evolution. *Proc. Natl. Acad. Sci. USA* **2012**, *109*, 18488–18492. [CrossRef] [PubMed]
38. Şimşek, E.; Kim, M. Power-law tail in lag time distribution underlies bacterial persistence. *Proc. Natl. Acad. Sci. USA* **2019**, *116*, 17635–17640. [CrossRef] [PubMed]
39. Rebelo, J.S.; Domingues, C.P.F.; Monteiro, F.; Nogueira, T.; Dionisio, F. Bacterial persistence is essential for susceptible cell survival in indirect resistance, mainly for lower cell densities. *PLoS ONE* **2021**, *16*, e0246500. [CrossRef] [PubMed]
40. Brockmann, D.; Hufnagel, L.; Geisel, T. The scaling laws of human travel. *Nature* **2006**, *439*, 462–465. [CrossRef]
41. Gonzalez, M.C.; Hidalgo, C.A.; Barabasi, A.L. Understanding individual human mobility patterns. *Nature* **2008**, *453*, 779–782. [CrossRef]
42. Pastor-Satorras, R.; Vespignani, A. Epidemic Spreading in Scale-Free Networks. *Phys. Rev. Lett.* **2001**, *86*, 3200–3203. [CrossRef]
43. Boguñá, M.; Pastor-Satorras, R.; Vespignani, A. Absence of Epidemic Threshold in Scale-Free Networks with Connectivity Correlations. *Phys. Rev. Lett.* **2003**, *90*, 28701. [CrossRef]
44. Schlosser, F.; Maier, B.F.; Jack, O.; Hinrichs, D.; Zachariae, A.; Brockmann, D. COVID-19 lockdown induces disease-mitigating structural changes in mobility networks. *Proc. Natl. Acad. Sci. USA* **2020**, *117*, 32883–32890. [CrossRef]
45. Klemm, P.; Schembri, M.A. Bacterial adhesins: Function and structure. *Int. J. Med. Microbiol.* **2000**, *290*, 27–35. [CrossRef]
46. Modi, R.I.; Adams, J. Coevolution in bacterial-plasmid populations. *Evolution* **1991**, *45*, 656–667. [CrossRef] [PubMed]
47. Levin, B.R.; Lipsitch, M.; Perrot, V.; Schrag, S.; Antia, R.; Simonsen, L.; Walker, N.M.; Stewart, F.M. The Population Genetics of Antibiotic Resistance. *Clin. Infect. Dis.* **1997**, *24*, S9–S16. [CrossRef] [PubMed]
48. Schrag, S.J.; Perrot, V.; Levin, B.R. Adaptation to the fitness costs of antibiotic resistance in *Escherichia coli*. *Proc. R. Soc. B Biol. Sci.* **1997**, *264*, 1287–1291. [CrossRef] [PubMed]
49. Björkman, J.; Nagaev, I.; Berg, O.G.; Hughes, D.; Andersson, D.I. Effects of Environment on Compensatory Mutations to Ameliorate Costs of Antibiotic Resistance. *Science* **2000**, *287*, 1479–1482. [CrossRef]
50. Dahlberg, C.; Chao, L. Amelioration of the Cost of Conjugative Plasmid Carriage in *Eschericha coli* K12. *Genetics* **2003**, *165*, 1641–1649. [CrossRef]
51. Maisnier-Patin, S.; Andersson, D.I. Adaptation to the deleterious effects of antimicrobial drug resistance mutations by compensatory evolution. *Res. Microbiol.* **2004**, *155*, 360–369. [CrossRef]
52. Dionisio, F.; Conceição, I.; Marques, A.C.; Fernandes, L.; Gordo, I. The evolution of a conjugative plasmid and its ability to increase bacterial fitness. *Biol. Lett.* **2005**, *1*, 250–252. [CrossRef]
53. Nilsson, A.I.; Zorzet, A.; Kanth, A.; Dahlström, S.; Berg, O.G.; Andersson, D.I. Reducing the fitness cost of antibiotic resistance by amplification of initiator tRNA genes. *Proc. Natl. Acad. Sci. USA* **2006**, *103*, 6976–6981. [CrossRef]
54. Hall, J.P.J.; Wright, R.C.T.; Guymer, D.; Harrison, E.; Brockhurst, M.A. Extremely fast amelioration of plasmid fitness costs by multiple functionally diverse pathways. *Microbiology* **2020**, *166*, 56–62. [CrossRef]
55. Sørensen, M.E.S.; Wood, A.J.; Cameron, D.D.; Brockhurst, M.A. Rapid compensatory evolution can rescue low fitness symbioses following partner switching. *Curr. Biol.* **2021**, *31*, 3721–3728.e4. [CrossRef]
56. Brockhurst, M.A.; Harrison, E. Ecological and evolutionary solutions to the plasmid paradox. *Trends Microbiol.* **2022**, *30*, 534–543. [CrossRef] [PubMed]
57. Trindade, S.; Sousa, A.; Xavier, K.B.; Dionisio, F.; Ferreira, M.G.; Gordo, I. Positive Epistasis Drives the Acquisition of Multi-drug Resistance. *PLoS Genet.* **2009**, *5*, e1000578. [CrossRef] [PubMed]
58. Silva, R.F.; Mendonça, S.C.M.; Carvalho, L.M.; Reis, A.M.; Gordo, I.; Trindade, S.; Dionisio, F. Pervasive Sign Epistasis between Conjugative Plasmids and Drug-Resistance Chromosomal Mutations. *PLoS Genet.* **2011**, *7*, e1002181. [CrossRef] [PubMed]
59. Millan, A.S.; Heilbron, K.; MacLean, R.C. Positive epistasis between co-infecting plasmids promotes plasmid survival in bacterial populations. *ISME J.* **2014**, *8*, 601–612. [CrossRef] [PubMed]
60. Gama, J.A.; Zilhão, R.; Dionisio, F. Co-resident plasmids travel together. *Plasmid* **2017**, *93*, 24–29. [CrossRef] [PubMed]
61. Gama, J.A.; Zilhão, R.; Dionisio, F. Multiple plasmid interference—Pledging allegiance to my enemy's enemy. *Plasmid* **2017**, *93*, 17–23. [CrossRef]
62. Gama, J.A.; Zilhão, R.; Dionisio, F. Conjugation efficiency depends on intra and intercellular interactions between distinct plasmids: Plasmids promote the immigration of other plasmids but repress co-colonizing plasmids. *Plasmid* **2017**, *93*, 6–16. [CrossRef] [PubMed]

63. Gama, J.A.; Fredheim, E.G.A.; Cléon, F.; Reis, A.M.; Zilhão, R.; Dionisio, F. Dominance between Plasmids Determines the Extent of Biofilm Formation. *Front. Microbiol.* **2020**, *11*, 2070. [CrossRef]
64. Gama, J.A.; Zilhão, R.; Dionisio, F. Plasmid Interactions Can Improve Plasmid Persistence in Bacterial Populations. *Front. Microbiol.* **2020**, *11*, 2033. [CrossRef]
65. Zwanzig, M.; Harrison, E.; Brockhurst, M.A.; Hall, J.P.J.; Berendonk, T.U.; Berger, U. Mobile Compensatory Mutations Promote Plasmid Survival. *mSystems* **2019**, *4*, e00186-18. [CrossRef]
66. Valle, A.A.-D.; León-Sampedro, R.; Rodríguez-Beltrán, J.; DelaFuente, J.; Hernández-García, M.; Ruiz-Garbajosa, P.; Cantón, R.; Peña-Miller, R.; Millán, A.S. Variability of plasmid fitness effects contributes to plasmid persistence in bacterial communities. *Nat. Commun.* **2021**, *12*, 2653. [CrossRef] [PubMed]
67. Dionisio, F.; Nogueira, T.; Carvalho, L.M.; Mendes-Soares, H.; Mendonça, S.C.; Domingues, I.; Moreira, B.; Reis, A.M. What Maintains Plasmids among Bacteria. In *Horizontal Gene Transfer in Microorganisms*; Caister Academic Press: Norwich, UK, 2012; pp. 131–154.
68. Domingues, C.P.F.; Rebelo, J.S.; Monteiro, F.; Nogueira, T.; Dionisio, F. Harmful behaviour through plasmid transfer: A successful evolutionary strategy of bacteria harbouring conjugative plasmids. *Philos. Trans. R. Soc. B Biol. Sci.* **2022**, *377*, 20200473. [CrossRef] [PubMed]
69. Ghigo, J.-M. Natural conjugative plasmids induce bacterial biofilm development. *Nature* **2001**, *412*, 442–445. [CrossRef] [PubMed]
70. Reisner, A.; Höller, B.M.; Molin, S.; Zechner, E.L. Synergistic Effects in Mixed *Escherichia coli* Biofilms: Conjugative Plasmid Transfer Drives Biofilm Expansion. *J. Bacteriol.* **2006**, *188*, 3582–3588. [CrossRef]
71. Davies, J.; Davies, D. Origins and Evolution of Antibiotic Resistance. *Microbiol. Mol. Biol. Rev.* **2010**, *74*, 417–433. [CrossRef]
72. Escudeiro, P.; Pothier, J.; Dionisio, F.; Nogueira, T. Antibiotic Resistance Gene Diversity and Virulence Gene Diversity Are Correlated in Human Gut and Environmental Microbiomes. *mSphere* **2019**, *4*, e00135-19. [CrossRef]
73. Beceiro, A.; Tomás, M.; Bou, G. Antimicrobial Resistance and Virulence: A Successful or Deleterious Association in the Bacterial World? *Clin. Microbiol. Rev.* **2013**, *26*, 185–230. [CrossRef]
74. Deng, Y.; Xu, L.; Liu, S.; Wang, Q.; Guo, Z.; Chen, C.; Feng, J. What drives changes in the virulence and antibiotic resistance of *Vibrio harveyi* in the South China Sea? *J. Fish Dis.* **2020**, *43*, 853–862. [CrossRef]
75. Pan, Y.; Zeng, J.; Li, L.; Yang, J.; Tang, Z.; Xiong, W.; Li, Y.; Chen, S.; Zeng, Z. Coexistence of Antibiotic Resistance Genes and Virulence Factors Deciphered by Large-Scale Complete Genome Analysis. *mSystems* **2020**, *5*, e00821-19. [CrossRef]
76. Cantón, R. Antibiotic resistance genes from the environment: A perspective through newly identified antibiotic resistance mechanisms in the clinical setting. *Clin. Microbiol. Infect.* **2009**, *15*, 20–25. [CrossRef]
77. Martinez, J.L. The role of natural environments in the evolution of resistance traits in pathogenic bacteria. *Proc. R. Soc. B Biol. Sci.* **2009**, *276*, 2521–2530. [CrossRef] [PubMed]
78. Allen, H.K.; Donato, J.; Wang, H.H.; Cloud-Hansen, K.A.; Davies, J.; Handelsman, J. Call of the wild: Antibiotic resistance genes in natural environments. *Nat. Rev. Microbiol.* **2010**, *8*, 251–259. [CrossRef] [PubMed]
79. Castanon, J.I.R. History of the Use of Antibiotic as Growth Promoters in European Poultry Feeds. *Poult. Sci.* **2007**, *86*, 2466–2471. [CrossRef]
80. Darmancier, H.; Domingues, C.P.F.; Rebelo, J.S.; Amaro, A.; Dionísio, F.; Pothier, J.; Serra, O.; Nogueira, T. Are Virulence and Antibiotic Resistance Genes Linked? A Comprehensive Analysis of Bacterial Chromosomes and Plasmids. *Antibiotics* **2022**, *11*, 706. [CrossRef] [PubMed]
81. Cho, I.; Blaser, M.J. The human microbiome: At the interface of health and disease. *Nat. Rev. Genet.* **2012**, *13*, 260–270. [CrossRef]
82. Domingues, C.P.F.; Rebelo, J.S.; Pothier, J.; Monteiro, F.; Nogueira, T.; Dionisio, F. The Perfect Condition for the Rising of Superbugs: Person-to-Person Contact and Antibiotic Use Are the Key Factors Responsible for the Positive Correlation between Antibiotic Resistance Gene Diversity and Virulence Gene Diversity in Human Metagenomes. *Antibiotics* **2021**, *10*, 605. [CrossRef] [PubMed]
83. Valentino, V.; Sequino, G.; Cobo-Díaz, J.F.; Álvarez-Ordóñez, A.; De Filippis, F.; Ercolini, D. Evidence of virulence and antibiotic resistance genes from the microbiome mapping in minimally processed vegetables producing facilities. *Food Res. Int.* **2022**, *162*, 112202. [CrossRef] [PubMed]
84. Carr, W.; Kurbatova, E.; Starks, A.; Goswami, N.; Allen, L.; Winston, C. Interim Guidance: 4-Month Rifapentine-Moxifloxacin Regimen for the Treatment of Drug-Susceptible Pulmonary Tuberculosis—United States. *MMWR. Morb. Mortal. Wkly. Rep.* **2022**, *71*, 285–289. [CrossRef]
85. Chambers, H.F.; DeLeo, F.R. Waves of resistance: Staphylococcus aureus in the antibiotic era. *Nat. Rev. Microbiol.* **2009**, *7*, 629–641. [CrossRef]
86. Smith, H.W.; Halls, S. Observations on infective drug resistance in Britain. *Br. Med. J.* **1966**, *1*, 266–269. [CrossRef]

Disclaimer/Publisher's Note: The statements, opinions and data contained in all publications are solely those of the individual author(s) and contributor(s) and not of MDPI and/or the editor(s). MDPI and/or the editor(s) disclaim responsibility for any injury to people or property resulting from any ideas, methods, instructions or products referred to in the content.

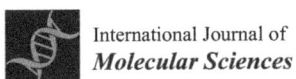

Review

The Connection between Gut and Lung Microbiota, Mast Cells, Platelets and SARS-CoV-2 in the Elderly Patient

Giovanna Traina

Department of Pharmaceutical Sciences, University of Perugia, Via Romana, 06126 Perugia, Italy; giovanna.traina@unipg.it

Abstract: The human coronavirus SARS-CoV-2 or COVID-19 that emerged in late 2019 causes a respiratory tract infection and has currently resulted in more than 627 million confirmed cases and over 6.58 million deaths worldwide up to October 2022. The highest death rate caused by COVID-19 is in older people, especially those with comorbidities. This evidence presents a challenge for biomedical research on aging and also identifies some key players in inflammation, including mast cells and platelets, which could represent important markers and, at the same time, unconventional therapeutic targets. Studies have shown a decrease in the diversity of gut microbiota composition in the elderly, particularly a reduced abundance of butyrate-producing species, and COVID-19 patients manifest faecal microbiome alterations, with an increase in opportunistic pathogens and a depletion of commensal beneficial microorganisms. The main purpose of this narrative review is to highlight how an altered condition of the gut microbiota, especially in the elderly, could be an important factor and have a strong impact in the lung homeostasis and COVID-19 phenomenon, jointly to the activation of mast cells and platelets, and also affect the outcomes of the pathology. Therefore, a targeted and careful control of the intestinal microbiota could represent a complementary intervention to be implemented for the management and the challenge against COVID-19.

Keywords: SARS-CoV-2; inflammation; intestinal microbiota; immune protection; mast cells; platelets; aging

1. Introduction

The human coronavirus SARS-CoV-2 or COVID-19 that emerged in late 2019 causes a respiratory tract infection of the COVID-19 disease and, according to the official website of the Ministry of Health, which reports World Health Organization data, has currently resulted in more than 627 million confirmed cases and over 6.58 million deaths worldwide up to October 2022.

The characteristic symptoms presented by patients affected by SARS-CoV-2 led to the belief that it was a pneumonia with an interstitial component, very often bilateral, associated with respiratory symptoms which in the early phase are generally limited, but which can subsequently lead to progressive clinical instability with respiratory failure. The phenomenon of the so-called "silent hypoxemia", characterized by low blood oxygenation values in the absence of subjective feeling of dyspnea, is characteristic of this phase of the disease. This scenario, in a number of people, can evolve towards a worsening clinical picture dominated by a cytokine storm, the excessive immune response from the uncontrolled release of a series of interleukins, chemokines, interferons, and tumour necrosis factors and the consequent hyperinflammatory state, which determines local and systemic consequences. Such a response represents a negative prognostic factor producing, at the pulmonary level, pictures of arterial and venous thrombi of small vessels and evolution towards severe and sometimes permanent pulmonary lesions (pulmonary fibrosis) [1]. In particular, vascular permeability is increased, resulting in a large amount of fluid and blood cells entering the alveoli, causing dyspnoea and even respiratory failure, desquamation

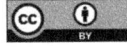

of alveolar cells and hyaline membrane formation. A mass of fluid similar to mucus accumulates in the lungs, and this accumulation is caused by an excessive immune response due to signalling molecules, in particular interleukin-(IL)-6, IL-8, and tumour necrosis factor (TNFα) [1–4]. Cytokine overproduction and cytokine storm induce clinically relevant extrapulmonary effects on various key organs such as heart, kidney, liver and intestine and dysbiosis [3]. The final stages of this very severe clinical picture can lead to multi-organ failure, with cardiovascular, gastrointestinal, haematological, respiratory, neurological and renal complications [5].

1.1. SARS-CoV-2: An Overview

Coronaviruses (CoVs) belong to the coronaviridae family, which comprises a group of positive-enveloped single-stranded RNA viruses. These viruses have the largest genome among RNA viruses, and morphologically they appear as surrounded by a corona under the electron microscope [6].

Like other coronaviruses, SARS-CoV-2 has four structural proteins, known as: protein S (ear or spinule), E (envelope), M (membrane) and N (nucleocapsid); the N protein contains the RNA genome while the S, E and M proteins together create the viral capsid. Specifically, there are three protein components of the viral envelope. The most important of these is the S-glycoprotein (Spike), a very large transmembrane protein that mediates attachment to the receptor and the fusion of the cell membrane of the host cell with that of the virus. M-glycoprotein is the most abundant constituent of CoVs and shapes the virion envelope. Protein E is a small polypeptide, and due to its small size and limited amount, E was detected much later than other structural proteins [6].

1.2. Imbalance of Renin Angiotensin System

The renin angiotensin system (RAS) is a well-known physiological system responsible for controlling cardiovascular dynamics through the modulation of blood pressure. In particular, angiotensinogen is converted into angiotensin I by renin, produced in the kidneys. Angiotensin I is transformed into angiotensin II by an extracellular angiotensin converting enzyme (ACE). Angiotensin II binds to the G protein-coupled receptor (GPCR), angiotensin II type 1 receptor (AT1R) in order to initiate its physiological functions. In general, the activation of AT1R by angiotensin II causes several physiologically important events including vasoconstriction, inflammation, thrombosis and production of reactive oxygen species (ROS). Angiotensin II is further degraded into angiotensin 1–7 by the action of the ACE2 enzyme. Angiotensin 1–7 binds to another GPCR and induces physiological events essentially opposite to those induced by AT1R activation, which include vasodilation, anti-inflammatory, antifibrosis, antithrombosis and ROS neutralization. ACE2 plays a key role as a negative regulator in the overall RAS pathway, exerting protective functions in various RAS-based models of pathogenesis. ACE2 also limits the expression by macrophages of several proinflammatory cytokines.

In the pulmonary phase of COVID-19, SARS-CoV-2 enters the type 2 pneumocyte by inducing the internalization of ACE2 and resulting in down-regulation and deficiency of ACE2. SARS-CoV-2-induced ACE2 deficiency reduces the conversion of angiotensin II to angiotensinogen 1–7 and increases the availability of angiotensin II. Excessive angiotensin II causes AT1R to over-activate, resulting in an imbalance of RAS. However, it should be remembered that SARS-CoV-2 invades host cells via two receptors: ACE2 and through cluster of differentiation 147 (CD147) transmembrane protein mediated endocytosis [7].

Although it has a lower affinity for the COVID-19 virus than ACE2, CD127 specifically accounts for the increase in blood glucose in infected patients, the risk of delayed COVID-19 in women, the increased susceptibility in geriatrics, and the increased susceptibility to T lymphocyte infections [8].

1.3. COVID-19 and Inflammation in the Elderly

Inflammation is a complex and multifactorial phenomenon that involves several trigger mechanisms. An inflammatory state underlies a wide variety of diseases, pain, stress, and depression, and an exacerbated inflammatory response may drive the deleterious consequences of the infection [9,10].

Since pre-existing chronic inflammatory conditions such as hypertension, diabetes, obesity, cardiovascular disease, as well as autoimmune diseases also activate the RAS pathway, COVID-19 patients show a significant association between ACE2 deficiency and the clinical severity of these comorbidities. In addition, a decrease in ACE2 expression with age has clinical implications for the poor prognosis of elderly COVID-19 patients. Since the ACE2 gene is located on the X chromosome, the high male mortality rate in COVID-19 patients has been hypothesized to be related to the lower levels of ACE2 gene expression in male patients, so much so that the restoration of SARS-CoV-2-induced RAS imbalance has been suggested as an ideal clinical approach to slow the early progression of COVID-19 pathogenesis [11]. In addition, IL-6, which is one of the cytokines most expressed in the COVID-19 patient, is a multi-effective cytokine with both anti-inflammatory and pro-inflammatory roles. Elevated IL-6 level in COVID-19 patients is a predictor of higher mortality rates [10]. Moreover, IL-6 has been reported to facilitate CD147 expression [12].

In general, proinflammatory cytokines increase the expression of cell adhesion molecules on the surface of neutrophils and endothelial cells. This promotes intercellular interactions. Furthermore, the increased permeability of the pulmonary endothelium and the reduction in barrier protection attracts more neutrophils to the site of infection through endothelial penetration. Such dysregulation of the inflammatory immune response prevents the activation of the adaptive immune response [13,14].

In this perspective, it is very important to characterize the host–pathogen relationship, including immunoprotection correlates, such as COVID-19 virus-specific antibodies that limit disease and correlates of immune dysregulation, such as overproduction of cytokines that can promote disease.

It is known that a patient in old age suffers stressogenic conditions, both those linked to the action of the virus and those attributable to the awareness of the pathology, as well as the physiological conditions linked to the elderly state. Due to an age-altered immune system but also from rather frequent nutritional deficiencies, elderly people are particularly exposed to the risk of infection [15]. In addition, studies reported that visceral fat increases with age, and visceral fat inflammation increases the risk of COVID-19- related complications [16,17].

The semeiology of infections is sometimes atypical in the elderly and the signs and symptoms appear more discreetly than in young adults, leading to diagnostic and therapeutic delay that further aggravates the prognosis of infectious diseases in elderly patients.

Innate immunity serves at the first line of antiviral defence and the largest number of immune cells reside in the intestinal system. However, impaired immune responses in the elderly are responsible for many diseases, as well as increased susceptibility to infections. The response to COVID-19 includes various innate and adaptive traits, such as changes in the composition of dendritic cells and B cells and deeply altered T cell phenotypes that could impair immunoprotective T cells immunity [18]. Recent studies have highlighted the role of adaptive immunity like T cells and B cells in COVID-19. Laing et al. [18] showed reduced T cell immunity in COVID-19 patients. It has been suggested that immunological interventions targeting early predictive inflammatory markers would be more beneficial than those that block the late cytokine-related storm and therefore, very importantly, personalized therapeutic intervention would be required for each patient. Yet, an excessive quantity of neutrophils is associated with the course and severity of COVID-19 [19,20].

Recognition of pathogen-associated molecular patterns (PAMPs) by host pattern recognition receptors (PRRs) is the first step in activating the innate immune system against viral infection. These receptors include, among others, nucleotide-binding oligomerization domain-like receptors (NODs), and toll-like receptors (TLRs). This virus-derived PAMP recognition by innate immune receptors activates a series of signalling cascades that ultimately lead to the activation of transcription factors such as nuclear factor-kappa B (NF-kB) and interferon regulatory factors.

COVID-19 patients show general lymphopenia, which is a significant reduction in the overall number of circulating lymphocytes in the blood [21]. In contrast, the monocyte-macrophage system is significantly upregulated by SARS-CoV-2 infection. In general, monocytes are innate immune cells that participate in inflammatory responses, phagocytosis, antigen presentation, and a variety of other immune processes. Circulating monocytes pour into peripheral tissues to differentiate into macrophages or dendritic cells during inflammation. Thus, the upregulation of monocytes by SARS-CoV-2 infection may contribute to the improvement of proinflammatory processes. Neutrophils are also recruited to the site of infection through the circulation and permeabilization of the endothelial membranes adjacent to the site of infection [1–3]. However, due to lymphopenia, COVID-19 patients are more vulnerable to microbial infection. It has been speculated that the inability to eradicate SARS-CoV-2 infection due to its innate immune response antagonism hyper-inflates the innate immune system. This causes an excessive release of inflammatory cytokines to compensate for the depletion of the immune system due to SARS-CoV-2-induced lymphopenia. Finally, the overproduction of cytokines increases the membrane permeability of the capillary walls around the infected alveoli, causing pulmonary oedema, dyspnoea and hypoxemia. The introduction of plasma fluid into the alveoli as well as the loss of elasticity due to the reduced production of surfactant cause complications.

Importantly, SARS-CoV-2 primarily enters through the respiratory tract to infect humans, but it can also enter through the gastrointestinal tract [22].

2. Intestinal Microbiota and Systemic Protection

In this context, the involvement of the gut microbiota could play an important role in the COVID-19 phenomenon perhaps not yet sufficiently considered. From a clinical point of view, the elderly patient presents a dysregulation of microbial homeostasis and neurodegeneration that can lead to a condition of greater fragility. This condition manifests itself as a reduced functional reserve, reduced resistance to stress, increased susceptibility to disease, mood, and increased risk of adverse health outcomes [23]. The gut could serve as a reservoir for acute respiratory syndrome COVID-19. Evidence reported that the intestinal microbiota is really altered in SARS-CoV-2 infection [24,25]. In addition, Zuo et al. found that the loss of beneficial species in SARS-CoV-2 persists for a long time in most patients suggesting that exposure to SARS-CoV-2 infection and/or hospitalization may be associated with lasting damage to the intestinal microbiota [25]. In particular, a condition of dysbiosis, perturbations in the structural and, therefore, functional dynamics of the intestinal microbiota, could have a crucial role in COVID-19 disease. Physiologically, the microbiota protects the intestine from colonization of exogenous pathogens and potentially dangerous autochthonous microorganisms. Man has evolved side by side with microbes. The mammalian intestine is colonized by trillions of microorganisms, and most of these are bacteria that evolved together with the host in a symbiotic relationship, ensuring the state of immunosurveillance of the organism. It is well-known that the microbiota can modulate the innate and the adaptive immune system [26–28].

Aging implies an imbalanced immunological response to microbial infection associated with elevated levels of several cytokines, including IL-1, IL-6 and TNFα [29,30]. In addition, changes in the expression of PRRs, activation of such receptors by endogenous ligands associated with cellular damage, and unusual downstream signalling events of PRRs activation have evolved to induce a chronic cytokine secretion [31].

The conditions of the intestinal microbiota and pulmonary changes are closely related to immune responses [32]. Interestingly, SARS-CoV-2 leverages the ACE2 receptor to access the host, and this receptor is expressed in both the respiratory and gut tracts [33]. ACE2 is involved in controlling intestinal inflammation. The direct colonization of intestinal

ACE2 receptors through ingestion of the virus is potentially responsible for a range of gastrointestinal tract symptoms associated with COVID-19 [34,35]. Chronic obstructive pulmonary disease is often concomitant with chronic diseases of the gastrointestinal tract. Yet, there is a higher risk of allergic diseases of the airways and use of antibiotics and alteration in the composition of the gut microbiota [36]. Finally, a crosstalk pattern between Bacillus and Lactobacillus in the gut has recently been reported, revealing the extremely complicated interactions of multiple bacterial species in the gut microbiota [37].

The central role of the intestinal microbiota in the development of mucosal immunity is not surprising, as multiple interactions with the external environment take place in the gut and the intestinal epithelial barrier must tolerate the intestinal microbiota which constitutes the majority of the antigens presented to the resident immune cells [38]. Despite this condition, there is no strong activation of a local or systematic immune response. This condition occurs because tolerance is induced due to intestinal epithelial cells (ICE) which are in close contact with the intestinal microbiota and are constantly exposed to a large number of antigens [32,38]. In order to minimize the toxic potential of these antigens, ICEs adopt a number of strategies, such as reducing their TLRs, and modifying the antigenic fractions of the microbiota, to make them less immunogenic. The important role of the gut microbiota in the development of the systemic immune system has been assessed by studies conducted in the model of germ-free mice, i.e., without microbiota, born and kept in sterile conditions. These mice have various immune disorders, abnormal numbers of different types of immune cells, altered cytokines, as well as deficits in the local and systemic lymphoid structure [39].

The gut microbiota is a physical barrier to incoming pathogens through competitive exclusion, i.e., resistance to colonization, via mechanisms such as the occupation of attachment sites, the consumption of nutrients and the production of antimicrobial substances [40]. The interactions between antimicrobial peptides and microbiota are bidirectional. Gut bacteria secrete and consume a wide variety of neuromodulators and neurotransmitters, including serotonin, dopamine, gamma-aminobutyric acid, epinephrine and noradrenaline [41]. In this context, blood levels of serotonin, a metabolite of tryptophan independent of the kynurenine pathway, are lower in patients with severe COVID-19 than in healthy controls, suggesting that during SARS-CoV2 infection tryptophan is facilitated to take the kynurenine route [42].

A plethora of microbiota-derived compounds are produced as intermediates or final products of microbial metabolism and can influence biological functions both in the peripheral and the central nervous system (CNS) through nerve activation, cytokine production, neurotransmitters, and via systemic circulation [41,43]. The metabolites produced by the intestine not only modulate gastrointestinal immunity, but also affect distant organs, such as lung and brain.

A relevant response of the host's immune system following microbial colonization of the gut is the production of immunoglobulin (Ig)A by gut-associated lymphoid tissues. IgA plays a vital role in mucosal homeostasis in the intestine and functions as the dominant antibody [43,44].

2.1. Inflammation and Dysbiosis of the Elderly Patient

The gut microbiota shows a great inter-individual variation and the human intestinal microbiome, i.e., the community that includes the genetic heritage and environmental interactions of all microorganisms, is very diverse and complex and continues to fluctuate during the various stages of life [43]. Furthermore, the intestinal microbiome is closely associated with various characteristics of integrity of the intestinal barrier, anti-inflammatory balance, immune and cardio-metabolic health, as well as the intestine–brain axis [41,44]. A loss of microbiota stability has been frequently observed in the elderly. The disruption of the intestinal barrier integrity as well as a condition of intestinal dysbiosis can further complicate the state of severity in SARS-CoV-2 [45,46]. In severe cases of SARS-CoV-2, elevated zonulin levels are a marker related to increased mortality. Measurement of LPS binding protein, a marker of inflammation, revealed a significant increase in more severe cases, supporting the association between severe COVID-19 and loss of intestinal barrier integrity and microbial translocation [47].

The excessive accumulation of senescent cells present in aging and age-related diseases can contribute to chronic silent inflammation and tissue and organic dysfunction. Furthermore, old-age problems could contribute to a greater predisposition to various infectious and associated diseases of the intestine causing alterations in the microbiota of the elderly [30,48,49].

Studies have shown a decrease in the diversity of gut microbiota composition in the elderly, and COVID-19 patients manifest faecal microbiome alterations, with an increase in opportunistic pathogens and a depletion of commensal beneficial microorganisms [14,15]. Older people are known to have a less diverse gut microbiota and a noticeable decrease in beneficial microorganisms such as *Bifidobacterium*. Since diet, drug intake and the composition of the gut microbiome undergo substantial changes during aging, the intestinal metabolic environment, and therefore the levels of microbial metabolites, are influenced by age. Gut microbial-derived metabolites play a key role in inflammatory signalling by interacting with host immune cells. Some bacterial species, such as *Faecalibacterium prausnitzii*, *Roseburia intestinalis*, and *Anaerostipes butyraticus* are able to digest complex carbohydrates by fermentation, generating short-chain fatty acids (SCFA), fatty acids with fewer than six carbon atoms, consisting mainly of acetate, propionate and butyrate [32,50,51]. The elderly has lower SCFA levels than young subjects. A decrease in SCFA production in the colon has been linked to lower fibre intake and antibiotic treatments in the elderly by regulating expression of pro-inflammatory cytokines including IL-6, IL-12 and TNF-α [52]. SCFAs are important for their ability to reduce intestinal inflammation, protect against pathogenic invasion and maintain barrier integrity primarily by activating G-protein-coupled receptors (GPCRs) or inducing their suppressive effects on histone deacetylase (HDAC), and by affecting gene expression. The genesis of the cytokine storm could take place in the gastrointestinal tract [41]. SCFAs maintain the physiology of the intestinal epithelium by regulating cell turnover and barrier functions. SCFAs constitute a key regulatory system for the activation, recruitment and differentiation of immune cells, including neutrophils, macrophages, dendritic cells (DCs) and T lymphocytes [41,50]. A reduced abundance of butyrate-producing species is found in COVID-19 patients [51] and it has been suggested that the use of butyrate-producing species in COVID-19 patients in order to maintain the integrity of epithelium at the level of tight junctions could likely help reduce invasion of SARS-CoV-2 [52].

The intestinal microbiota plays a crucial role in gastrointestinal physiology by providing, among other activities, the synthesis of endogenous vitamins, such as vitamin K and most of the components of the vitamin B complex [41]. In particular, vitamin B constitutes an important support for the correct activation of the immune response, and interestingly, it improves respiratory function, maintains the integrity of the endothelium and prevents hypercoagulability. A dysbiotic condition could lead to a vitamin B deficiency and could significantly impair immune function. Therefore, B vitamins could be a crucial aid in the treatment of SARS-CoV-2 [52].

Another interesting aspect of diet in the elderly is the consumption of proteins, and in particular a diet that includes an excessive amount of proteins can be responsible for an increase in the intestinal production of potentially deleterious bacterial metabolites. The requirement for a higher dose of protein in elderly subjects is suggested in order to compensate for the lower sensitivity to anabolic stimulus. However, the very amount of protein in the diet and additional amino acids can influence the onset and progression of inflammation [53–55]. This condition could also, in turn, affect epithelial repair since some bacterial metabolites inhibit respiration of colon epithelial cells, cell proliferation and/or the influence of barrier function.

Another element that characterizes the elderly subject is greater constipation leading to the use of laxatives, whose prolonged consumption has harmful effects on the entire intestinal ecosystem, loss of colon tone and a dangerous condition of habit [56,57]. There can be multiple causes of constipation, including eating disorders and dehydration, as well as pathological conditions, gastrointestinal pathologies, neurological or psychological causes [58].

Evidence suggests that age-related intestinal dysbiosis may contribute to unhealthy aging [59–63]. Since the gut microbiota communicates with the host through various biomolecules, pathways independent of the signalling of nutrients and epigenetic mechanisms, an alteration of these communication pathways related to age-related intestinal dysbiosis can heavily influence the health and life span of the host and trigger an innate immune response [45]. The circulation of bacterial compounds in the host is probably due to the breakdown of the intestinal epithelial barrier caused by the silent chronic inflammation state, and greater intestinal permeability has been suggested as a potential source of age-related inflammation [64–66].

The link between intestinal dysbiosis, chronic inflammation and fragility has been highlighted with intestinal permeability biomarkers [65]. These factors can lead to greater adherence and loss of various microbes and microbial derivatives and increase the host's susceptibility to various local but also systemic disorders through the gut-brain axis, the gut- liver axis, the gut-lung axis [67]. Therefore, in this context, microbial metabolites play an important role in human longevity. However, it is not clear whether the condition of intestinal dysbiosis is a cause or rather a consequence of aging and associated inflammatory disorders. The composition of the gut microbiota is related to circulating cytokine levels and health indicators in the elderly [12]. If the gut microbiota is an age-associated inflammation factor, this would mean that age-related changes in the gut microbiota represent a form of microbial dysbiosis.

A physiological translocation of microbial products is present throughout life; however, with aging, this microbial translocation increases and favours dysbiosis conditions. This feed-forward process increases over the years. In conditions of alteration of the epithelial barrier, the COVID-19 virus finds a fertile ground. Age-associated inflammation is a strong risk factor for mortality in the elderly. Patients with higher levels of inflammatory markers are more likely to be hospitalized, and have higher mortality rates, are fragile, are less independent and are more likely to experience late disease [64,67]. Finally, inflammation in the elderly increases the susceptibility to pneumococcal infection, and is associated with a rise in disease severity and reduced survival [68].

Current research confirms that the intestinal microbiota is significantly altered in SARS-CoV-2 infection, highlighting the crucial role of microbiota in modulating the human response to SARS-CoV-2 infection [25,28]. Interestingly, the alterations are characterized by an opportunistic growth of pathogens while, at the same time, there is a dramatic decrease in beneficial commensal microorganisms [25].

Studies have reported the intimate relationship between infection and gut microbiota dysbiosis and have shown that infection is associated not only with gut bacteria but also with resident viruses. A study reported that treatment with *Lactobacillus brevis* OW38 to aged mice reduced the lipopolysaccharide (LPS) level in colon fluid and blood. Administration of *Lactobacillus brevis* OW38 reduced the ratio of Firmicutes or Proteobacteria to Bacteroidetes. In addition, this lactic acid bacterium was able to inhibit the expression of inflammatory markers, such as myeloperoxidase, TNF, and IL-1β, and inhibited NF-κB activation [69].

2.2. Microbiota and Lung

The lung microbiota is less relevant in quantity than the gastrointestinal microbiota; however, it is originally colonized by the oropharynx and by microaspirations of the gastrointestinal tract. The predominant bacterial phyla both in the lungs and gut are the same, Firmicutes and Bacteroidetes [70]. The fungal component is also prominent, which is known to communicate with bacteria. The gut and lung microbiota are in parallel throughout life, although dietary changes affect not only the gut microbiota but also the lung microbiome [71,72]. Bidirectional crosstalk has been demonstrated in animal experiments [73]. Members of the gut microbiome induce immune tolerance and block the colonization of pathogens through the activation of the immune system and the direct and indirect actions of the microbiota. When the immune system "learns" to recognize the enemy from the microbiome, the effect can also occur in a distant organ [74]. Various studies have shown that lung infections are associated and mutually influenced with a change in the gut microbiota [75] (Figure 1).

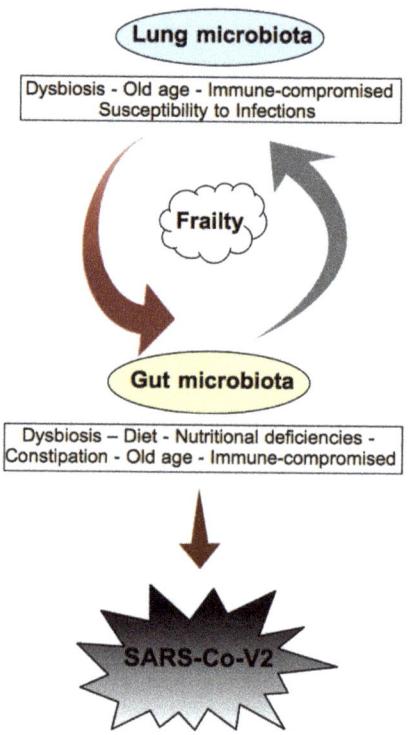

Figure 1. Schematic representation of the bidirectional link between lung and gut. The gut microbiota influences lung health through a cross dialogue between the gut microbiota and the lungs, the "gut–lung axis". The functional state of the elderly, dysbiotic condition, immune compromise, nutritional deficiencies constitute as a whole, a condition of extreme vulnerability.

COVID-19 represents a further aggravation of the inflammatory problem as age-associated inflammation causes macrophage dysfunction and tissue damage. An increase in circulating bacterial toxins implies a reduction in the gene expression of tight junctions and lethal lung damage [71]. Aging is characterized by a particular condition, the so-called "chronic age-related inflammation". This condition is genetically preordained and is a chronic inflammatory process with a shift in the profile of proinflammatory cytokines at the level of the various districts with the presence of greater amounts of histamine, IL-1 and TNF cytokines and chemotactic factors. In the elderly, it is a consequence of the long-term antigenic load with a continuous involvement of the immune system. The functional degradation of the immune system that occurs with aging is linked to changes in immune-competitive cells and other cells. The changes affect the size of cells, but also their functions and population size. In the elderly, chemotaxis, phagocytosis and antigen presentation worsen in a context of high level of proinflammatory cytokines. Excessive cytokine production leads to chronic overstimulation of the immune system [72].

Like the gastrointestinal tract, lungs are at the forefront of immunity as they are constantly attacked by a wide variety of external environmental stimuli. The microbiome of the lungs plays a crucial role in shaping and harmonizing lung immunity. As in the intestine, the lung microbiota has the task of strengthening innate and adaptive immunity, releasing factors that support respiratory functions and defend the lungs from pathogens [75]. Intestinal dysbiosis has been implicated in various lung diseases, such as asthma and cystic fibrosis. Diet alters the microbiome. So, an altered lung microbiome predicts disease progression in interstitial lung disease [76,77].

Studies have reported the role of fibre-rich diets in modulating innate immunity, supported by a reduction in inflammatory marker levels [77]. A diet rich in fibre influences and modifies not only the intestinal microbiota, but also the lung microbiota, supporting the role of nutrition on lung immunity [77–79].

The depletion of some species of the intestinal microbiota due to the intake of antibiotics influences lung diseases and allergic inflammation [80,81]. In mice it has been observed that influenza virus infection in the respiratory tract increases Enterobacteriaceae and reduces Lactobacilli and Lactococci in the gut microbiota [82]. Dysbiosis in the lung microbiota after LPS administration is accompanied by disorders of the intestinal microbiota due to the movement of bacteria from their lung into the bloodstream [83].

Lactobacilli and Bifidobacteria are beneficial probiotics that exert a trophic effect on the intestinal mucosa. They can promote host defence against infections and reduce hypersensitivity reactions to commensal bacteria and antigens. Specific selected probiotic strains are capable of modulating the expression of proinflammatory molecules and anti-inflammatory properties. The anti-inflammatory and preventive abilities of specific probiotic mixtures have been described [84–86]. Interestingly, M1 macrophages, which produce proinflammatory cytokines, such as IL-6, and M2 macrophages which produce anti-inflammatory cytokines, such as IL-10, can be modulated by specific probiotic treatments [85]. Finally, already various studies have reported that respiratory viral infections can affect the gut microbiome condition, including pulmonary influenza virus and respiratory syncytial infections [73,87].

3. Focus on Mast Cells, SARS-CoV-2 and Microbiota

In the context of the wide variety of cells involved in SARS-CoV-2, two types of cells that are at the forefront of the pathogenesis are mast cells (MCs) and platelets, and a control over them could represent biomarkers and targets at the same time for an interesting therapeutic strategy.

MCs are innate immunity cells present in mucous membranes and connective tissue, strategically located at the interface with the external environment such as the skin, lungs and intestines, where they act as gatekeepers for attack of pathogens [70,88], and they play, themselves, pathogenic roles in many inflammatory responses. MCs organize the inflammatory response and are crucial early participants in responses to viral infection. Once activated, in a very short time MCs release mediators classified as dependent or independent of degranulation. These molecules contribute to inflammation and changes at the site of infection. Mast cells also can be activated by a variety of both bacterial and viral products, and, consequently, to release a very wide spectrum of proinflammatory and immuno-regulatory molecules. In addition, many studies have analysed the ability of MCs to contract common viruses and release molecules such as histamine and leukotrienes [89,90]. MCs are resistant to productive infection with respiratory syncytial virus but have a protective response that includes the production of cytokines and chemokines that promote the recruitment of antiviral effector cells [89]. MCs can be activated directly by active viral infection or by contact with viral particles. Activation of MCs leads to the production of a variety of mediators, including large amounts of interferons (IFNs) by human virus-infected cells. In addition to initiating an antiviral state in neighbouring cells, a storm of chemokines and cytokines promote the local recruitment of effector cells. IFN also acts in an autocrine manner to further promote the production of MCs. The molecules released by MCs also act by improving lymph nodes hypertrophy. Furthermore, the involvement of local dendritic cells promotes the development of a subsequent acquired immune response [91]. Mast cells can influence T cell proliferation and cytokine production [92]. In addition, MCs produce proteases that are increased in COVID-19 sera and lung districts [93]. Mast cells contain the serine protease ACE2 [94].

MCs play a leading role in many pathophysiological conditions, in which there is a condition of chronic silent inflammation. IL-1β, IL-6 and IL-8 are typical of silent chronic inflammation and MCs are both producers and effectors of these cytokines. Furthermore, MCs are involved in inflammatory responses and psychological stress [70]. MCs are about 2–3% of the immune cellular pool of the lamina propria, and in the muscular and serous layers (3000–25,000 MCs/mm^3) [10]. Variations in the number of MCs are observed in the elderly, as with aging there are changes in connective and mucous tissues as well as other changes closely related to CNS disorders, including depression and anxiety [95]. An increase in the number of MCs during aging has also been observed in human organs and organs of other mammals and vertebrate animals.

MCs play a crucial role in host–microbiota communication, as they can help influence microbiota status and host conditions by modifying their activation [10,96]. MCs can contribute to the maintenance of intestinal homeostasis and their activation is linked to a variety of factors, motor abnormalities and dysfunctions of the intestinal epithelial barrier [10,26]. MCs establish functional signalling pathways with the nervous system and nerves in the gut. Their activation induces sensitization of the nerves, and these, in turn, can condition the release of mediators from MCs. This crosstalk is critical in the generation of symptoms or in the pathogenesis of inflammatory disorders [97,98].

MC responses to virus and other pathogens provide excellent tools for modifying local immune responses and could represent an attractive target for COVID-19 treatment, vaccination, and other immunotherapeutic uses. As is known, MCs can be activated by PAMPS through TLRs. Interestingly, MCs have been shown to express the renin–angiotensin system, the angiotensin 2 converting enzyme ectoprotease required for binding of SARS-CoV-2 and serine proteases [70,99]. This could lead to the secretion of proinflammatory mediators in a targeted and selective manner, without release of histamine or tryptase, as has already been described for the release of IL-6 in response to IL-1β from human MC cultures [70].

MCs could be a potential target to control SARS–CoV-2, for example employing known MC stabilizing agents [96]. Interestingly, some specific probiotic strains are able to stabilize MCs, especially *L. rhamnosus* GG [100]. Oral administration with *L. rhamnosus* JB-1 induces inhibition of peritoneal MC degranulation [101].

Relationships established between gut microbiota composition, cytokine storm, and MC activation in SARS-CoV-2 patients suggest that the gut microbiome is extremely involved in the severity of the pathology. Finally, an intestinal dysbiosis condition could then contribute to the condition of feeding those persistent symptoms that characterize the outcomes of SARS-CoV-2.

4. Focus on Platelets, Microbiota and SARS-CoV-2

Platelets play an important role in a variety of regulatory and degenerative processes [102]. Platelets participate in inflammation by producing a variety of pro-inflammatory molecules [103]. COVID-19 is associated with increased production of large immature platelets, as megakaryocytes respond to increased platelet consumption. Circulating IL-1β, IL-6 and IL-8 are not regulated in chronic systemic and silent inflammation and also have receptors on platelets [103]. Platelet hyperactivation is observed in aging. And it is unclear whether such hyperactivity is the cause or effect of various other vascular disorders in the elderly [104]. Platelets can interact with viruses through a variety of receptors, including TLRs. The role of platelets in haemostasis is well known, and hypercoagulability is an important sign of inflammation. In particular, IL-1β, IL-6 and IL-8 are critically involved in the formation of abnormal clots, erythrocyte pathology and platelet hyperactivation. The most relevant changes were detected when all three cytokines caused platelet hyperactivation and spread with vessel damage and thrombogenic effects [105]. Interestingly, a metabolite of the gut microbiota, called phenylacetylglutamine, was recently identified as being able to enhance platelet activation-related phenotypes, thus favouring platelet hyperactivation. This metabolite could therefore increase the thrombotic capacity and increase the risk of cardiovascular complications [106]. In this context, a targeted control of the microbiota could counter the development of such cardiovascular diseases.

Numerous cases of thrombocytopenia have been detected in patients with COVID-19 and three mechanisms have been hypothesized to explain the phenomenon: (i) the virus can directly infect bone marrow cells and inhibit platelet synthesis. The cytokine storm destroys progenitor cells and leads to reduced platelet production; (ii) the immune system destroys platelets; (iii) platelets aggregate in the lungs, resulting in the consumption of micro-thrombi and platelets [107]. The production of cytokines induced by a dysbiotic microbiota, the activating effect that inflammatory stimuli exert on platelets, MCs and astrocytes, allow the release of further pro-inflammatory molecules, involving an amplification of the harmful effect, micro-thrombi and, considering the location of MCs near the nerves, even possible neurological and brain damage, up to psychopathological conditions, anxiety and depressive syndromes [108]. Finally, it has recently been shown that the lung contributes to platelet biogenesis [109]. Therefore, platelets play a crucial role in the pathogenesis of SARS-CoV-2, as they release various types of molecules through the different stages of the disease. Platelets may have important potential to contribute to the thrombus-inflammation that occurs in SARS-CoV-2, and an inhibition of pathways related to platelet activation could significantly improve outcomes during COVID-19. It has been shown that *L. plantarum*, *L. rhamnosus* and *L. acidophilus* can control any platelet activation [110] (Figure 2).

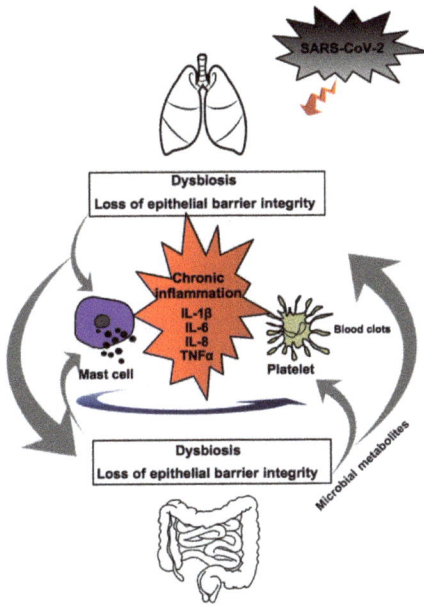

Figure 2. Drawing illustrating the crosstalk between the various players discussed in the paper. In the elderly subject there is a state of fragility of the lung and intestinal microbiota, with loss of the integrity of the epithelial barriers, and chronic silent inflammatory state. Activated mast cells produce a wide variety of cytokines, chemokines and other inflammatory mediators that extensively influence and condition the gut and lung microbiota composition in a vicious cycle; these mediators also affect platelets which, in turn, are affected by microbial metabolites.

5. Interventions with Antiviral Bacteria

Gut microbiota control could have distal protective effects on antiviral responses. There is evidence of the role of inflammasome activation in immune defence against influenza virus infection [111,112].

The commensal respiratory bacteria, *Corynebacterium pseudodiphtheriticum* modulates the TLR3 antiviral response against respiratory syncytial virus, enhancing the production of TNFα, IL-6, IFNγ and IFNβ by increasing the T cell subpopulations that produce these cytokines [113]. The protective role of commensal bacteria, mainly probiotics, is now well established. Specific probiotics such as lactic bacteria, are actually considered friendly bacteria, and secrete antiviral substances during their growth [113,114]. A dialogue is established between the intestinal microbiota and that of the airways through the intestine-lung axis and it could explain how gut bacteria are able to enhance antiviral immunity as gut microbial metabolites could stimulate immune cells that, in turn, could move distally and mediate an antiviral response [112,114].

Lactobacillus paracasei and *L. plantarum* were able to reduce the inflammatory response in the lungs by increasing IL-10, and thus controlling the antiviral response [115,116]. Studies have shown the action of *L. gasseri* in various viral infections, including respiratory infections. Recent reports indicate *L. gasseri* SBT2055 is a promising probiotic useful for the prevention of human respiratory syncytial virus [117]. Finally, other nutritional interventions for coronavirus infection control have also been suggested, such as reducing the consumption of purine food sources [118], as it has been suggested that coronaviruses use purine nucleotides to promote synthesis of RNA [119].

Some possible mechanisms of antiviral activity mediated by bacteria could be the following: (i) bacteria could prevent the adsorption and cellular internalization of the virus by trapping it; (ii) bacteria could establish a link with cells to organize antiviral protection; (iii) microbial metabolites could have a direct antiviral effect.

Interestingly, some probiotic strains show antiviral activity against some coronaviruses [120]. Selective probiotic strains are able to control the levels of type I interferons, increase the number and activity of antigen presenting cells, NK cells, T lymphocytes, specific antibody levels in the lungs [119]. Specific probiotic strains are also capable of modifying the dynamic balance between proinflammatory and immunoregulatory cytokines that allow viral clearance while minimizing lung damage mediated by the immune response. *Bifidobacterium longum* SP 07/3, *L. gasseri* PA 16/8, and *Bifidobacterium bifidum* MF 20/5 contribute to reducing the duration of common cold episodes but also days with fever [121]. This could be especially important in preventing COVID-19 complications. A randomized clinical trial with *L. plantarum* DR7 showed suppression of plasma proinflammatory cytokines, such as IFN-γ, TNF-α in adult patients and potentiation of anti-inflammatory cytokines in young adults, along with a reduction in oxidative stress levels [122].

Strategies could be developed to alter the gut microbiome in order to manage the gastrointestinal effects of the virus in elderly COVID-19 patients and also to control the lung microbiota.

6. Conclusions

Over a century ago, in his book, Metchnikoff [123] suggested that the manipulation of the gut microbiota could prolong life. A dysregulated immune response may cause lung immunopathology. Strategies to combat multifaceted COVID-19 could be to reduce age-associated inflammation, delay the onset of disease inflammation and prolong life. The functional state of the elderly, their dysbiotic condition, immune-compromised with nutritional deficiencies constitutes as a whole, a condition of extreme vulnerability.

Intestinal microbiota dysbiosis is strongly associated with the pathogenesis of several metabolic and inflammatory diseases and the control of the intestinal microbiota could represent a certain challenge to COVID-19, now and even later, in the consequences that SARS-CoV-2 will bring on the general population.

Changes in the microbial population of the elderly and the associated decline in intestinal tissue function can fuel a chronic state of inflammation, resulting in a vicious cycle that further affects host–microbiome interactions and amplifies the frailty of the elderly. On the other hand, chronic immune stimulation as a consequence of silent systemic inflammation and changes in the metabolome and microbial stimuli contribute to immune senescence.

Funding: This research received no external funding.

Institutional Review Board Statement: Not applicable.

Informed Consent Statement: Not applicable.

Conflicts of Interest: The author declares no conflict of interests.

References

1. Zhang, C.; Wu, Z.; Li, J.-W.; Zhao, H.; Wang, G.Q. Cytokine Release Syndrome in Severe COVID-19: Interleukin-6 Receptor Antagonist Tocilizumab may be the Key to Reduce Mortality. *Int. J. Antimicrob. Agents* **2020**, *55*, 105954. [CrossRef] [PubMed]
2. Shi, Y.; Wang, Y.; Shao, C.; Huang, J.; Gan, J.; Huang, X.; Bucci, E.; Piacentini, M.; Ippolito, G.; Melino, G. COVID-19 infection: The perspectives on immune responses. *Cell Death Differ.* **2020**, *27*, 1451–1454. [CrossRef] [PubMed]
3. Xu, Z.; Shi, L.; Wang, Y.; Zhang, J.; Huang, L.; Zhang, C.; Liu, S.; Zhao, P.; Liu, H.; Zhu, L.; et al. Pathological findings of COVID-19 associated with acute respiratory distress syndrome. *Lancet Respir. Med.* **2020**, *8*, 420–422. [CrossRef] [PubMed]
4. Zhang, W.; Zhao, Y.; Zhang, F.; Wang, Q.; Li, T.; Liu, Z.; Wang, J.; Qin, Y.; Zhang, X.; Yan, X.; et al. The use of anti-inflammatory drugs in the treatment of people with severe coronavirus disease 2019 (COVID-19): The Perspectives of clinical immunologists from China. *Clin. Immunol.* **2020**, *214*, 108393. [CrossRef] [PubMed]
5. Conte, C. Possible Link between SARS-CoV-2 Infection and Parkinson's Disease: The Role of Toll-Like Receptor 4. *Int. J. Mol. Sci.* **2021**, *22*, 7135. [CrossRef] [PubMed]
6. Liu, Y.-C.; Kuo, R.-L.; Shih, S.-R. COVID-19: The first documented coronavirus pandemic in history. *Biomed. J.* **2020**, *43*, 328–333. [CrossRef]
7. Fenizia, C.; Galbiati, S.; Vanetti, C.; Vago, R.; Clerici, M.; Tacchetti, C.; Daniele, T. SARS-CoV-2 Entry: At the Crossroads of CD147 and ACE2. *Cells* **2021**, *10*, 1434. [CrossRef]
8. Behl, T.; Kaur, I.; Aleya, L.; Sehgal, A.; Singh, S.; Sharma, N.; Bhatia, S.; Al-Harrasi, A.; Bungau, S. CD147-spike protein interaction in COVID-19: Get the ball rolling with a novel receptor and therapeutic target. *Sci. Total Environ.* **2021**, *808*, 152072. [CrossRef]
9. Channappanavar, R.; Perlman, S. Pathogenic human coronavirus infections: Causes and consequences of cytokine storm and immunopathology. *Semin. Immunopathol.* **2017**, *39*, 529–539. [CrossRef]
10. Traina, G. Mast Cells in Gut and Brain and Their Potential Role as an Emerging Therapeutic Target for Neural Diseases. *Front. Cell. Neurosci.* **2019**, *13*, 345. [CrossRef]
11. Lee, C.; Choi, W.J. Overview of COVID-19 inflammatory pathogenesis from the therapeutic perspective. *Arch. Pharmacal Res.* **2021**, *44*, 99–116. [CrossRef]
12. Hu, J.; Lei, L.; Wang, Y.; Wang, K.; Hu, X.; Wang, A.; Vanderkerken, K. Interleukin-6 drives multiple myeloma progression by up-regulating of CD147/emmprin expression. *Blood* **2016**, *128*, 5632. [CrossRef]
13. Mitroulis, I.; Alexaki, V.I.; Kourtzelis, I.; Ziogas, A.; Hajishengallis, G.; Chavakis, T. Leukocyte integrins: Role in leukocyte recruitment and as therapeutic targets in inflammatory disease. *Pharmacol. Ther.* **2015**, *147*, 123–135. [CrossRef] [PubMed]
14. Tay, M.Z.; Poh, C.M.; Rénia, L.; Macary, P.A.; Ng, L.F.P. The trinity of COVID-19: Immunity, inflammation and intervention. *Nat. Rev. Immunol.* **2020**, *20*, 363–374. [CrossRef] [PubMed]
15. Zhou, F.; Yu, T.; Du, R.; Fan, G.; Liu, Y.; Liu, Z.; Xiang, J.; Wang, Y.; Song, B.; Gu, X.; et al. Clinical course and risk factors for mortality of adult inpatients with COVID-19 in Wuhan, China: A retrospective cohort study. *Lancet* **2020**, *395*, 1054–1062. [CrossRef] [PubMed]
16. Hunter, G.R.; Gower, B.A.; Kane, B.L. Age Related Shift in Visceral Fat. *Int. J. Body Compos. Res.* **2010**, *8*, 103–108.
17. Colleluori, G.; Graciotti, L.; Pesaresi, M.; Di Vincenzo, A.; Perugini, J.; Di Mercurio, E.; Caucci, S.; Bagnarelli, P.; Zingaretti, C.M.; Nisoli, E.; et al. Visceral fat inflammation and fat embolism are associated with lung's lipidic hyaline membranes in subjects with COVID-19. *Int. J. Obes.* **2022**, *46*, 1009–1017. [CrossRef]
18. Laing, A.G.; Lorenc, A.; del Molino del Barrio, I.; Das, A.; Fish, M.; Monin, L.; Muñoz-Ruiz, M.; McKenzie, D.R.; Hayday, T.S.; Francos-Quijorna, I.; et al. A dynamic COVID-19 immune signature includes associations with poor prognosis. *Nat. Med.* **2020**, *26*, 16231635. [CrossRef]
19. Qun, S.; Wang, Y.; Chen, J.; Huang, X.; Guo, H.; Lu, Z.; Wang, J.; Zheng, C.; Ma, Y.; Zhu, Y.; et al. Neutrophil-to-Lymphocyte Ratios Are Closely Associated with the Severity and Course of Non-mild COVID-19. *Front. Immunol.* **2020**, *11*, 2160. [CrossRef]
20. Park, J.H.; Lee, H.K. Re-analysis of Single Cell Transcriptome Reveals That the NR3C1-CXCL8-Neutrophil Axis Determines the Severity of COVID-19. *Front. Immunol.* **2020**, *11*, 2145. [CrossRef]
21. Tavakolpour, S.; Rakhshandehroo, T.; Wei, E.X.; Rashidian, M. Lymphopenia during the COVID-19 infection: What it shows and what can be learned. *Immunol. Lett.* **2020**, *225*, 31–32. [CrossRef] [PubMed]

22. Chen, J.; Vitetta, L.; Henson, J.D.; Hall, S. The intestinal microbiota and improving the efficacy of COVID-19 vaccinations. *J. Funct. Foods* **2021**, *87*, 104850. [CrossRef] [PubMed]
23. Maggini, S.; Pierre, A.; Calder, P.C. Immune Function and Micronutrient Requirements Change over the Life Course. *Nutrients* **2018**, *10*, 1531. [CrossRef] [PubMed]
24. Claesson, M.J.; Jeffery, I.B.; Conde, S.; Power, S.E.; O'Connor, E.M.; Cusack, S.; Harris, H.M.B.; Coakley, M.; Lakshminarayanan, B.; O'Sullivan, O.; et al. Gut microbiota composition correlates with diet and health in the elderly. *Nature* **2012**, *488*, 178–184. [CrossRef] [PubMed]
25. Zuo, T.; Zhang, F.; Lui, G.C.Y.; Yeoh, Y.K.; Li, A.Y.L.; Zhan, H.; Wan, Y.; Chung, A.C.K.; Cheung, C.P.; Chen, N.; et al. Alterations in Gut Microbiota of Patients With COVID-19 During Time of Hospitalization. *Gastroenterology* **2020**, *159*, 944–955.e948. [CrossRef]
26. Thaiss, C.A.; Zmora, N.; Levy, M.; Elinav, E. The microbiome and innate immunity. *Nature* **2016**, *535*, 65–74. [CrossRef]
27. Honda, K.; Littman, D.R. The microbiota in adaptive immune homeostasis and disease. *Nature* **2016**, *535*, 75–84. [CrossRef]
28. Yeoh, Y.K.; Zuo, T.; Lui, G.C.-Y.; Zhang, F.; Liu, Q.; Li, A.Y.; Chung, A.C.; Cheung, C.P.; Tso, E.Y.; Fung, K.S.; et al. Gut microbiota composition reflects disease severity and dysfunctional immune responses in patients with COVID-19. *Gut* **2021**, *70*, 698–706. [CrossRef]
29. Bettelli, E.; Carrier, Y.; Gao, W.; Korn, T.; Strom, T.B.; Oukka, M.; Weiner, H.L.; Kuchroo, V.K. Reciprocal developmental pathways for the generation of pathogenic effector TH17 and regulatory T cells. *Nature* **2006**, *441*, 235–238. [CrossRef]
30. Goldstein, D.R. Aging, imbalanced inflammation and viral infection. *Virulence* **2010**, *1*, 295–298. [CrossRef]
31. Sanada, F.; Taniyama, Y.; Muratsu, J.; Otsu, R.; Shimizu, H.; Rakugi, H.; Morishita, R. Source of Chronic Inflammation in Aging. *Front. Cardiovasc. Med.* **2018**, *5*, 12. [CrossRef] [PubMed]
32. Belkaid, Y.; Hand, T.W. Role of the Microbiota in Immunity and Inflammation. *Cell* **2014**, *157*, 121–141. [CrossRef] [PubMed]
33. Shang, J.; Ye, G.; Shi, K.; Wan, Y.; Luo, C.; Aihara, H.; Geng, Q.; Auerbach, A.; Li, F. Structural basis of receptor recognition by SARS-CoV-2. *Nature* **2020**, *581*, 221–224. [CrossRef] [PubMed]
34. Hindson, J. COVID-19: Faecal–oral transmission? *Nat. Rev. Gastroenterol. Hepatol.* **2020**, *17*, 259. [CrossRef]
35. Gu, J.; Han, B.; Wang, J. COVID-19: Gastrointestinal Manifestations and Potential Fecal–Oral Transmission. *Gastroenterology* **2020**, *158*, 1518–1519. [CrossRef]
36. Budden, K.F.; Gellatly, S.L.; Wood, D.L.A.; Cooper, M.A.; Morrison, M.; Hugenholtz, P.; Hansbro, P.M. Emerging pathogenic links between microbiota and the gut–lung axis. *Nat. Rev. Microbiol.* **2017**, *15*, 55–63. [CrossRef]
37. Yu, T.; Kong, J.; Zhang, L.; Gu, X.; Wang, M.; Guo, T. New crosstalk between probiotics Lactobacillus plantarum and Bacillus subtilis. *Sci. Rep.* **2019**, *9*, 13151. [CrossRef]
38. Neish, A.S. Mucosal Immunity and the Microbiome. *Ann. Am. Thorac. Soc.* **2014**, *11* (Suppl. 1), S28–S32. [CrossRef]
39. Wu, H.J.; Wu, E. The role of gut microbiota in immune homeostasis and autoimmunity. *Gut Microbes* **2012**, *3*, 4–14. [CrossRef]
40. Garcia-Gutierrez, E.; Mayer, M.J.; Cotter, P.D.; Narbad, A. Gut microbiota as a source of novel antimicrobials. *Gut Microbes* **2018**, *10*, 1–21. [CrossRef]
41. Conte, C.; Sichetti, M.; Traina, G. Gut–Brain Axis: Focus on Neurodegeneration and Mast Cells. *Appl. Sci.* **2020**, *10*, 1828. [CrossRef]
42. Thomas, T.; Stefanoni, D.; Reisz, J.A.; Nemkov, T.; Bertolone, L.; Francis, R.O.; Hudson, K.E.; Zimring, J.C.; Hansen, K.C.; Hod, E.A.; et al. COVID-19 infection alters kynurenine and fatty acid metabolism, correlating with IL-6 levels and renal status. *JCI Insight* **2020**, *5*, e140327. [CrossRef] [PubMed]
43. Mostov, K.E. Transepithelial transport of immunoglobulins. *Annu. Rev. Immunol.* **1994**, *12*, 63–84. [CrossRef] [PubMed]
44. Kim, S.; Jazwinski, S.M. Quantitative measures of healthy aging and biological age. *Healthy Aging Res.* **2015**, *4*, 26. [CrossRef] [PubMed]
45. van Tongeren, S.P.; Slaets, J.P.J.; Harmsen, H.J.M.; Welling, G.W.; Viterbo, A.; Harel, M.; Horwitz, B.A.; Chet, I.; Mukherjee, P.K. Fecal Microbiota Composition and Frailty. *Appl. Environ. Microbiol.* **2005**, *71*, 6241–6246. [CrossRef]
46. Sharma, L.; Riva, A. Intestinal Barrier Function in Health and Disease—Any role of SARS-CoV-2? *Microorganisms* **2020**, *8*, 1744. [CrossRef]
47. Giron, L.B.; Dweep, H.; Yin, X.; Wang, H.; Damra, M.; Goldman, A.R.; Gorman, N.; Palmer, C.S.; Tang, H.Y.; Shaikh, M.W.; et al. Severe COVID-19 Is Fueled by Disrupted Gut Barrier Integrity. *MedRxiv* **2020**. [CrossRef]
48. Jackson, M.A.; Jeffery, I.B.; Beaumont, M.; Bell, J.T.; Clark, A.G.; Ley, R.E.; O'Toole, P.W.; Spector, T.D.; Steves, C.J. Signatures of early frailty in the gut microbiota. *Genome Med.* **2016**, *8*, 8. [CrossRef]
49. Maffei, V.J.; Kim, S.; Blanchard, E.; Luo, M.; Jazwinski, S.M.; Taylor, C.M.; Welsh, D.A. Biological Aging and the Human Gut Microbiota. *J. Gerontol. Ser. A* **2017**, *72*, 1474–1482. [CrossRef]
50. Venegas, D.P.; Marjorie, K.; Landskron, G.; González, M.J.; Quera, R.; Dijkstra, G.; Harmsen, H.J.; Faber, K.N.; Hermoso, M.A. Short chain fatty acids (SCFAs)-mediated gut epithelial and immune regulation and its relevance for inflammatory bowel diseases. *Front. Immunol.* **2019**, *43*, 629–631.
51. Archer, D.L.; Kramer, D.C. The Use of Microbial Accessible and Fermentable Carbohydrates and/or Butyrate as Supportive Treatment for Patients with Coronavirus SARS-CoV-2 Infection. *Front. Med.* **2020**, *7*, 292. [CrossRef]
52. Zhang, L.; Liu, Y. Potential interventions for novel coronavirus in China: A systematic review. *J. Med. Virol.* **2020**, *92*, 479–490. [CrossRef]

53. Kamada, N.; Seo, S.-U.; Chen, G.Y.; Núñez, G. Role of the gut microbiota in immunity and inflammatory disease. *Nat. Rev. Immunol.* **2013**, *13*, 321–335. [CrossRef]
54. Vidal-Lletjós, S.; Beaumont, M.; Tomé, D.; Benamouzig, R.; Blachier, F.; Lan, A. Dietary Protein and Amino Acid Supplementation in Inflammatory Bowel Disease Course: What Impact on the Colonic Mucosa? *Nutrients* **2017**, *9*, 310. [CrossRef]
55. Scott, N.A.; Andrusaite, A.; Andersen, P.; Lawson, M.; Alcon-Giner, C.; LeClaire, C.; Caim, S.; Le Gall, G.; Shaw, T.; Connolly, J.P.R.; et al. Antibiotics induce sustained dysregulation of intestinal T cell immunity by perturbing macrophage homeostasis. *Sci. Transl. Med.* **2018**, *10*, eaao4755. [CrossRef]
56. de Giorgio, R.; Ruggeri, E.; Stanghellini, V.; Eusebi, L.H.; Bazzoli, F.; Chiarioni, G. Chronic constipation in the elderly: A primer for the gastroenterologist. *BMC Gastroenterol.* **2015**, *15*, 130. [CrossRef]
57. Schuster, B.G.; Kosar, L.; Kamrul, R. Constipation in older adults: Stepwise approach to keep things moving. *Can. Fam. Physician* **2015**, *61*, 152–158.
58. Kau, A.L.; Ahern, P.P.; Griffin, N.W.; Goodman, A.L.; Gordon, J.I. Human nutrition, the gut microbiome and the immune system. *Nature* **2011**, *474*, 327–336. [CrossRef]
59. Tiihonen, K.; Ouwehand, A.; Rautonen, N. Human intestinal microbiota and healthy ageing. *Ageing Res. Rev.* **2010**, *9*, 107–116. [CrossRef]
60. Tang, L.; Gu, S.; Gong, Y.; Li, B.; Lu, H.; Li, Q.; Zhang, R.; Gao, X.; Wu, Z.; Zhang, J.; et al. Clinical Significance of the Correlation between Changes in the Major Intestinal Bacteria Species and COVID-19 Severity. *Engineering* **2020**, *6*, 1178–1184. [CrossRef]
61. Chiu, L.; Bazin, T.; Truchetet, M.-E.; Schaeverbeke, T.; Delhaes, L.; Pradeu, T. Protective Microbiota: From Localized to Long-Reaching Co-Immunity. *Front. Immunol.* **2017**, *8*, 1678. [CrossRef] [PubMed]
62. Rehman, T. Role of the gut microbiota in age-related chronic inflammation. *Endocr. Metab. Immune Disord. Drug Targets* **2012**, *12*, 361–367. [CrossRef] [PubMed]
63. Nicoletti, C. Age-associated changes of the intestinal epithelial barrier: Local and systemic implications. *Expert Rev. Gastroenterol. Hepatol.* **2015**, *9*, 1467–1469. [CrossRef] [PubMed]
64. Thevaranjan, N.; Puchta, A.; Schulz, C.; Naidoo, A.; Szamosi, J.; Verschoor, C.P.; Loukov, D.; Schenck, L.P.; Jury, J.; Foley, K.P.; et al. Age-Associated Microbial Dysbiosis Promotes Intestinal Permeability, Systemic Inflammation, and Macrophage Dysfunction. *Cell Host Microbe* **2017**, *21*, 455–466.e4. [CrossRef]
65. Qi, Y.; Goel, R.; Kim, S.; Richards, E.M.; Carter, C.S.; Pepine, C.J.; Raizada, M.K.; Buford, T.W. Intestinal Permeability Biomarker Zonulin is Elevated in Healthy Aging. *J. Am. Med. Dir. Assoc.* **2017**, *18*, 810.e1–810.e4. [CrossRef]
66. di Vito, R.; Conte, C.; Traina, G. A Multi-Strain Probiotic Formulation Improves Intestinal Barrier Function by the Modulation of Tight and Adherent Junction Proteins. *Cells* **2022**, *11*, 2617. [CrossRef]
67. de Gonzalo-Calvo, D.; de Luxán-Delgado, B.; Rodríguez-González, S.; García-Macia, M.; Suárez, F.M.; Solano, J.J.; Rodríguez-Colunga, M.J.; Coto-Montes, A. Interleukin 6, soluble tumor necrosis factor receptor I and red blood cell distribution width as biological markers of functional dependence in an elderly population: A translational approach. *Cytokine* **2012**, *58*, 193–198. [CrossRef]
68. Yende, S.; Tuomanen, E.; Wunderink, R.; Kanaya, A.; Newman, A.B.; Harris, T.; De Rekeneire, N.; Kritchevsky, S.B. Preinfection Systemic Inflammatory Markers and Risk of Hospitalization Due to Pneumonia. *Am. J. Respir. Crit. Care Med.* **2005**, *172*, 1440–1446. [CrossRef]
69. Jeong, J.-J.; Kim, K.; Hwang, Y.-J.; Han, M.; Kim, D.-H. Anti-inflammaging effects of *Lactobacillus brevis* OW38 in aged mice. *Benef. Microbes* **2016**, *7*, 707–718. [CrossRef]
70. Theoharides, T.C. COVID-19, pulmonary mast cells, cytokine storms, and beneficial actions of luteolin. *BioFactors* **2020**, *46*, 306–308. [CrossRef]
71. Ji, Y.; Sun, S.; Goodrich, J.K.; Kim, H.; Poole, A.C.; Duhamel, G.E.; Ley, R.E.; Qi, L. Diet-induced alterations in gut microflora contribute to lethal pulmonary damage in TLR2/TLR4-deficient mice. *Cell Rep.* **2014**, *8*, 137–149. [CrossRef] [PubMed]
72. Ye, Q.; Wang, B.; Mao, J. The pathogenesis and treatment of the 'Cytokine Storm' in COVID-19. *J. Infect.* **2020**, *80*, 607–613. [CrossRef]
73. Dumas, A.; Bernard, L.; Poquet, Y.; Lugo-Villarino, G.; Neyrolles, O. The role of the lung microbiota and the gut-lung axis in respiratory infectious diseases. *Cell. Microbiol.* **2018**, *20*, e12966. [CrossRef] [PubMed]
74. Groves, H.T.; Cuthbertson, L.; James, P.; Moffatt, M.F.; Cox, M.J.; Tregoning, J.S. Respiratory Disease following Viral Lung Infection Alters the Murine Gut Microbiota. *Front. Immunol.* **2018**, *9*, 182. [CrossRef] [PubMed]
75. Khatiwada, S.; Subedi, A. Lung microbiome and coronavirus disease 2019 (COVID-19): Possible link and implications. *Hum. Microbiome J.* **2020**, *17*, 100073. [CrossRef] [PubMed]
76. Salisbury, M.L.; Han, M.K.; Dickson, R.P.; Molyneaux, P.L. Microbiome in interstitial lung disease: From pathogenesis to treatment target. *Curr. Opin. Pulmon. Med.* **2017**, *23*, 404–410. [CrossRef] [PubMed]
77. Halnes, I.; Baines, K.J.; Berthon, B.S.; Macdonald-Wicks, L.K.; Gibson, P.G.; Wood, L.G. Soluble fibre meal challenge reduces airway inflammation and expression of GPR43 and GPR41 in asthma. *Nutrients* **2017**, *9*, 57. [CrossRef]
78. King, D.E.; Egan, B.M.; Woolson, R.F.; Mainous, A.G., 3rd; Al-Solaiman, Y.; Jesri, A. Effect of a high-fiber diet vs. a fiber-supplemented diet on C-reactive protein level. *Arch. Intern. Med.* **2007**, *167*, 502–506. [CrossRef]

79. Trompette, A.; Gollwitzer, E.S.; Yadava, K.; Sichelstiel, A.K.; Sprenger, N.; Ngom-Bru, C.; Blanchard, C.; Junt, T.; Nicod, L.P.; Harris, N.L.; et al. Gut microbiota metabolism of dietary fiber influences allergic airway disease and hematopoiesis. *Nat. Med.* **2014**, *20*, 159–166. [CrossRef]
80. Russell, S.L.; Gold, M.J.; Willing, B.P.; Thorson, L.; McNagny, K.M.; Finlay, B.B. Perinatal antibiotic treatment affects murine microbiota, immune responses and allergic asthma. *Gut Microbes* **2013**, *4*, 158–164. [CrossRef]
81. Metsälä, J.; Lundqvist, A.; Virta, L.J.; Kaila, M.; Gissler, M.; Virtanen, S.M. Prenatal and post-natal exposure to antibiotics and risk of asthma in childhood. *Clin. Exp. Allergy* **2014**, *45*, 137–145. [CrossRef] [PubMed]
82. Looft, T.; Allen, H.K. Collateral effects of antibiotics on mammalian gut microbiomes. *Gut Microbes* **2012**, *3*, 463–467. [CrossRef] [PubMed]
83. Sze, M.; Tsuruta, M.; Yang, S.-W.J.; Oh, Y.; Man, S.F.P.; Hogg, J.C.; Sin, D.D. Changes in the Bacterial Microbiota in Gut, Blood, and Lungs following Acute LPS Instillation into Mice Lungs. *PLoS ONE* **2014**, *9*, e111228. [CrossRef] [PubMed]
84. De Marco, S.; Sichetti, M.; Muradyan, D.; Piccioni, M.; Traina, G.; Pagiotti, R.; Pietrella, D. Probiotic Cell-Free Supernatants Exhibited Anti-Inflammatory and Antioxidant Activity on Human Gut Epithelial Cells and Macrophages Stimulated with LPS. *Evid -Based Complement. Altern. Med.* **2018**, *2018*, 1756308. [CrossRef] [PubMed]
85. Sichetti, M.; De Marco, S.; Pagiotti, R.; Traina, G.; Pietrella, D. Anti-inflammatory effect of multi-strain probiotics formulation (*L. rhamnosus*, *B. lactis* and *B. longum*). *Nutrition* **2018**, *53*, 95–102. [CrossRef]
86. Traina, G.; Menchetti, L.; Rappa, F.; Casagrande-Proietti, P.; Barbato, O.; Leonardi, L.; Carini, F.; Piro, F.; Brecchia, G. Probiotic mixture supplementation in the preventive management of trinitrobenzenesulfonic acid-induced inflammation in a murine model. *J. Biol. Regul. Homeost. Agents* **2016**, *30*, 895–901.
87. Yildiz, S.; Mazel-Sanchez, B.; Kandasamy, M.; Manicassamy, B.; Schmolke, M. Influenza A virus infection impacts systemic microbiota dynamics and causes quantitative enteric dysbiosis. *Microbiome* **2018**, *6*, 9. [CrossRef]
88. Traina, G. The role of mast cells in the gut and brain. *J. Integr. Neurosci.* **2021**, *20*, 185–196. [CrossRef]
89. Marshall, J.S.; Portales-Cervantes, L.; Leong, E. Mast cell responses to virus and pathogen products. *Int. J. Mol. Sci.* **2019**, *20*, 4241. [CrossRef]
90. Oymar, K.; Halvorsen, T.; Aksnes, L. Mast cells activation and leukotriene secretion in wheezing infants. Relation to respiratory syncytial virus and outcome. *Pediatr. Allergy Immunol.* **2006**, *17*, 37–42. [CrossRef]
91. Kapsenberg, M.L. Dendritic-cell control of pathogen-driven T-cell polarization. *Nat. Rev. Immunol.* **2003**, *3*, 984–993. [CrossRef]
92. Nakae, S.; Suto, H.; Kakurai, M.; Sedgwick, J.D.; Tsai, M.; Galli, S.J. Mast cells enhance T cell activation: Importance of mast cell-derived TNF. *Proc. Natl. Acad. Sci. USA* **2005**, *102*, 6467–6472. [CrossRef]
93. Gebremeskel, S.; Schanin, J.; Coyle, K.M.; Butuci, M.; Luu, T.; Brock, E.C.; Xu, A.; Wong, A.; Leung, J.; Korver, W.; et al. Mast Cell and Eosinophil Activation Are Associated With COVID-19 and TLR-Mediated Viral Inflammation: Implications for an Anti-Siglec-8 Antibody. *Front. Immunol.* **2021**, *12*, 650331. [CrossRef]
94. Caughey, G.H.; Raymond, W.W.; Wolters, P.J. Angiotensin II generation by mast cell alpha- and beta-chymases. *Biochim. Biophys. Acta* **2000**, *1480*, 245–257. [CrossRef]
95. Kutukova, N.A.; Nazarov, P.G.; Kudryavtseva, G.V.; Shishkin, V.I. Mast cells and aging. *Adv. Gerontol.* **2017**, *7*, 68–75. [CrossRef]
96. De Zuani, M.; Secco, C.D.; Frossi, B. Mast cells at the crossroads of microbiota and IBD. *Eur. J. Immunol.* **2018**, *48*, 1929–1937. [CrossRef]
97. Traina, G. Mast cells in the brain—Old cells, new target. *J. Integr. Neurosci.* **2017**, *16(s1)*, S69–S83. [CrossRef]
98. Traina, G.; Cocchi, M. Mast Cells, Astrocytes, Arachidonic Acid: Do They Play a Role in Depression? *Appl. Sci.* **2020**, *10*, 3455. [CrossRef]
99. Martinez, M.A. Compounds with Therapeutic Potential against Novel Respiratory 2019 Coronavirus. *Antimicrob. Agents Chemother.* **2020**, *64*, e00399-20. [CrossRef]
100. Oksaharju, A.; Kankainen, M.; Kekkonen, R.A.; Lindstedt, K.A.; Kovanen, P.T.; Korpela, R.; Miettinen, M. Probiotic Lactobacillus rhamnosus downregulates FCER1 and HRH4 expression in human mast cells. *World J. Gastroenterol.* **2011**, *17*, 750–759. [CrossRef]
101. Forsythe, P.; Wang, B.; Khambati, I.; Kunze, W.A. Systemic Effects of Ingested Lactobacillus Rhamnosus: Inhibition of Mast Cell Membrane Potassium (IKCa) Current and Degranulation. *PLoS ONE* **2012**, *7*, e41234. [CrossRef] [PubMed]
102. Leiter, O.; Walker, T.L. Platelets in neurodegenerative conditions- Friend of foe? *Front. Immunol.* **2020**, *11*, 747. [PubMed]
103. Ponomarev, E.D. Fresh Evidence for Platelets as Neuronal and Innate Immune Cells: Their Role in the Activation, Differentiation, and Deactivation of Th1, Th17, and Tregs during Tissue Inflammation. *Front. Immunol.* **2018**, *9*, 406. [CrossRef] [PubMed]
104. Le Blanc, J.; Lordkipanidzé, M. Platelet Function in Aging. *Front. Cardiovasc. Med.* **2019**, *6*, 109. [CrossRef] [PubMed]
105. Bester, J.; Pretorius, E. Effects of IL-1β, IL-6 and IL-8 on erythrocytes, platelets and clot viscoelasticity. *Sci. Rep.* **2016**, *6*, 32188. [CrossRef] [PubMed]
106. Nemet, I.; Saha, P.P.; Gupta, N.; Zhu, W.; Romano, K.A.; Skye, S.M.; Cajka, T.; Mohan, M.L.; Li, L.; Wu, Y.; et al. A Cardiovascular Disease-Linked Gut Microbial Metabolite Acts via Adrenergic Receptors. *Cell* **2020**, *180*, 862–877.e22. [CrossRef]
107. Xu, P.; Zhou, Q.; Xu, J. Mechanism of thrombocytopenia in COVID-19 patients. *Ann. Hematol.* **2020**, *99*, 1205–1208. [CrossRef]
108. Cocchi, M.; Traina, G. Tryptophan and Membrane Mobility as Conditioners and Brokers of Gut–Brain Axis in Depression. *Appl. Sci.* **2020**, *10*, 4933. [CrossRef]

109. Lefrançais, E.; Ortiz-Muñoz, G.; Caudrillier, A.; Mallavia, B.; Liu, F.; Sayah, D.M.; Thornton, E.E.; Headley, M.B.; David, T.; Coughlin, S.R.; et al. The lung is a site of platelet biogenesis and a reservoir for haematopoietic progenitors. *Nature* **2017**, *544*, 105–109. [CrossRef]
110. Azizpour, K.; Van Kessel, K.; Oudega, R.; Rutten, F. The Effect of Probiotic Lactic Acid Bacteria (LAB) Strains on the Platelet Activation: A Flow Cytometry-Based Study. *J. Probiotics Health* **2017**, *5*, 2. [CrossRef]
111. Allen, I.C.; Scull, M.A.; Moore, C.B.; Holl, E.K.; McElvania-TeKippe, E.; Taxman, D.J.; Guthrie, E.H.; Pickles, R.J.; Ting, J.P.-Y. The NLRP3 Inflammasome Mediates In Vivo Innate Immunity to Influenza A Virus through Recognition of Viral RNA. *Immunity* **2009**, *30*, 556–565. [CrossRef] [PubMed]
112. Domínguez-Díaz, C.; García-Orozco, A.; Riera-Leal, A.; Padilla-Arellano, J.R.; Fafutis-Morris, M. Microbiota and Its Role on Viral Evasion: Is It with Us or Against Us? *Front. Cell. Infect. Microbiol.* **2019**, *9*, 256. [CrossRef] [PubMed]
113. Kanmani, P.; Clua, P.; Vizoso-Pinto, M.G.; Rodriguez, C.; Alvarez, S.; Melnikov, V.; Takahashi, H.; Kitazawa, H.; Villena, J. Respiratory Commensal Bacteria Corynebacterium pseudodiphtheriticum Improves Resistance of Infant Mice to Respiratory Syncytial Virus and Streptococcus pneumoniae Superinfection. *Front. Microbiol.* **2017**, *8*, 1613. [CrossRef] [PubMed]
114. Botić, T.; Klingberg, T.D.; Weingartl, H.; Cencic, A. A novel eukaryotic cell culture model to study antiviral activity of potential probiotic bacteria. *Int. J. Food Microbiol.* **2007**, *115*, 227–234. [CrossRef]
115. Park, M.-K.; Ngo, V.; Kwon, Y.-M.; Lee, Y.-T.; Yoo, S.; Cho, Y.-H.; Hong, S.-M.; Hwang, H.S.; Ko, E.-J.; Jung, Y.-J.; et al. Lactobacillus plantarum DK119 as a probiotic confers protection against influenza virus by modulating innate immunity. *PLoS ONE* **2013**, *8*, e75368. [CrossRef]
116. Belkacem, N.; Serafini, N.; Wheeler, R.; Derrien, M.; Boucinha, L.; Couesnon, A.; Cerf-Bensussan, N.; Boneca, I.G.; Di Santo, J.P.; Taha, M.-K.; et al. Lactobacillus paracasei feeding improves immune control of influenza infection in mice. *PLoS ONE* **2017**, *12*, e0184976. [CrossRef]
117. Eguchi, K.; Fujitani, N.; Nakagawa, H.; Miyazaki, T. Prevention of respiratory syncytial virus infection with probiotic lactic acid bacterium *Lactobacillus gasseri* SBT2055. *Sci. Rep.* **2019**, *9*, 4812. [CrossRef]
118. Morais, A.H.A.; Passos, T.S.; Maciel, B.L.L.; da Silva-Maia, J.K. Can Probiotics and Diet Promote Beneficial Immune Modulation and Purine Control in Coronavirus Infection? *Nutrients* **2020**, *12*, 1737. [CrossRef]
119. Ahn, D.-G.; Choi, J.-K.; Taylor, D.R.; Oh, J.-W. Biochemical characterization of a recombinant SARS coronavirus nsp12 RNA-dependent RNA polymerase capable of copying viral RNA templates. *Arch. Virol.* **2012**, *157*, 2095–2104. [CrossRef]
120. Baud, D.; Dimopoulou Agri, V.; Gibson, G.R.; Reid, G.; Giannoni, E. Using Probiotics to Flatten the Curve of Coronavirus Disease COVID-2019 Pandemic. *Front. Public Health* **2020**, *8*, 186. [CrossRef]
121. de Vrese, M.; Winkler, P.; Rautenberg, P.; Harder, T.; Noah, C.; Laue, C.; Ott, S.; Hampe, J.; Schreiber, S.; Heller, K.; et al. Effect of *Lactobacillus gasseri* PA 16/8, *Bifidobacterium longum* SP 07/3, *B. bifidum* MF 20/5 on common cold episodes: A double blind, randomized, controlled trial. *Clin Nutr.* **2005**, *24*, 48. [CrossRef] [PubMed]
122. Chong, H.-X.; Yusoff, N.A.A.; Hor, Y.Y.; Lew, L.C.; Jaafar, M.H.; Choi, S.-B.; Yusoff, M.S.; Wahid, N.; Bin Abdullah, M.F.I.L.; Zakaria, N.; et al. *Lactobacillus plantarum* DR7 improved upper respiratory tract infections via enhancing immune and inflammatory parameters: A randomized, double-blind, placebo-controlled study. *J. Dairy Sci.* **2019**, *102*, 4783–4797. [CrossRef] [PubMed]
123. Metchnikoff, E. *The Prolongation of Life: Optimistic Studies*; Putnam: New York, NY, USA, 1907.

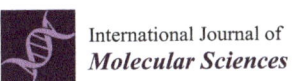

Review

Gut Microbiota and *Clostridium difficile*: What We Know and the New Frontiers

Andrea Piccioni [1], Federico Rosa [2], Federica Manca [2], Giulia Pignataro [1], Christian Zanza [3], Gabriele Savioli [4], Marcello Covino [1,2], Veronica Ojetti [2], Antonio Gasbarrini [1,2], Francesco Franceschi [1,2] and Marcello Candelli [1,*]

1. Department of Emergency Medicine, Fondazione Policlinico Universitario A. Gemelli IRCCS, 00168 Rome, Italy
2. Facoltà di Medicina e Chirurgia, Università Cattolica del Sacro Cuore, 00168 Rome, Italy
3. Foundation of Ospedale Alba-Bra, Department of Anesthesia, Critical Care and Emergency Medicine, Michele and Pietro Ferrero Hospital, 12060 Verduno, Italy
4. Emergency Department, Policlinico Universitario San Matteo, IRCCS, 27100 Pavia, Italy
* Correspondence: marcello.candelli@policlinicogemelli.it

Abstract: Our digestive system, particularly our intestines, harbors a vast amount of microorganisms, whose genetic makeup is referred to as the microbiome. *Clostridium difficile* is a spore-forming Gram-positive bacterium, which can cause an infection whose symptoms range from asymptomatic colonization to fearsome complications such as the onset of toxic megacolon. The relationship between gut microbiota and *Clostridium difficile* infection has been studied from different perspectives. One of the proposed strategies is to be able to specifically identify which types of microbiota alterations are most at risk for the onset of CDI. In this article, we understood once again how crucial the role of the human microbiota is in health and especially how crucial it becomes, in the case of its alteration, for the individual's disease. *Clostridium difficile* infection is an emblematic example of how a normal and physiological composition of the human microbiome can play a very important role in immune defense against such a fearsome disease.

Keywords: gut microbiota; *Clostridium difficile* infection; microbiome

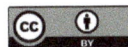

1. The Gut Microbiota

Our digestive system, particularly our intestines, harbors a vast amount of microorganisms including bacteria, archaea, bacteriophages, eukaryotic viruses, and fungi called the microbiota [1], whose genetic makeup is referred to as the microbiome.

The number of these microorganisms inhabiting the human gastrointestinal tract is extremely high, reaching, according to some estimates, a ratio of equality (about 1:1) vis-à-vis all cells in the human body, while the genetic material of these microorganisms appears to have at least 100 times more genetic diversity than that of the entire human genome [2,3].

A "superorganism" is defined as the set of the host and all the microorganisms that colonize it [2].

In terms of their composition, most of these bacteria belong to the *Firmicutes* phyla (64%), followed by *Bacteroidetes* (23%) and *Proteobacteria* (8%) to Gram-negative bacteria such as *E. coli* and *H. pylori* [4] (Figure 1).

The various gastrointestinal regions, because of their different characteristics, represent different microenvironments, in which specific microorganisms grow [5].

The stomach has special characteristics, such as its acidic ph, so most of the microorganisms that colonize it are acid resistant.

The most important microorganism residing in the gastric lumen is Helicobacter pylori, which influences the growth of other secondary species, which may play a mutualistic or pathogenic role [6].

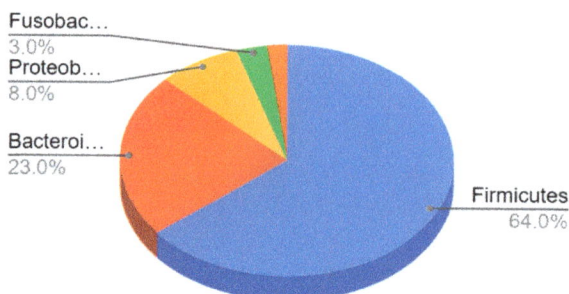

Figure 1. Composition of the gut microbiota. The most represented phyla are Firmicutes (64%) and Bacteroidetes (23%), followed by Proteobacteria (8%), Fusobacteria, verrucomicrobia, and actinobacteria (3%).

Regarding the small intestine, it is characterized by the presence of oxygen, rapid luminal flow, and bactericidal secretions such as bile acids.

In the duodenum, the predominant phyla are Firmicutes and Actinobacteria [7].

The colon, on the other hand, is in a condition of anaerobiosis, where the slower passage of food, absorption of water, and fermentation of undigested food take place.

For these reasons, the most common microorganisms are *Bacteroides, Bifidobacterium, Streptococcus, Enterobacteriaceae, Enterococcus, Clostridium, Lactobacillus,* and *Ruminococcus* [8] (Table 1).

Table 1. Summary of the predominant microorganisms in the various tracts of the digestive system with their basic characteristics.

Gastrointestinal Tract	Characteristics	Predominant Microorganisms
Stomach	Acidic environment	*Helicobacter pylori*
Small intestine	Plenty of oxygen, secretion of bactericidal substances, and rapid luminal flow	*Firmicutes* and *Actinobacteria*
Colon	Slow transit of food, anaerobic condition, site of water absorption, and fermentation of undigested food	*Bacteroides, Bifidobacterium, Streptococcus, Enterobacteriaceae, Enterococcus, Clostridium, Lactobacillus,* and *Ruminococcus*

This type of complex mutualistic interaction between these microorganisms and their host appears to have evolved over thousands of years [2].

In fact, the ingestion of germs that will later go on to contribute to the formation of human intestinal flora has been known since ancestral times, traces of which have been found in cave paintings, dating as far back as the Neolithic age [3].

The interaction between diet, microbiota, and the human host has fascinated researchers since the turn of the last century when Metchnikoff tried to link this complex interaction and senescence [4].

One of the controversial aspects that characterize this topic, is that in the early days, it was not very clear whether it was the microbiota that predisposed toward certain pathological conditions or whether the opposite was the case [9], while currently, most researchers argue that it is an alteration of the gut microbiota that predisposes toward the onset of certain diseases.

Most of these microorganisms play a commensal role with their host [9].

In fact, this complex host–individual interaction could become so long-lived only by bringing, most of the time, benefits to both parties.

In recent years, more and more efforts are being made to investigate certain aspects that characterize the microbiome, and one of these is to understand its interindividual diversity.

The mechanism by which each individual develops his or her own microbiome appears to be multifactorial in origin, with several factors being called into play, some genetic and others environmental such as those related to childbirth and early life, followed by the type of infant feeding, medications taken, and lifestyle [9].

We have seen how the gut microbiota is greatly affected by environmental influences.

An interesting line of research is on strategies to maintain good health through the homeostasis of the gut microbiota.

Some authors suggest practicing a vegetarian diet, while wheat gluten, red meat, and alcohol are related to dysbiosis that can trigger a chronic inflammatory response [10].

The very fact that so many factors come into play therefore makes it very arduous to know about each one.

Another fascinating field of study in recent years is trying to identify and understand the many functions performed by the microbiome.

The roles played by the gut microbiota are multiple, going on to act on food digestion, drug metabolism, and regulation of intestinal endocrine function, and going as far as being involved in host immune defense mechanisms (Table 2) [1].

Table 2. Gut microbiota functions.

	Gut Microbiota Functions
Influences	Development and function of the immune system, bone density, pathogen growth, gut endocrine functions, neurologic signaling.
Biosynthesis	Vitamins, steroid hormones, neurotransmitters
Metabolism	Drugs, xenobiotics, bile salts, food components, amino acids

The roles played by the microbiota are indeed multifaceted; in fact, it is not surprising to learn that some researchers are focusing on the possible role of microorganisms in fighting cancer, a new frontier with little evidence at the moment but very promising [11].

Again, the real challenge is to try to disentangle all these different functions that are performed in different individuals.

In our case, we will see how crucial its protective function is in the healthy individual and how disastrous its lack is in patients who will develop *Clostridium difficile* infection.

2. *Clostridium difficile*

Clostridium difficile is a spore-forming Gram-positive bacterium, which can cause an infection whose symptoms range from asymptomatic colonization to fearsome complications such as the onset of toxic megacolon [12].

It is this broad spectrum of clinical manifestations that makes this disease so insidious.

Detection of *C. difficile* without evidence of clinical signs is termed colonization, while *Clostridium difficile* infection (CDI) is referred to when *C. difficile* is present associated with its characteristic clinical manifestations [13].

CDI is a clinical condition that doctors in different specialties very often struggle with. CDI is one of the most common nosocomial infections [8,14].

By some estimates, CDI affects about 460,000 people a year in the US [15].

These important data help us understand why this disease is increasingly proving to be one of the big public health topics.

The main risk factors for CDI appear to be older age (above 65 years), antibiotic use, and nosocomial exposure [16].

Several considerations can be drawn from these data.

One is purely epidemiological: with the inevitable increase in the geriatric population, these numbers are unfortunately bound to increase.

Another, however, is that all three of the conditions mentioned are acquired.

It is precisely these observations that underlie the involvement of the microbiome in the pathogenesis of this disease.

The onset of CDI occurs as a result of the oro-fecal transmission of sufficient numbers of spores of a toxin-producing strain of C. difficile within the colon of the host, accompanied by their overgrowth at the expense of normal commensal microorganisms [17].

The occurrence of *Clostridium difficile* infection is thus associated with an alteration in the gut microbiota by antibiotics that are not active against C. difficile, which thus cause uncontrolled growth [18].

A great many antibiotics are therefore associated with the occurrence of CDI, and those with a higher risk appear to be more commonly used antibiotics including penicillins such as amoxicillin and ampicillin, as well as cephalosporins, clindamycin, and fluoroquinolones [14]. Thus, the main risk factor for CDI appears to be exposure to broad-spectrum antibiotics, precisely because of the changes they make to the normal human microbiome [19] (Figure 2). Asymptomatic colonization on admission to the hospital is estimated to have a prevalence of 0.6–13% [20].

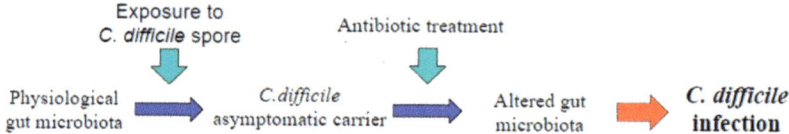

Figure 2. Pathogenesis of *Clostridium difficile* infection (CDI). One of the most accepted theories to explain the onset of CDI is the administration of antibiotics in a healthy *C. difficile carrier* patient. Antibiotic treatment, by generating a dysbiosis in the gut microbiota, causes a loss of its defense function, leading to the onset of CDI.

These data seem to explain such a high incidence of CDI, the genesis of which is multifactorial.

Thus, the factors at play are asymptomatic colonization, associated with antibiotic therapy that brings an imbalance to the microbiome, which may then promote the onset of CDI.

This is why CDI is often considered the best example of the symbiotic relationship between the individual and the host and how its imbalance can lead to disastrous consequences.

C. difficile is rarely invasive, and its mechanism of intestinal damage appears to be mediated by its potent exotoxins: toxin A and toxin B [21].

Treatment of CDI therefore relies on the use of antibiotics such as fidaxomicin, vancomycin, and metronidazole [22].

Fidaxomicin has proven to be the most selective antibiotic against C. difficile [23] and has been shown to be a highly effective treatment against this disease, although more data are needed regarding safety and efficacy in children and adults [24].

Vancomycin appears to be less selective than fidaxomicin against other intestinal bacteria [23] and continues to be the cornerstone treatment of CDI along with fidaxomicin.

Previously, metronidazole was considered along with vancomycin to be the pivotal treatment for CDI, until new guidelines in 2017 considered it to be of lower efficacy than fidaxomicin and vancomycin, which thus became the main antibiotics for the treatment of CDI [25].

Prolonged use of metronidazole is also burdened by important side effects such as neurotoxicity [26].

As antibiotic treatment is burdened with an important risk of relapse, new therapeutic strategies to cope with CDI are under investigation, which we will discuss later [25].

It should also not be forgotten that for very severe patients, those with a "fulminant" form of *C.m difficile* colitis who present with major symptoms such as shock, hypotension, and megacolon, surgical therapy is also considered [27].

Precisely because CDI is such a complex disease, it can require such diverse treatments.

However, as we shall see, even when a CDI is appropriately treated with the use of antibiotics, the serious problem of recurrence can arise, which is particularly significant for this disease.

The risk of recurrence remains significant, ranging from 12 to 64 percent, with a median of 22 percent [28].

Recurrence is said to occur when, after treatment accompanied by a total disappearance of clinical symptoms, there is a recurrence of CDI within two to eight weeks after discontinuing therapy [27].

Treatment of some of these forms of this recurrent colitis relies on the use of fecal microbiota transplantation (FMT), which is the installation of treated feces collected from a healthy donor into a patient with CDI [29,30].

Regarding FMT, there are some aspects that differ in different centers, such as the most effective dose and preparation time, while some aspects are absolutely shared, such as donor exclusion criteria.

In fact, one of the crucial aspects of this treatment is the careful selection of the donor, as there is a potential risk of pathogens through the FMT procedure.

Thus, patients who carry or are at risk of transmitting infectious diseases, those with gastrointestinal diseases, or who may have recently taken certain medications (antibiotics, immunosuppressants, etc.) that alter the composition of the gut microbiota are excluded [31].

Regarding the safety of this procedure, some data show that adverse effects occurred in 9.2% of patients, including death (3.5%), infection (2.5%), and recurrence of intestinal bowel disease (0.6%) [32].

There are many routes of administration of FMT: oral capsules, procedures involving the upper gastrointestinal tract such as the nasojejunal and nasoduodenal tube, and those of the lower gastrointestinal tract such as colonoscopy or enema.

The lower route of administration appears to be more effective than the upper route, although further studies are needed in this regard [33].

The use of FMT has also been considered for the treatment of fulminant colitis supported by several pieces of evidence, including a retrospective study of 199 patients, in which FMT was associated with reduced mortality and colectomy rates [34].

Meanwhile, evidence on the use of FMT for the treatment of recurrent CDI comes from both randomized trials [35] and meta-analyses [36].

FMT represents one of the latest frontiers of CDI treatment and is an ever-evolving field, in which the role of the microbiome is of paramount importance (Figure 3).

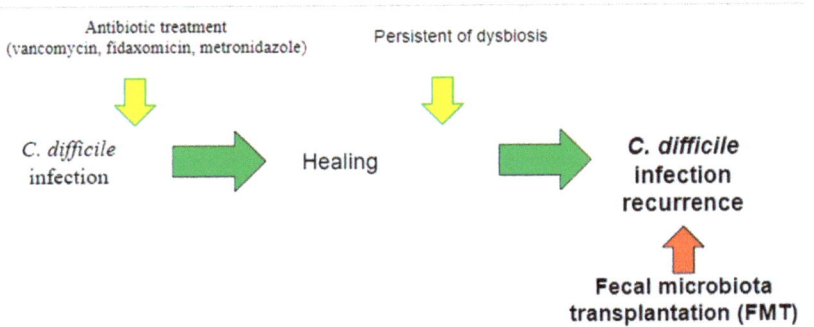

Figure 3. Use of fecal microbiota transplantation (FMT). Currently, the use of FMT is indicated for the treatment of recurrent CDI, in which recurrent infections occur due to the persistence of dysbiosis. The aim of this treatment is precisely to intervene by restoring the balance of the gut microbiota.

3. Interactions between the Gut Microbial Communities and *Clostridium difficile* Infection

3.1. What We Know

The relationship between gut microbiota and *Clostridium difficile* infection has been studied from different perspectives (Table 3).

Table 3. Summary of some existing interactions between microbiome and the occurrence of *Clostridium difficile* infection.

Relationship between Gut Microbiota and *Clostridium difficile* Infection
Healthy carriers—Up to 17.5% of adults are healthy carriers of *Clostridium difficile*, who do not develop the disease protected by commensal bacterial flora.
Colonization in infants—In fecal samples from newborns and infants, the presence of *Clostridium difficile* rates around 70%; the infant gut appears to be resistant to *Clostridium difficile* toxins.
Disruption of the microbiome and CDI risk factors—Alterations in the microbiota can lead to the onset of CDI. Risk factors that can lead to this include antibiotic use, age, PPI use, and presence of IBD, while having been affected by CDI is a serious risk factor for recurrence.
Fecal microbiota transplantation in CDI—Used for some relapsed forms, precisely because this therapy aims to resolve the dysbiosis that led to the onset of the infection.

C. difficile grows in the digestive tract of infants, where it does not develop an infection but rather a colonization, until during growth when new microbial species take over, providing protection against *C. difficile* itself, although any new imbalance may again stimulate its growth [37].

The composition of the gut microbiota then, after a rapid change in early life, remains nearly stable throughout adulthood, until undergoing new changes with advancing age.

Colonization resistance refers to the peculiar ability on the part of the gut microbiome to resist colonization against pathogenic organisms, including *C. difficile*.

Several mechanisms underlying this resistance to colonization against *C. difficile* have been hypothesized, ranging from stimulation of host immune defenses, competition for nutrients, production of a protective physical barrier against the intestinal mucosa to production of inhibitory substances such as secondary bile acids and bacteriocins [38].

3.2. Healthy Carriers

Asymptomatic colonization of *C. difficile* without any signs of disease has been described in many studies on both human beings and animals [39].

The literature suggests that the range of intestinal *C. difficile* colonization of healthy adults can rate from 2.4% to 17.5% [40], and it can be associated with the composition of intestinal microbial communities but also with other extrinsic factors, such as the living environment as well as the host immune state.

Ozaki et al. reported that *C. difficile* colonization was relatively common among healthy individuals. A healthy asymptomatic carrier has no major difference regarding the gut microbial community compared to a healthy subject. Therefore, Rea MC et al. suggested that the commensal flora in such subjects could protect the host by preventing potentially pathogenic *C. difficile* colonization, multiplication, and toxin production [41].

However, unlike a healthy person with a negative culture, the carrier subject can develop CDI because of the changes in the microbiome that may contribute and favor the growth of the microbe and eventually CDI such as antibiotic treatment, diet, age, host immune state, environment, and hospital admission.

The presence of *C. difficile* in healthy carriers is one of the most important pieces of evidence of one of the many roles played by normal commensal flora.

In this case, the microbiome performs its physiological and essential immune regulatory function, thus succeeding in curbing even a dreaded condition such as *CDI*.

3.3. Colonization in Infants

In fecal samples from newborns and infants, the presence of *C. difficile* rates around 70% [42].

Environment, hospitalization, and prematurity have been associated with the colonization of the bacterium. Some studies showed that vaginal delivery and maternal genital tract are not a risk for newborn acquisition. Vaginal swabs of mothers just before delivery have been examined, and they were all negative for *C. difficile* by culture, but their infants were positive.

Penders et al. [43] associated increased colonization with *C. difficile* with birth by cesarean delivery. The newborns had lower numbers of Bifidobacterium and Bacteroidetes and were more often colonized with *C. difficile* compared with vaginal delivery infants.

Rousseau et al. observed that some microbial taxa such as *Bifidobacterium longum* were protective and negatively correlated to *C. difficile* colonization. In contrast, *Ruminococcus gravus* and *Klebsiella pneumoniae* were susceptible microbial taxa [44].

Plus, the feeding method used has been reported as a factor that can influence *C. difficile* colonization. Breast milk is a more protective factor than formula milk. That can be explained, as some studies showed, by an increase in the acidity in the intestine contents, which may facilitate sporulation and reduce vegetative forms [45].

All of this evidence only reiterates how the gut microbiota begins to form and perform its functions from the earliest days of life, and again, there are multiple factors involved in the development and regulation of the microbiome.

Proteins of human milk play an inhibitory role in toxin TcdA [46].

Moreover, secretory IgA has shown neutralizing activity against toxin A [47].

On the other hand, formula-fed infants are often colonized with *Escherichia coli*, *C. difficile*, Bacteroides, and Lactobacilli compared with breast-fed infants [43].

What is important to underline is that toxigenic and non-toxigenic *C. difficile* has been isolated in infants with a higher percentage of the non-toxigenic one. However, even with the presence of toxigenic strains, colonization seems not to be associated with CDI.

So, the infant gut appears to be resistant to CD toxins. That could be explained by the absence of toxin receptors, poorly developed cellular signaling pathways because of the immature gut mucosa, or the presence of protective factors in the infantile gut that remains at the moment unknown [47].

As we have just seen, this fundamental interaction plays an essential and delicate role from an early age.

4. *Clostridium difficile* Infection

4.1. Disruption of the Microbiome and Clostridium difficile Infection Risk Factors

Clearly, the most well-known risk factor for developing *CDI* is antibiotic use, both short- and long-term because of its impact on microbiota diversity. In fact, a healthy microbial community gut is capable of interfering with *C. difficile* spores, and it does not necessarily result in disease. However, every change in the microbial environment could bring spore germination, CD growth, and toxin production [48].

Another known risk factor is increasing age. In elderly people, the structure of the microbiome undergoes changes, is less diverse, and shows a decrease in protective species such as *Bifidobacteria* and some *Firmicutes*, as well as an increase in *Bacteroidetes* and *Proteobacteria* [49].

That change also influences the immune system of an elderly person which becomes weaker and more fragile. As a matter of fact, the rate of *C. difficile* infection is higher for people aged 65. Advancing age is also associated with hospitalization, use of antibiotics, and development of different diseases [50–54].

Another risk factor is proton pump inhibitors (PPIs), which increase the gastric pH and modulate microbiota, influencing above all *Lactobacillus* [51].

Gastrointestinal pathologies such as inflammatory bowel disease (IBD) may impact *C. difficile* susceptibility. As some studies show, we observed in subjects suffering from IBD a decreased diversity of *Firmicutes* and *Bacteroidetes* and the presence of pathogenic bacteria such as the *Proteobacteria* phylum [52].

Moreover, its inflammatory products in IBD (antimicrobial peptides lipocalin-2 and calprotectin) potentially impact the growth of surrounding microbes [53].

Differently, as a protective factor, we can safely say that a good composition of microbial communities' gut and a strong immune response could be useful against CDI.

Serum IgG antibodies against toxins A and B have been associated with protection in some studies [54].

So immunization, both active and passive, could be a good strategy to study for CDI treatment [55].

Therefore, a full understanding of all these risk factors is of paramount importance for the development of new preventive strategies to avoid the occurrence of this dangerous infection.

4.2. Recurrent Clostridium difficile Infection and the Incomplete Recovery of the Microbiota

The most common complication of CDI is incomplete recovery and recurrent infection. The rates are about 20.30% after an initial infection and up to 60% after three infections [56].

Some studies notice that each episode of CDI brings an increasing chance of recurrence, also due to an increase in antibiotic use and disease severity [57].

However, it is also hypothesized that antibiotic treatment interferes with the ability of the gut microbiota to recover fully and re-establish colonization resistance in some individuals. Alternatively, recurrence could reflect the failure of the host to mount a protective immune response against *C. difficile* [58].

This is how an imbalance, an acquired rupture of this delicate balance between the host and the individual, can degenerate into an almost irreparable situation.

We can safely assert that being able to prevent one of the most frequent complications, namely the recurrence of this widespread infection, is one of the great challenges of public health.

4.3. Fecal Microbiota Transplantation in Clostridium difficile Infection

More recent work has studied fecal microbiota transplantation (FMT) for recurrent *Clostridium difficile* infection.

Patients with severe CDI refractory to traditional antibiotic treatment have had success with FMT, which restores colon homeostasis by reintroducing bacteria from healthy donor stool. The success rate for FMT is greater than 90% for those who had recurrent CDI, but the mechanism behind this treatment is partially unknown [59].

Successful fecal microbiota transplantation is correlated with a dysbiosis resolution by the replenishment of *Roseburia* and *Bacteroidetes*, which are also involved in butyrate production. After fecal transplantation, studies reported the presence of an increase in richness and diversity, an eradication of *Proteobacteria* species, and a restoration of *Firmicutes* and *Bacteroidetes* species [60].

They also found that the patients' gut communities were completely restored within three days following fecal transplantation, with stability in species for at least four months and indistinguishable from that of the donor [61].

Following FMT, *Bacteroidetes* increased and *Proteobacteria* decreased. Some others observed protective microbial taxa are *Alistipes, Ruminococcaceae, Lachnospiraceae, Peptostreptococcaceae,* and *Verrucomicrobiaceae*. All the species are negatively correlated to *C. difficile* colonization [62] (Figure 4).

This is an emblematic example of how by being able to re-establish that fundamental relationship between the host and gut microbiota, one of its most important functions, namely that of immune regulation, can be recovered.

All these new discoveries undoubtedly make it one of the most promising and steadily growing fields in all of medicine.

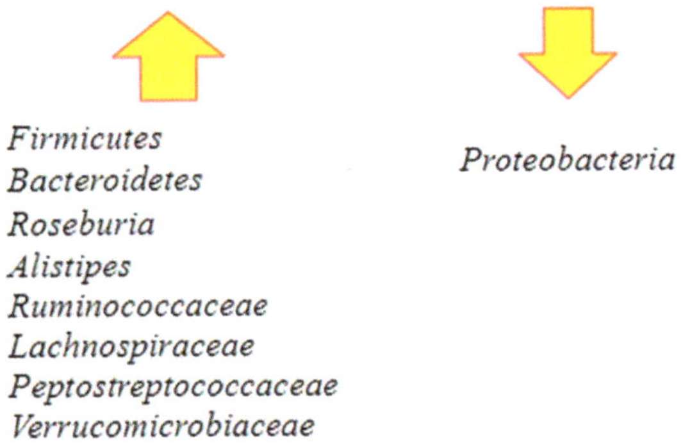

Firmicutes
Bacteroidetes   *Proteobacteria*
Roseburia
Alistipes
Ruminococcaceae
Lachnospiraceae
Peptostreptococcaceae
Verrucomicrobiaceae

Figure 4. Major changes in the gut microbiota following fecal microbiota transplantation (FMT) [60,62]. After the procedure, there is an increase in the richness and diversity of the microbiome and the restoration of *Bacteroidetes* and *Roseburia*, which are involved in butyrate production. There is also restoration of *Firmicutes* and other protective microbial taxa such as *Alistipes*, *Ruminococcaceae*, *Lachnospiraceae*, *Peptostreptococcaceae*, and *Verrucomicrobiaceae*. At the same time, an important decrease in Proteobacteria occurs.

5. New Therapeutic Strategies

With this close link between the microbiome and the onset of *Clostridium difficile* infection, several lines of research are currently underway aimed at developing new therapeutic strategies (Table 4).

Despite all this new evidence, there is currently still not full unanimity on defining the microbial species associated with asymptomatic colonization versus those related to the onset of CDI, which remains one of the current challenges to be addressed [47,63].

One of the proposed strategies is to be able to specifically identify which types of microbiota alterations are most at risk for the onset of *CDI* [38].

This field is particularly promising due to the fact that we are increasingly witnessing significant technological development, with reduced sequencing costs.

In this case, it is the evolution of science in a broad sense, understood as the development of new technologies that are increasingly within the reach of researchers that could also prove decisive in this specific area of study.

Other authors, on the other hand, suggest how diet may influence the composition of the microbiota and consequently its interaction with various pathological conditions, including CDI, thus looking for a correlation between diet and the development of this disease [64].

This aspect also appears to be much studied for other diseases such as metabolic syndrome and chronic inflammatory bowel disease, less so for CDI.

From the pathophysiological point of view, the connection between diet and the microbiome is very clear.

However, the occurrence of *CDI*, as we have seen, also calls into question several other factors, and that is why it makes this field of study very difficult, albeit very promising.

Meanwhile, new therapeutic frontiers make use of probiotics and prebiotics.

Probiotics are "Live microorganisms that, when administered in adequate amounts, confer a health benefit upon the host" [65], while prebiotics are "A selectively fermented ingredient that allows specific changes, both in the composition and/or activity in the gastrointestinal microflora that confers benefits upon host well-bring and health" [66].

Meanwhile, "synbiotic" means the administration of a prebiotic together with a specific probiotic to enhance the engraftment and development of that specific microbe [67].

A study was recently conducted in which treatment with live purified Firmicutes bacterial spores was successfully proposed for patients with recurrent CDI [68].

An increase in the concentration of secondary bile acids compared to primary bile acids is one of the factors inhibiting the germination of CD spores.

For this very reason, spore-forming *Firmicutes* bacteria were grafted with the specific purpose of increasing the concentration of secondary bile acids to thus inhibit spore germination and subsequent CD growth [68].

Here, we have an important finding of how an accurate understanding of this complex individual–host interaction can provide us with important new therapeutic weapons.

Some of the latest research involves in vitro experiments and makes use of synbiotics, bacterial secreted compounds that inhibit the activity of *C. difficile* toxins [67].

These research studies, though currently relegated to the early stages, appear to be very promising.

Live recombinant biotherapeutic products (LBPs) are defined as microorganisms that have been genetically modified by the targeted addition, deletion, or modification of genetic material [69].

Several clinical trials on CDI are currently underway: one is biotherapeutic, whose potential use in CDI relapses is being studied [70], while another one involves the use of Gram-positive selective-spectrum antimicrobials [71] for *CDI* patients.

Again, efforts are being made to counteract this disease by looking at the factors that regulate host immunity.

Other researchers have focused on studying the interaction between the onset of CDI and the presence of valerate, a short-chain fatty acid produced by amino acid fermentation in the microbiota.

Valerate appears to be one of the factors that inhibit the growth of *C. difficile*; in fact, its levels increase after fecal microbiota transplantation [72].

Some of the most surprising research involves the use of bacteriophages.

Bacteriophages are viruses that can go to specific targets, going on to infect and replicate within the designated host [69].

Their potential and undisputed strength would be to go against *C. difficile* without the use of antibiotics [3,69].

There has also been speculation that this particular therapeutic weapon could be used against *C. difficile*, but without obtaining important evidence at present.

A very promising paper was recently published, in which ADS024, a newly characterized strain of *Bacillus velezensis*, was identified that appears to have strong activity against *C. difficile* with negligible impact on the rest of the bacterial flora, and also having protease activity directed against TcdA and TcdB toxins which we have seen to be responsible for the clinical manifestations of this disease [73].

We fully share the enthusiasm shown by Khanna [74] in a recent article in which he summarized the four ongoing trials of capsule therapies (CP101, RBX7455, SER-109, VE303) plus the one based on the use of enema (RBX2660), again related to remodeling the microbiota to cope with *CDI*.

In conclusion, we also point out an excellent paper by Rusha et al. [75] who expounded an excellent summary of probiotic strains used in human clinical trials to treat CDAD.

Table 4. New strategies for the prevention of *Clostridium difficile* infection through its interaction with the gut microbiota.

New Therapeutic Strategies	
Aim in the future for increasingly accurate identification of microbiota alterations responsible for the onset of CDI	(Revolinski et al., 2018) [38]
Investigating the relationship between diet, microbiome, and the development of CDI	(Shaji et al., 2022) [64]
Oral administration of pore-forming *Firmicutes* bacteria to prevent recurrence of CDI (phase 3, double-blind, randomized, placebo-controlled study of 182 patients, with a safety profile similar to placebo; has superior efficacy for prevention of recurrent infections)	(Feuerstadt et al., 2022) [68]
Use of symbionts (in vitro studies)	(Mills et al., 2018) [67]

Table 4. Cont.

New Therapeutic Strategies	
Biotherapeutic and Gram-positive selective-spectrum antimicrobials (clinical trials in progress)	(Orenstein et al., Garey et al., 2022) [70,71]
Identify products of the human microbiota that counteract the occurrence of *Clostridium difficile* infection	(McDonald et al., 2018) [72]
Counteracting *Clostridium difficile* without the use of antibiotics by using bacteriophages	(Zhang et al., 2022) [69]
Identification of ADS024, a new potential therapeutic bacterium directed against *Clostridium difficile*	(O'Donnell, et al. 2022) [73]

6. Conclusions

In this article, we carefully explored aspects concerning the complex interaction between *C. difficile* and gut microbiota.

The microbiome is a complex system whose fundamental importance we understand more and more, both for the health and disease of the individual.

It will still take a long time to fully understand it, for multiple reasons, including its extreme variability in different individuals and its involvement in so many different functions.

C. difficile infection is one of the great public health challenges.

It is one of the most frequent infections, where the role of its interaction with the microbiota is crucial.

From these assumptions, several therapeutic strategies to deal with CDI have arisen and are being studied.

The most intuitive one is to go after the microorganisms themselves that cause this disease, as is currently done with the use of antibiotics, or by experimenting with new and different innovative methods, such as bacteriophages.

The other strategy, on the other hand, is to work on the substrate that promotes the pathogenesis of CDI.

In this regard, we mentioned fecal microbiota transplantation and all the other numerous therapeutic strategies that are still being researched or tested.

We also saw how it is not enough to eliminate the bacteria that cause CDI since in the absence of a protective substrate from the microbiome, the risk of recurrence is extremely high.

It is precisely in order to prevent these recurrences that the use of fecal transplantation, one of the latest therapeutic frontiers involving the gut microbiota, is being employed.

As we discussed extensively, research on these issues is more alive than ever, and we hope it will continue to be so that we can have new therapeutic weapons against this infection.

Author Contributions: Conceptualization, A.P. and M.C. (Marcello Candelli); methodology, A.P. and F.R.; software, F.M. and C.Z.; validation, A.G., F.F. and V.O.; formal analysis, A.P. and G.S.; investigation, F.R., F.M. and G.P.; resources, G.P.; data curation, F.M., C.Z. and G.S.; writing original draft preparation, A.P., F.R. and F.M.; writing—review and editing, M.C. (Marcello Covino), F.F. and A.G.; visualization, M.C. (Marcello Covino) and V.O.; supervision, A.G., F.F. and M.C. (Marcello Candelli). All authors have read and agreed to the published version of the manuscript.

Funding: This research received no external funding.

Institutional Review Board Statement: The study was conducted according to the guidelines of the Declaration of Helsinki. Ethical review and approval were waived for this study because it is a review.

Informed Consent Statement: Not applicable.

Data Availability Statement: Not applicable.

Conflicts of Interest: The authors declare no conflict of interest.

References

1. Lynch, S.V.; Pedersen, O. The Human Intestinal Microbiome in Health and Disease. *N. Engl. J. Med.* **2016**, *375*, 2369–2379. [CrossRef] [PubMed]
2. Thursby, E.; Juge, N. Introduction to the human gut microbiota. *Biochem. J.* **2017**, *474*, 1823–1836. [CrossRef] [PubMed]
3. Gasbarrini, G.; Mosoni, C. The gut microbiota: Its history, characterization and role in different ages and environmental conditions and in gastrointestinal, metabolic and neurodegenerative pathologies. *Microb. Health Dis.* **2019**, *1*, e143.
4. Abenavoli, L.; Scarpellini, E.; Colica, C.; Boccuto, L.; Salehi, B.; Sharifi-Rad, J.; Aiello, V.; Romano, B.; De Lorenzo, A.; Izzo, A.A.; et al. Gut Microbiota and Obesity: A Role for Probiotics. *Nutrients* **2019**, *11*, 2690. [CrossRef] [PubMed]
5. Hollister, E.B.; Gao, C.; Versalovic, J. Compositional and functional features of the gastrointestinal microbiome and their effects on human health. *Gastroenterology* **2014**, *146*, 1449–1458. [CrossRef]
6. Bik, E.M.; Eckburg, P.B.; Gill, S.R.; Nelson, K.E.; Purdom, E.A.; Francois, F.; Perez-Perez, G.; Blaser, M.J.; Relman, D.A. Molecular analysis of the bacterial microbiota in the human stomach. *Proc. Natl. Acad. Sci. USA* **2006**, *103*, 732–737. [CrossRef]
7. El Aidy, S.; van den Bogert, B.; Kleerebezem, M. The small intestine microbiota, nutritional modulation and relevance for health. *Curr. Opin. Biotechnol.* **2015**, *32*, 14–20. [CrossRef]
8. Kazor, C.E.; Mitchell, P.M.; Lee, A.M.; Stokes, L.N.; Loesche, W.J.; Dewhirst, F.E.; Paster, B.J. Diversity of Bacterial Populations on the Tongue Dorsa of Patients with Halitosis and Healthy Patients. *J. Clin. Microbiol.* **2003**, *41*, 558–563. [CrossRef]
9. Fan, Y.; Pedersen, O. Gut microbiota in human metabolic health and disease. *Nat. Rev. Microbiol.* **2021**, *19*, 55–71. [CrossRef]
10. Rishi, P.; Thakur, K.; Vij, S.; Rishi, L.; Singh, A.; Kaur, I.P.; Patel, S.K.S.; Lee, J.-K.; Kalia, V.C. Diet, Gut Microbiota and COVID-19. *Indian J. Microbiol.* **2020**, *60*, 420–429. [CrossRef]
11. Kalia, V.C.; Patel, S.K.S.; Cho, B.K.; Wood, T.K.; Lee, J.K. Emerging applications of bacteria as antitumor agents. *Semin Cancer Biol.* **2021**. Epub ahead of print. [CrossRef] [PubMed]
12. Lee, H.S.; Plechot, K.; Gohil, S.; Le, J. Clostridium difficile: Diagnosis and the Consequence of Over Diagnosis. *Infect. Dis. Ther.* **2021**, *10*, 687–697. [CrossRef] [PubMed]
13. Crobach, M.J.T.; Vernon, J.J.; Loo, V.G.; Kong, L.Y.; Péchiné, S.; Wilcox, M.H.; Kuijper, E.J. Understanding Clostridium difficile Colonization. *Clin. Microbiol. Rev.* **2018**, *31*, e00021-17. [CrossRef] [PubMed]
14. Leffler, D.A.; Lamont, J.T. Clostridium difficile Infection. *N. Engl. J. Med.* **2015**, *372*, 1539–1548. [CrossRef] [PubMed]
15. Guh, A.Y.; Mu, Y.; Winston, L.G.; Johnston, H.; Olson, D.; Farley, M.M.; Wilson, L.E.; Holzbauer, S.M.; Phipps, E.C.; Dumyati, G.K.; et al. Trends in U.S. Burden of *Clostridioides difficile* Infection and Outcomes. *N. Engl. J. Med.* **2020**, *382*, 1320–1330. [CrossRef]
16. Kelly, C.R.; Fischer, M.; Allegretti, J.R.; LaPlante, K.; Stewart, D.B.; Limketkai, B.N.; Stollman, N.H. ACG Clinical Guidelines: Prevention, Diagnosis, and Treatment of Clostridioides difficile Infections. *Am. J. Gastroenterol.* **2021**, *116*, 1124–1147, Erratum in *Am. J. Gastroenterol.* **2022**, *117*, 358. [CrossRef]
17. Burnham, C.A.; Carroll, K.C. Diagnosis of Clostridium difficile infection: An ongoing conundrum for clinicians and for clinical laboratories. *Clin. Microbiol. Rev.* **2013**, *26*, 604–630.
18. Sun, X.; Hirota, S.A. The roles of host and pathogen factors and the innate immune response in the pathogenesis of Clostridium difficile infection. *Mol. Immunol.* **2015**, *63*, 193–202. [CrossRef]
19. Theriot, C.M.; Bowman, A.A.; Young, V.B. Antibiotic-Induced Alterations of the Gut Microbiota Alter Secondary Bile Acid Production and Allow for Clostridium difficile Spore Germination and Outgrowth in the Large Intestine. *mSphere* **2016**, *1*, e00045-15. [CrossRef]
20. Alasmari, F.; Seiler, S.M.; Hink, T.; Burnham, C.-A.D.; Dubberke, E.R. Prevalence and Risk Factors for Asymptomatic Clostridium difficile Carriage. *Clin. Infect. Dis.* **2014**, *59*, 216–222. [CrossRef]
21. Voth, D.E.; Ballard, J.D. Clostridium difficile toxins: Mechanism of action and role in disease. *Clin. Microbiol. Rev.* **2005**, *18*, 247–263. [CrossRef] [PubMed]
22. Johnson, S.; Lavergne, V.; Skinner, A.M.; Gonzales-Luna, A.J.; Garey, K.W.; Kelly, C.P.; Wilcox, M.H. Clinical Practice Guideline by the Infectious Diseases Society of America (IDSA) and Society for Healthcare Epidemiology of America (SHEA): 2021 Focused Update Guidelines on Management of Clostridioides difficile Infection in Adults. *Clin. Infect. Dis.* **2021**, *73*, e1029–e1044. [CrossRef] [PubMed]
23. Tannock, G.W.; Munro, K.; Taylor, C.; Lawley, B.; Young, W.; Byrne, B.; Emery, J.; Louie, T. A new macrocyclic antibiotic, fidaxomicin (OPT-80), causes less alteration to the bowel microbiota of Clostridium difficile-infected patients than does vancomycin. *Microbiology* **2010**, *156 Pt 11*, 3354–3359. [CrossRef] [PubMed]
24. Guery, B.; Menichetti, F.; Anttila, V.-J.; Adomakoh, N.; Aguado, J.M.; Bisnauthsing, K.; Georgopali, A.; Goldenberg, S.D.; Karas, A.; Kazeem, G.; et al. Extended-pulsed fidaxomicin versus vancomycin for Clostridium difficile infection in patients 60 years and older (EXTEND): A randomised, controlled, open-label, phase 3b/4 trial. *Lancet Infect. Dis.* **2018**, *18*, 296–307. [CrossRef]
25. Czepiel, J.; Dróżdż, M.; Pituch, H.; Kuijper, E.J.; Perucki, W.; Mielimonka, A.; Goldman, S.; Wultańska, D.; Garlicki, A.; Biesiada, G. Clostridium difficile infection: Review. *Eur. J. Clin. Microbiol. Infect. Dis.* **2019**, *38*, 1211–1221. [CrossRef]
26. Godfrey, M.; Finn, A.; Zainah, H.; Dapaah-Afriyie, K. Metronidazole-induced encephalopathy after prolonged metronidazole course for treatment of C. difficile colitis. *BMJ Case Rep.* **2015**, *16*, bcr2014206162. [CrossRef]
27. McDonald, L.C.; Gerding, D.N.; Johnson, S.; Bakken, J.S.; Carroll, K.C.; Coffin, S.E.; Dubberke, E.R.; Garey, K.W.; Gould, C.V.; Kelly, C.; et al. Clinical Practice Guidelines for Clostridium difficile Infection in Adults and Children: 2017 Update by the Infectious Diseases Society of America (IDSA) and Society for Healthcare Epidemiology of America (SHEA). *Clin. Infect. Dis.* **2018**, *66*, e1–e48. [CrossRef]

28. Chakra, C.N.A.; Pepin, J.; Sirard, S.; Valiquette, L. Risk factors for recurrence, complications and mortality in Clostridium difficile infection: A systematic review. *PLoS ONE* **2014**, *9*, e98400, Erratum in *PLoS ONE* **2014**, *9*, e107420.
29. Mullish, B.H.; Quraishi, M.N.; Segal, J.P.; McCune, V.L.; Baxter, M.; Marsden, G.L.; Moore, D.J.; Colville, A.; Bhala, N.; Iqbal, T.H.; et al. The use of faecal microbiota transplant as treatment for recurrent or refractory Clostridium difficile infection and other potential indications: Joint British Society of Gastroenterology (BSG) and Healthcare Infection Society (HIS) guidelines. *Gut* **2018**, *67*, 1920–1941. [CrossRef]
30. Mullish, B.H.; Alexander, J.L.; Segal, J.P. Microbiota and faecal microbiota transplant. *Microb. Health Dis.* **2021**, *3*, e586.
31. Bakken, J.S.; Borody, T.; Brandt, L.J.; Brill, J.V.; Demarco, D.C.; Franzos, M.A.; Kelly, C.; Khoruts, A.; Louie, T.; Martinelli, L.P.; et al. Treating Clostridium difficile infection with fecal microbiota transplantation. *Clin. Gastroenterol. Hepatol.* **2011**, *9*, 1044–1049. [CrossRef] [PubMed]
32. Wang, S.; Xu, M.; Wang, W.; Cao, X.; Piao, M.; Khan, S.; Yan, F.; Cao, H.; Wang, B. Systematic Review: Adverse Events of Fecal Microbiota Transplantation. *PLoS ONE* **2016**, *11*, e0161174. [CrossRef] [PubMed]
33. Quraishi, M.N.; Widlak, M.; Bhala, N.; Moore, D.; Price, M.; Sharma, N.; Iqbal, T.H. Systematic review with meta-analysis: The efficacy of faecal microbiota transplantation for the treatment of recurrent and refractory Clostridium difficile infection. *Aliment. Pharmacol. Ther.* **2017**, *46*, 479–493. [CrossRef]
34. Cheng, Y.W.; Phelps, E.; Nemes, S.; Rogers, N.; Sagi, S.; Bohm, M.; El-Halabi, M.; Allegretti, J.R.; Kassam, Z.; Xu, H.; et al. Fecal Microbiota Transplant Decreases Mortality in Patients with Refractory Severe or Fulminant Clostridioides difficile Infection. *Clin. Gastroenterol. Hepatol.* **2020**, *18*, 2234–2243.e1. [CrossRef] [PubMed]
35. Hvas, C.L.; Dahl Jørgensen, S.M.; Jørgensen, S.P.; Storgaard, M.; Lemming, L.; Hansen, M.M.; Erikstrup, C.; Dahlerup, J.F. Fecal Microbiota Transplantation Is Superior to Fidaxomicin for Treatment of Recurrent Clostridium difficile Infection. *Gastroenterology* **2019**, *156*, 1324–1332.e3. [CrossRef] [PubMed]
36. Tariq, R.; Pardi, D.S.; Bartlett, M.G.; Khanna, S. Low Cure Rates in Controlled Trials of Fecal Microbiota Transplantation for Recurrent Clostridium difficile Infection: A Systematic Review and Meta-analysis. *Clin. Infect. Dis.* **2019**, *68*, 1351–1358. [CrossRef]
37. Sehgal, K.; Khanna, S. Gut microbiome and Clostridioides difficile infection: A closer look at the microscopic interface. *Therap. Adv. Gastroenterol.* **2021**, *14*, 1756284821994736. [CrossRef]
38. Revolinski, S.L.; Munoz-Price, L.S. Clostridium difficile Exposures, Colonization, and the Microbiome: Implications for Prevention. *Infect. Control Hosp. Epidemiol.* **2018**, *39*, 596–602. [CrossRef]
39. Ozaki, E.; Kato, H.; Kita, H.; Karasawa, T.; Maegawa, T.; Koino, Y.; Matsumoto, K.; Takada, T.; Nomoto, K.; Tanaka, R.; et al. Clostridium difficile colonization in healthy adults: Transient colonization and correlation with enterococcal colonization. *J. Med. Microbiol.* **2004**, *53 Pt 2*, 167–172. [CrossRef]
40. Zhang, L.; Dong, D.; Jiang, C.; Li, Z.; Wang, X.; Peng, Y. Insight into alteration of gut microbiota in Clostridium difficile infection and asymptomatic C. difficile colonization. *Anaerobe* **2015**, *34*, 1–7. [CrossRef]
41. Rea, M.C.; O'Sullivan, O.; Shanahan, F.; O'Toole, P.W.; Stanton, C.; Ross, R.P.; Hill, C. Clostridium difficile carriage in elderly subjects and associated changes in the intestinal microbiota. *J. Clin. Microbiol.* **2012**, *50*, 867–875. [CrossRef] [PubMed]
42. Al-Jumaili, I.J.; Shibley, M.; Lishman, A.H.; Record, C.O. Incidence and origin of Clostridium difficile in neonates. *J. Clin. Microbiol.* **1984**, *19*, 77–78. [CrossRef] [PubMed]
43. Penders, J.; Thijs, C.; Vink, C.; Stelma, F.F.; Snijders, B.; Kummeling, I.; Van den Brandt, P.A.; Stobberingh, E.E. Factors influencing the composition of the intestinal microbiota in early infancy. *Pediatrics* **2006**, *118*, 511–521. [CrossRef] [PubMed]
44. Rousseau, C.; Levenez, F.; Fouqueray, C.; Doré, J.; Collignon, A.; Lepage, P. Clostridium difficile colonization in early infancy is accompanied by changes in intestinal microbiota composition. *J. Clin. Microbiol.* **2011**, *49*, 858–865. [CrossRef]
45. Stark, P.L.; Lee, A. The microbial ecology of the large bowel of breast-fed and formula-fed infants during the first year of life. *J. Med. Microbiol.* **1982**, *15*, 189–203. [CrossRef]
46. Rolfe, R.D.; Song, W. Immunoglobulin and non-immunoglobulin components of human milk inhibit Clostridium difficile toxin A-receptor binding. *J. Med. Microbiol.* **1995**, *42*, 10–19. [CrossRef]
47. Jangi, S.; Lamont, J.T. Asymptomatic colonization by Clostridium difficile in infants: Implications for disease in later life. *J. Pediatr. Gastroenterol. Nutr.* **2010**, *51*, 2–7. [CrossRef]
48. Seekatz, A.M.; Young, V.B. Clostridium difficile and the microbiota. *J. Clin. Invest.* **2014**, *124*, 4182–4189. [CrossRef]
49. Claesson, M.J.; Cusack, S.; O'Sullivan, O.; Greene-Diniz, R.; De Weerd, H.; Flannery, E.; Marchesi, J.R.; Falush, D.; Dinan, T.G.; Fitzgerald, G.F.; et al. Composition, variability, and temporal stability of the intestinal microbiota of the elderly. *Proc. Natl. Acad. Sci. USA* **2011**, *108* (Suppl. S1), 4586–4591. [CrossRef]
50. Simor, A.E.; Bradley, S.F.; Strausbaugh, L.J.; Crossley, K.; Nicolle, L.E.; SHEA Long-Term-Care Committee. Clostridium difficile in long-term-care facilities for the elderly. *Infect. Control Hosp. Epidemiol.* **2002**, *23*, 696–703. [CrossRef]
51. Vesper, B.J.; Jawdi, A.; Altman, K.W.; Haines, G.K., 3rd; Tao, L.; Radosevich, J.A. The effect of proton pump inhibitors on the human microbiota. *Curr. Drug Metab.* **2009**, *10*, 84–89. [CrossRef] [PubMed]
52. Berg, A.M.; Kelly, C.P.; Farraye, F. Clostridium difficile infection in the inflammatory bowel disease patient. *Inflamm. Bowel. Dis.* **2013**, *19*, 194–204. [CrossRef] [PubMed]
53. Faber, F.; Bäumler, A.J. The impact of intestinal inflammation on the nutritional environment of the gut microbiota. *Immunol. Lett.* **2014**, *162 Pt A*, 48–53. [CrossRef]

54. Kyne, L.; Warny, M.; Qamar, A.; Kelly, C.P. Association between antibody response to toxin A and protection against recurrent Clostridium difficile diarrhoea. *Lancet* **2001**, *357*, 189–193. [CrossRef]
55. Gerding, D.N.; Johnson, S. Management of Clostridium difficile infection: Thinking inside and outside the box. *Clin. Infect. Dis.* **2010**, *51*, 1306–1313. [CrossRef]
56. Cho, J.M.; Pardi, D.S.; Khanna, S. Update on Treatment of Clostridioides difficile Infection. *Mayo Clin. Proc.* **2020**, *95*, 758–769. [CrossRef] [PubMed]
57. Drekonja, D.M.; Amundson, W.H.; DeCarolis, D.D.; Kuskowski, M.A.; Lederle, F.A.; Johnson, J.R. Antimicrobial use and risk for recurrent Clostridium difficile infection. *Am. J. Med.* **2011**, *124*, 1081.e1–1081.e7. [CrossRef]
58. Chang, J.Y.; Antonopoulos, D.A.; Kalra, A.; Tonelli, A.; Khalife, W.T.; Schmidt, T.M.; Young, V.B. Decreased diversity of the fecal Microbiome in recurrent Clostridium difficile-associated diarrhea. *J. Infect. Dis.* **2008**, *197*, 435–438. [CrossRef]
59. Koenigsknecht, M.J.; Young, V.B. Faecal microbiota transplantation for the treatment of recurrent Clostridium difficile infection: Current promise and future needs. *Curr. Opin. Gastroenterol.* **2013**, *29*, 628–632. [CrossRef]
60. Shahinas, D.; Silverman, M.; Sittler, T.; Chiu, C.; Kim, P.; Allen-Vercoe, E.; Weese, S.; Wong, A.; Low, D.E.; Pillai, D.R. Toward an understanding of changes in diversity associated with fecal microbiome transplantation based on 16S rRNA gene deep sequencing. *mBio* **2012**, *3*, e00338-12. [CrossRef]
61. Shankar, V.; Hamilton, M.J.; Khoruts, A.; Kilburn, A.; Unno, T.; Paliy, O.; Sadowsky, M.J. Species and genus level resolution analysis of gut microbiota in Clostridium difficile patients following fecal microbiota transplantation. *Microbiome* **2014**, *2*, 13. [CrossRef] [PubMed]
62. Hamilton, M.J.; Weingarden, A.R.; Unno, T.; Khoruts, A.; Sadowsky, M.J. High-throughput DNA sequence analysis reveals stable engraftment of gut microbiota following transplantation of previously frozen fecal bacteria. *Gut Microbes* **2013**, *4*, 125–135. [CrossRef]
63. Martinez, E.; Taminiau, B.; Rodriguez, C.; Daube, G. Gut Microbiota Composition Associated with *Clostridioides difficile* Colonization and Infection. *Pathogens* **2022**, *11*, 781. [CrossRef] [PubMed]
64. Shaji, A.; Ruksar, S.S.; Manisha, T.; Mohanadas, R. Dietary impact on the gut microbiome and its effects on clostridium difficile, inflammaroty bowel disease and metabolic syndromes. *Exp. Clin. Med. Ga.* **2022**. [CrossRef]
65. Hill, C.; Guarner, F.; Reid, G.; Gibson, G.R.; Merenstein, D.J.; Pot, B.; Morelli, L.; Canani, R.B.; Flint, H.J.; Salminen, S.; et al. Expert consensus document. The International Scientific Association for Probiotics and Prebiotics consensus statement on the scope and appropriate use of the term probiotic. *Nat. Rev. Gastroenterol. Hepatol.* **2014**, *11*, 506–514. [CrossRef]
66. Slavin, J. Fiber and prebiotics: Mechanisms and health benefits. *Nutrients* **2013**, *5*, 1417–1435. [CrossRef]
67. Mills, J.; Rao, K.; Young, V.B. Probiotics for prevention of Clostridium difficile infection. *Curr. Opin. Gastroenterol.* **2018**, *34*, 3–10. [CrossRef]
68. Feuerstadt, P.; Louie, T.J.; Lashner, B.; Wang, E.E.; Diao, L.; Bryant, J.A.; Sims, M.; Kraft, C.S.; Cohen, S.H.; Berenson, C.S.; et al. SER-109, an Oral Microbiome Therapy for Recurrent Clostridioides difficile Infection. *N. Engl. J. Med.* **2022**, *386*, 220–229. [CrossRef]
69. Zhang, Y.; Fleur, A.S.; Feng, H. The development of live biotherapeutics against *Clostridioides difficile* infection towards reconstituting gut microbiota. *Gut Microbe* **2022**, *14*, 2052698. [CrossRef]
70. Orenstein, R.; Dubberke, E.R.; Khanna, S.; Lee, C.H.; Yoho, D.; Johnson, S.; Hecht, G.; DuPont, H.L.; Gerding, D.N.; Blount, K.F.; et al. Durable reduction of Clostridioides difficile infection recurrence and microbiome restoration after treatment with RBX2660: Results from an open-label phase 2 clinical trial. *BMC Infect. Dis.* **2022**, *22*, 245. [CrossRef]
71. Garey, K.W.; McPherson, J.; Dinh, A.Q.; Hu, C.; Jo, J.; Wang, W.; Lancaster, C.K.; Gonzales-Luna, A.J.; Loveall, C.; Begum, K.; et al. Efficacy, Safety, Pharmacokinetics, and Microbiome Changes of Ibezapolstat in Adults with Clostridioides difficile Infection: A Phase 2a Multicenter Clinical Trial. *Clin. Infect. Dis.* **2022**, *75*, 1164–1170. [CrossRef] [PubMed]
72. McDonald, J.A.K.; Mullish, B.H.; Pechlivanis, A.; Liu, Z.; Brignardello, J.; Kao, D.; Holmes, E.; Li, J.V.; Clarke, T.B.; Thursz, M.R.; et al. Inhibiting Growth of Clostridioides difficile by Restoring Valerate, Produced by the Intestinal Microbiota. *Gastroenterology* **2018**, *155*, 1495–1507.e15. [CrossRef] [PubMed]
73. O'Donnell, M.M.; Hegarty, J.W.; Healy, B.; Schulz, S.; Walsh, C.J.; Hill, C.; Ross, R.P.; Rea, M.C.; Farquhar, R.; Chesnel, L. Identification of ADS024, a newly characterized strain of *Bacillus velezensis* with direct *Clostriodes difficile* killing and toxin degradation bio-activities. *Sci. Rep.* **2022**, *12*, 9283. [CrossRef]
74. Khanna, S. Microbiota restoration for recurrent Clostridioides difficile: Getting one step closer every day! *J. Intern. Med.* **2021**, *290*, 294–309. [CrossRef] [PubMed]
75. Pal, R.; Athamneh, A.I.M.; Deshpande, R.; Ramirez, J.A.R.; Adu, K.T.; Muthuirulan, P.; Pawar, S.; Biazzo, M.; Apidianakis, Y.; Sundekilde, U.K.; et al. Probiotics: Insights and new opportunities for *Clostridioides difficile* intervention. *Crit. Rev. Microbiol.* **2022**, 1–21. [CrossRef] [PubMed]

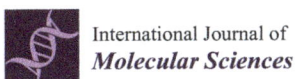

Review

The Role of the Human Microbiome in the Pathogenesis of Pain

Klaudia Ustianowska [1], Łukasz Ustianowski [1], Filip Machaj [1,2], Anna Gorący [3], Jakub Rosik [1,4], Bartosz Szostak [1], Joanna Szostak [5] and Andrzej Pawlik [1,*]

1. Department of Physiology, Pomeranian Medical University, 70-111 Szczecin, Poland
2. Department of Medical Biology, Medical University of Warsaw, 00-575 Warsaw, Poland
3. Independent Laboratory of Invasive Cardiology, Pomeranian Medical University, 70-111 Szczecin, Poland
4. Department of Chemistry, The University of Chicago, Chicago, IL 60637, USA
5. Department of Experimental and Clinical Pharmacology, Pomeranian Medical University, 70-111 Szczecin, Poland
* Correspondence: pawand@poczta.onet.pl

Abstract: Understanding of the gut microbiome's role in human physiology developed rapidly in recent years. Moreover, any alteration of this microenvironment could lead to a pathophysiological reaction of numerous organs. It results from the bidirectional communication of the gastrointestinal tract with the central nervous system, called the gut–brain axis. The signals in the gut–brain axis are mediated by immunological, hormonal, and neural pathways. However, it is also influenced by microorganisms in the gut. The disturbances in the gut–brain axis are associated with gastrointestinal syndromes, but recently their role in the development of different types of pain was reported. The gut microbiome could be the factor in the central sensitization of chronic pain by regulating microglia, astrocytes, and immune cells. Dysbiosis could lead to incorrect immune responses, resulting in the development of inflammatory pain such as endometriosis. Furthermore, chronic visceral pain, associated with functional gastrointestinal disorders, could result from a disruption in the gut microenvironment. Any alteration in the gut–brain axis could also trigger migraine attacks by affecting cytokine expression. Understanding the gut microbiome's role in pain pathophysiology leads to the development of analgetic therapies targeting microorganisms. Probiotics, FODMAP diet, and fecal microbiota transplantation are reported to be beneficial in treating visceral pain.

Keywords: microbiome; pain; IBS; neuropathy

1. Introduction

The gut has the most populous and diverse system of anaerobic and aerobic microorganisms in the human body [1–3]. It is composed mainly of bacteria. However, yeasts, archaea, or parasites living in the large area of the gastrointestinal tract often play a substantial role in this microenvironment [1,2,4,5]. The first years of life, including delivery, are crucial for the development of this complex system [6,7]. Especially at this time, selective pressure is induced by essential host and environmental factors such as breastfeeding or formula feeding, weaning age, diet, infections, and antibiotics [6,7].

The gut microbiota lives in homeostasis with its host. These interactions are regulated by an integral gut barrier and immune system [8,9]. The gastrointestinal tract communicates bidirectionally with the central nervous system via direct and indirect mechanisms [10]. This intricate interplay is called the gut–brain axis (GBA) [11] (Figure 1). Immunological, hormonal, and neural signals play vital roles in this interaction [10,12]. At the same time, the gastrointestinal response to central stimulation is influenced by microorganisms [11]. The microbiota participates in supplying the gut with necessary nutrients and maintaining its barrier integrity. Both terminals of the GBA use serotonin as a vital transmitter [13] Some behavioral changes regulated by serotoninergic transmission seem to depend on the microbiome [13]. Moreover, the GBA affects other systems [10,14–16].

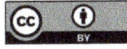

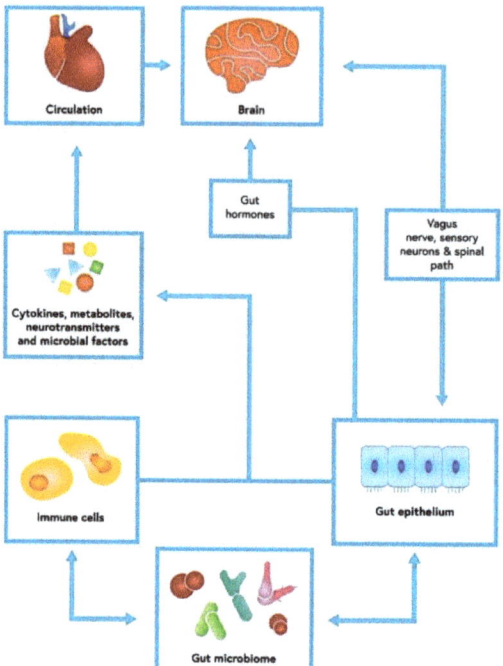

Figure 1. Gut–brain axis with an interconnected net of dependencies. The cerebral function could be modified by gut microbiome and its influence on gut epithelium and immune response. This bidirectional axis uses cytokines and other soluble factors, but also neuronal communication. The short-chain fatty acids (SCFAs) produced by fiber-fermenting bacteria probably have immunomodulatory functions. By binding to G-protein coupled receptors (GPR41, GPR43, and GPR109A), SCFAs exert an anti-inflammatory response in the gut mucosa [17,18].

Disrupted homeostasis in the GBA was first associated with gastrointestinal symptoms and disorders such as inflammatory bowel disease (IBD) or irritable bowel syndrome (IBS) [19]. Moreover, alterations in the composition of the commensal bacterial species populating the gastrointestinal tract are risk factors for a variety of diseases, including cancer [10,14,20–23]. A plant diet has an opposite effect promoting colonization of the gut by protective bacteria and inducing the production of short-chain fatty acids (SCFAs) by species such as *Faecalibacterium prausnitzii* or *Roseburia intestinalis* [24,25].

Subsequently, studies connecting the microbiota with elements of pain pathogenesis were performed. SCFAs are microbial metabolites that affect T-regulatory cells controlling inflammation [26]. Microorganisms produce neurotransmitters that, together with ingested nutrients, stimulate enteroendocrine cells to produce multiple hormones [27,28]. There is growing evidence relating the microbiome to stress, anxiety, neurological diseases, and depression [29–31]. Brain functions affected by microorganisms might augment nociceptive transmission [32–35].

Initiation of pain transmission is induced by nociceptors, which convert noxious stimuli into nerve impulses [36,37]. Then, the signal is modulated by multiple neurons of different types and functions or non-neuronal cells such as glia [36–39]. Nevertheless, sustained pain depends on emotional or cognitive experience [36,40]. It is regulated peripherally and centrally by substances whose production is affected by the microbiome. Pain should serve as protection from tissue damage [37]. Nonetheless, chronic pain leads to a lower quality of life [32,41]. Thus, a better understanding of its mechanism is crucial to improving the lives of millions of people worldwide. Moreover, targeting the gut microbiota seems to be a promising novel therapeutic approach for pain management.

As the aforementioned processes continue to receive increasing attention, we addressed the role of the gut microbiota in pain regulation and discussed the possibility of pain therapy by targeting the gut microbiota. In this narrative review, we collected results from in vitro and in vivo studies on the association between the GBA, pain, and its management.

2. Neuropathic Pain and Central Mechanisms of Pain Regulation

Neuropathic pain occurs as a result of nerve-damaging trauma or somatosensory nervous system disease, including its central and peripheral components [42]. Various conditions, such as diabetes, alcoholism, hypothyroidism, or spinal stenosis, contribute to the development of neuropathic symptoms [42]. This type of pain manifests as abnormal sensations usually felt by patients for the first time. They perceive areas of skin with a sensory deficit, paraesthesia, either spontaneous or evoked pain and thermal or mechanical hypersensitivity [42]. Some drugs used in chemotherapy treatment, such as platinum, vincristine, or toxoids, may cause chemotherapy-induced peripheral neuropathy (CIPN) [43]. Over 30% of patients fighting cancer suffer from such severe CIPN-related pain that they are not receiving sufficient treatment dosages [44].

The gastrointestinal tract consists of various microorganisms, which are reported to play a significant role in neuroinflammatory responses. Neuroimmune activation is considered one of the primary mechanisms determining the central sensitization of chronic pain. It was shown in recent studies that the periphery, including gastrointestinal cells, might arouse brain cells [45]. The gut microbiota particularly regulates microglial function [46]. By affecting the activity of different cells, such as astrocytes, endothelial cells, microglia, monocytes, macrophages, pericytes and T-cells, the gut microbiota may regulate neuroinflammation (Figure 2). When those cells are activated, they start to produce multiple pro-inflammatory mediators such as C–C motif chemokine ligand 2 (CCL2 or MCP-1), CXCL-1, interleukin-1β (IL-1β), interferon-γ (IFN-γ), MMP-2/9, and tumor necrosis factor-α (TNF-α) [12]. Cytokines and chemokines secreted by microglia or astrocytes influence synaptic neurotransmission by increasing glutamate and decreasing gamma-amino-butyric acid (GABA) levels, resulting in pain hypersensitivity [47,48]. Taking all the data under consideration, the gut microbiota can play a major role in central sensitization underlying chronic pain associated with neuroinflammation; hence, it may contribute to the development of diverse neurological diseases [49]. Ding et al., in their article, examined the influence of the gut microbiota on neuropathic pain in chronic-constriction injury of the sciatic nerve (CCI) and whether it is associated with T-cell immune responses. CCI is an animal model widely used to represent neuropathic pain. The study showed that the gut microbiota, via modulation of both pro- and anti-inflammatory T-cell responses, induces the development of neuropathic pain. Moreover, the gut microbiota also has an impact on nociceptive behavior in sciatic nerve CCI. The study found that changes in the gut microbiota caused by the administration of oral antibiotics reduced CCI neuropathic pain. It manifested as weakened mechanical allodynia and thermal hyperalgesia [50]. Another study reported that the gut microbiota might lead to peripheral nerve trauma-induced neuropathic pain. Yang et al. showed that rats with spared nerve injury (SNI) and gut microbial dysbiosis might be prone to neuropathic pain and depression-like phenotypes, including anhedonia [46]. By contrast, in the study by Huang et al. in rat models, no significant association between oral probiotics such as *L. reuteri* LR06 or *Bifidobacterium* BL5b and anti-nociceptive effects on CCI-induced neuropathic pain was demonstrated [51]. Recent studies showed that the gut microbiota is involved in the pathogenesis of CIPN pain and modifies the effects of chemotherapeutics on tumor growth [52,53]. Shen et al. found that the gut microbiota takes part in the evolution of mechanical hyperalgesia induced by chemotherapy. In their study, mice after antibiotic treatment and germ-free mice both experienced reduced mechanical hyperalgesia after oxaliplatin administration. Moreover, restoration of the germ-free mouse microbiota revoked the protective effect [54]. Another study reported that neuropathic pain induced by paclitaxel therapy might be relieved with a DSF probiotic (high concentration of *L. plantarum, S. thermophilus, B. breve, L. paracasei, L. delbrueckii, L. acidophilus, B. longum, B. infantis*). Castelli et al. implied that the use of a probiotic as an adjuvant during chemotherapy might be beneficial in counteracting pain associated with CINP [55].

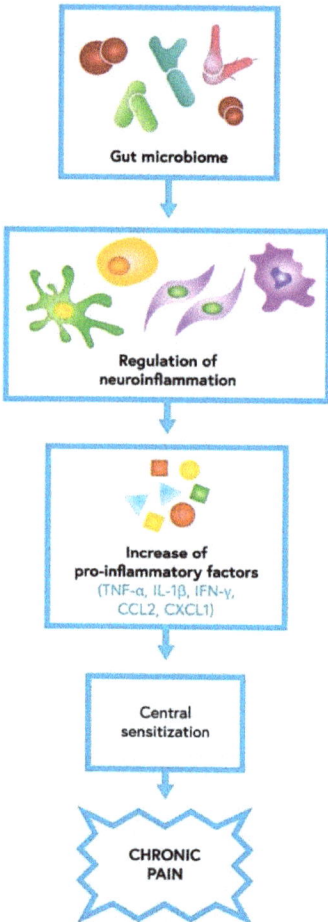

Figure 2. The role of gut microbiota in neuroinflammation which contributes to central sensitization underlying chronic pain; IL-1β—interleukin-1β, IFN-γ—interferon-γ, TNF-α—tumor necrosis factor-α, CCL2—C–C motif chemokine ligand 2, CXCL1—C-X-C motif chemokine 1 [12].

3. Inflammation and Inflammatory Pain

3.1. Endometriosis

Dysbiosis in the GI tract disrupts immune function, which leads to the elevation of inflammatory cytokines and alteration of immune cell profiles. Those factors may play a role in the connection between the GI tract and endometriosis, as both have a high prevalence in patients [56]. As the GI tract possesses an organized lymphoid structure with many immune cells, the gut microbiota stimulates its growth and function, as shown in a study by Hooper et al. [57]. They further showed that dysbiosis alters the composition of immune cells, triggering inflammation [56]. In the case of the vaginal microbiota, it has been shown that a non-Lactobacillus-dominant (NLD) microbiota is associated with overgrowth of pathogenic bacteria, causing bacterial vaginosis. This may decrease reproductive potency, and a vaginal microbiota rich in *Gardnerella*, *Prevotella*, and *Bacteroides* sp. may increase the risk of endometriosis or pelvic inflammatory disease (PID) [58–62]. In recent years, it was also discovered that the uterus, previously thought to be a sterile environment, has its own microbiota. A healthy woman's microbiota consists primarily of *Firmicutes*, *Bacteroides*, *Proteobacteria*, and *Actinobacteria*, according to a study by Baker et al., and a review by Moreno et al. identified the five most represented genera in the endometrial microbiota [62–64].

Ata et al. studied women with stage III/IV endometriosis and compared their microbiota from the gut, cervix, and vagina to that of a control group of healthy women. The cervical microbiota of women with endometriosis had an increased number of pathogenic species, and stool samples had higher *Shigella* and *Escherichia* concentrations [65]. Other studies also found a correlation between the increase in bacteria associated with bacterial vaginosis or opportunistic pathogens in the reproductive tract with endometriosis in women [61,65–74].

3.2. Chronic Pelvic Pain

Chronic pelvic pain (CPP) is a long-lasting pain that lowers quality of life, with many possible causes, such as endometriosis or chronic bacterial prostatitis [75,76]. Recent discoveries regarding the gut microbiome and visceral pain led to hypotheses about the correlation between CPP and the human microbiota. Shoskes et al. determined that patients with CPP had lower gut microbiota diversity than the control group, especially amongst *Prevotella* [77]. A study by Du et al. created a mouse model with experimental autoimmune prostatitis (EAP). EAP mice developed changes in the gut microflora, resulting in a distorted balance in Th17/Treg cells and decreased levels of short-chain fatty acids (SCFAs) in both serum and feces. Microbiota of healthy mice had notably fewer *Firmicutes*, *Nitrospirae*, or *Fusobacteria* than those with EAP. Additionally, the EAP mice had bacteria producing SCFAs, including *Bacteroides*, *Butyricicoccus*, and *Ruminococcaceae*. Changes in Th17/Treg balance were later reversed by supplementation of the SCFA propionate [78]. Their findings were consistent with other studies regarding chronic non-bacterial prostatitis [79,80]. Pelvic allodynia may also be caused by deficient lipase acyloxyacyl hydrolase (AOAH), an enzyme present in microglia. A study by Rahman-Enyart et al. suggests that AOAH plays a role in the modulation of pelvic pain, and its production is dependent on changes in the gut microbiome [81]. As new studies show, the microbiota is a crucial part of overall health, and its changes are correlated with many illnesses; however, further research is needed to make a comprehensive understanding of this topic possible.

4. Visceral Pain, Peripheral Mechanisms of Pain Regulation, and IBS

Visceral pain is a medical term for pain originating from the internal organs within the thorax or abdomen and is divided into acute and chronic pain. Acute visceral pain, caused by typically identifiable causes, is treated with appropriate therapeutic agents, including over the counter (OTC) medications such as non-steroidal anti-inflammatory drugs (NSAIDs) or acetaminophen, and is relatively easy to cure. On the other hand, chronic visceral pain can be difficult to treat even with opioids, and its unknown pathology led to the creation of the term functional gastrointestinal disorders (FGIDs), a collection of many disorders in pediatric and adult patients. FGID includes terms such as irritable bowel syndrome (IBS), infant colic and abdominal migraine, or functional dyspepsia. In the gastrointestinal tract (GI tract), nociceptor nerve endings are found throughout the layers of the GI tract. They respond to many stimuli from the tract and transfer them to their cell bodies in the dorsal horn of the spinal cord [82]. After being transferred to the contralateral side of the spinal cord, the signal is then transmitted to the limbic part of the brain via the spinothalamic tract. A response is then created, and a descending inhibitory circuitry is activated, causing a release of inhibitory neurotransmitters.

In recent years, scientists studied how the microbiome of the GI tract may influence the visceral pain response. The microbial population of a person stabilizes after the first 3 years of life and from then on is relatively stable [82]. Its greatest changes are noticed during disease states; however, while disorders affecting the GI tract are the more obvious causes, GI tract dysbiosis has been observed in many other illnesses. Non-intestinal disorders, such as obesity, allergy, asthma, or autoimmune diseases can also be a factor [82–85]. Additionally, the use of broad-spectrum antibiotic treatment changes the gut microbiota, and using such antibiotics without strong clinical purpose may become a factor in IBS. In a study by Vicentini et al., mice treated with broad-spectrum antibiotics showed effects on the structure and function of the GI tract, resulting in the loss of enteric neurons in enteric plexuses. Post-treatment supplementation of short-chain fatty acids (SCFAs), naturally produced by a healthy gut microbiome, restored neuronal loss in both submucosal and myenteric plexuses [86]. Similarly, a study by De Palma et al. focused on replicating IBS dysbiosis in rats. With fecal microbiota transplant in rats, visceral hypersensitivity increased when compared to gnotobiotic rats receiving a healthy microbiota, suggesting a link between IBS-associated hypersensitivity and the intestinal microbiota [87,88].

4.1. IBS

The influence of the gut microbiota and its dysbiosis on the pathophysiology of IBS was investigated in many studies that compared differences in the GI tract microbiome between IBS patients and controls [89–92]. Those studies showed that the intestinal microbiome of IBS patients had reduced amounts of *Bacteroides*, *Prevotella*, and *Parabacteroides* sp. Noor et al. and Maccaferi et al. showed that IBS patients had an increased population of *Bacillus*, *Bifidobacteria*, *Lactobacillus*, *Clostridium*, and *Eubacterium rectale* [93–95]. Those studies led to research about probiotic intervention and its benefits for IBS patients. In a study by Sisson et al., Symprove, a probiotic containing three *Lactobacillus* types and one Enterococcus, was shown to improve symptom severity in IBS [96]. In another study by Guglielmetti et al., *Bifidobacterium bifidum* MIMBb75 alleviated IBS symptomology by decreasing pain, discomfort, digestive upset, or bloating [97]. Further studies on probiotics for IBS presented another bacterial species with a positive influence on the relief of IBS symptoms [13,98]. Butyrate producers such as *Faecalibacterium* sp. have an anti-inflammatory impact on the GI tract, and *F. prausnitzii* is a source of serine protease that was shown to have anti-nociceptive activity by decreasing the excitability of dorsal root ganglia neurons [99–102]. Unknown IBS pathophysiology led to the creation of the term 'psychobiotics', referring to probiotics and bacterial metabolites that signal directly to the brain. In a randomized controlled trial (RCT) of 44 adults with IBS, patients were treated with *Bifidobacterium longum* NCC3001. Patients showed a significant reduction in depression and an increase in quality of life with no change in IBS symptom severity or the fecal microbiota profile. This suggested that there is some direct signaling of *B. longum* metabolites to the central nervous system (CNS) [103].

4.2. Peripheral Mechanism of Pain Regulation

The enteric nervous system (ENS) is formed by about 200–600 million neurons and is often referred to as the 'second brain'. This network plays a part in maintaining GI tract function and reaches the lamina propria of the mucosa. ENS neurons form the subserous, myenteric, and submucosal plexuses and carry impulses to and from the brain. Intrinsic primary afferent neurons (IPANs) initiate secretory, motor, and vasomotor reactions from stimuli within the mucosa and from the central nervous system (CNS) [104]. Enteric sensory neurons receive the information through neurotransmitters and hormones released by enteroendocrine (EEC) and enterochromaffin (EC) enteric cells.

Enteric hormones such as serotonin (5-HT), glucagon-like peptide 1 (GLP-1), or peptide YY (PYY) are thought to have an impact on visceral pain and its management [104]. 5-HT excreted by EC cells activates receptors on EC cells and extrinsic primary afferent nerve (EPAN) terminals. This triggers enteric reflexes such as secretion, peristalsis, and perception of pain and inflammation [105–107].

Microbes in the GI tract microbiome can synthesize various neurotransmitters and metabolites involved in gut–brain communication, as shown in recent studies [108–111]. This includes SCFAs, tryptophan metabolites, GABA, dopamine, and noradrenaline [104]. One of the SCFAs, butyrate, was proposed as an agent with an indirect effect on regulating inflammatory visceral pain. Its injection in rat and mouse brains stimulated the production of brain-derived neurotrophic factor (BDNF), which favors neurogenesis, memory formation, and mood stabilization [112–114].

Bacteria such as *Escherichia*, *Fusobacterium*, *Prevotella*, *Enterococcus casseliflavus*, or *Bacteroides* can produce tryptophan, which later passes the blood–brain barrier (BBB), influencing serotoninergic neurotransmission in the CNS. In a study by Agus et al., it was shown that during gut inflammation, an increase in tryptophan conversion to kynurenine may be responsible for the development of anxiety and mood shifts [115]. During inflammation, there is an enhanced plasma level of kynurenine, which may favor its passage through the BBB and later metabolism into kynurenic acid (KynA) and quinolinic acid (QuiA), the latter of which is described as a neurotoxic agent [111].

Another microbial product, glutamate, is produced by certain microbial strains in the healthy GI tract [116–119]. It is a major neurotransmitter in the CNS and acts as a neuroactive molecule. A recent study suggested that glutamate may also regulate gut sensory and motor functions via receptors in the ENS [120,121]. During stress-induced dysbiosis, glutamate receptor expression is altered. In antibiotic-treated mice with dysbiosis, there were decreased levels of hippocampal NMDA and BDNF, which were later restored by prebiotic treatment [31,122–124].

GABA is an important neurotransmitter in the brain. Bravo et al. studied its role in pain management and suggested that GABA can inhibit visceral hypersensitivity, altering abdominal pain [125]. Oral administration of *Lactobacillus rhamnosus* in mice increased GABA levels in the CNS. Additionally, in a study by Perez-Berezo et al., administration of the *E. coli* Nissle 1917 (EcN) strain showed an increase in analgesic lipopeptide production, activation of GABA receptors on IPANs, and inhibition of visceral hypersensitivity [126].

5. Headache and Its Association with Drugs

Headache is one of the most frequently reported symptoms [127], and various types have been described. Primary headaches can be divided into four groups: migraine, tension headache, trigeminal autonomic cephalgia, and other primary headache disorders [127]. Migraine, a neurological disorder characterized by headache, nausea, vomiting, and photophobia or phonophobia [128,129], is one of the most common types of headaches [17]. The hemicrania occurs due to hypothalamus activation and further pituitary adenylate cyclase-activating polypeptide (PACAP) secretion, which is responsible for vasodilatation [17]. Moreover, migraine is related to GI illnesses, which include celiac syndrome, irritable bowel syndrome, or infection by *Helicobacter pylori* [12,30]. There is also an association between the gut microbiome and the pathogenesis of migraine. The gut–brain axis triggers the migraine attack through pro-inflammatory factors, gut microbiome composition, neuropeptides, serotonin pathways, stress hormones, and nutritional substances. The physical or psychological stress factors may lead to gut microbiome changes such as dysbiosis [30]. This, in turn, causes an increase in calcitonin gene-related peptide (CGRP) secretion [17], which is correlated with migraine symptoms and has antibacterial effect on strains such as *E. coli*, *E. faecalis*, and *L. acidophilus* [17,30]. This particular type of headache is associated with pro-inflammatory factors. During migraine attacks, increased secretion of serum cytokines such as IL-1b, IL-6, IL-8, and TNF-a was observed. Moreover, Arzani et al. reported that in germ-free mice, the hypernociception induced by inflammatory mediators is reduced [30]. These could result from increased expression of IL-10 in germ-free mouse models [130]. This cytokine is an important regulator of inflammatory responsiveness [130]. These lines of evidence emphasize the importance of the gut microbiome in migraine and have prompted research on whether probiotic supplementation is a beneficial therapy for the condition [12]. The data on the efficacy of probiotic supplementation in migraine are incoherent. Sensenig et al. showed that most patients who were given probiotics, such as *L. bulgaricus, L. acidophilus, E. faecium*, and *B. bifidum*, reported an improvement in quality of life [131]. By contrast, another study showed no significant differences between a group of patients who suffered from migraine and were supplemented with probiotics and the one that was not supplemented with probiotics [12,132].

To summarize, the association between the gut microbiome and migraine is clear. Studies show not only a correlation in pathogenesis but also a possible way of treating migraine with probiotics. However, there is still a lot to be discovered [12].

Opioid Tolerance

Opioids are known for their anti-nociceptive, anti-tussive and anti-diarrheal properties. They are the major drugs used in cancer and post-surgical pain treatment [133], although their severe side effects, such as tolerance, dependence, emesis, or constipation, lead to significant restrictions in their use [12]. GI symptoms associated with these drugs are known as opioid bowel dysfunction (OBD) and are the result of the stimulation of opioid receptors in the GI tract [134]. The research shows that chronic use of opioids may result in dysbiosis [12,135], damage to the gut barrier, bacterial translocation, and secretion of pro-inflammatory factors. Opioid tolerance was associated with a lack of *Bifidobacteria* and *Lactobacillaceae* in mice [12,25]. The enteric glia are responsible for the proper functioning of the GI tract [12]. Furthermore, they are also relevant to the development of the ectypal inflammatory reaction to long-term use of opioid drugs [136]. The bacterial product bacterial lipopolysaccharide (LPS) was reported to be associated with the production of pro-inflammatory cytokines during long-term opioid treatment [136]. Due to the chronic use of morphine, we can observe increased activity in enteric glia of the P2X receptor [12,136], a calcium-permeable ion channel activated by ATP and associated with cytokine secretion by enteric glia [25]. This leads to an enhanced inflammatory reaction [25]. LPS is also related to the intensified expression of connexin 43 (Cx43), a gap junction protein that mediates the secretion of ATP [136]. Cx43 can be blocked by non-specific connexin inhibitor (CBX), which results in a decreased inflammatory response [136].

Another study showed that administration of broad-spectrum antibiotics prevents GI side effects and tolerance to opioid-related drugs with long-term use of morphine [137]. Analgesic tolerance can be avoided by oral vancomycin due to its active properties against Gram-positive bacteria, the translocation of which is significant in the tolerance process [12,25,137]. Furthermore, germ-free mice have reduced morphine tolerance, which can be reclaimed by gut microbiome reconstitution [138]. In addition, opioid tolerance can be a result of the inactivation of tetrodotoxin-resistant (TTX-R) Na+ channels in dorsal root ganglia (DGR) neurons, which can be reversed by oral vancomycin administration [139]. In conclusion, the above-described studies prove the importance of the gut microbiota in opioid tolerance occurrence. They show the role of the gut flora in the genesis of morphine tolerance and indicate how the side effects of opioid drug use may enhance the entire process.

6. The Gut Microbiota as a Therapeutic Target in Chronic Pain

6.1. Probiotics and Prebiotics

Probiotics are living microorganisms that can provide health benefits to the host [140]. A growing body of research supports the thesis that probiotics are effective in modifying the balance of the gut microbiota [141,142]. Some of their proven beneficial effects include improved digestion, boosted immunity, and decreased cholesterol levels [143]. Some of the more recent studies suggest that probiotics might be effective in alleviating the symptoms of chronic intestinal disorders, such as Crohn's disease [144].

Several preclinical animal studies have demonstrated the beneficial effects of probiotics on visceral pain [145–147]. In multiple studies, probiotics exerted beneficial effects on visceral hypersensitivity. In rats, probiotic VSL#3 decreased visceral hypersensitivity potentially through the mast cell-PAR2-TRPV1 pathway, which then affects the release of potent mediators that affect the enteric nerves and smooth muscles [145]. Moreover, supplementation with *Clostridium butyricum*, a commensal bacterium, may inhibit colonic inflammation in a mouse model of IBS through its action on nod-like receptor pyrin domain-containing protein 6 [146]. In a similar model, *Roseburia hominis* alleviated visceral hypersensitivity and prevented the expression of occludin from decreasing [147]. Moreover, in rats, *B. infantis* 35624 significantly reduced visceral pain, suggesting that it may be effective in treating symptoms of IBS [148].

Several human studies have also revealed the benefits of using probiotics for chronic pain. A randomized, double-blind study on 101 pediatric patients suffering from IBS (NCT01180556) revealed that a 4-week supplementation of *L. reuteri* DSM 17938 reduced both the frequency and the intensity of abdominal pain in children [149]. Moreover, a probiotic mixture of *Bifidobacterium infantis* M-63, breve M-16V, and longum BB536 (NCT02566876) was successful in attenuating the symptoms of abdominal pain in IBS but not in functional dyspepsia. Likewise, the intervention group noted the markedly higher quality of life improvement in comparison with a placebo (48% vs. 17%, $p = 0.001$) [150]. A 2009 review by Newlove-Delgado et al. retrospectively investigating the use of probiotics in children with recurrent abdominal pain suggested that those preparations are likely to improve pain symptoms in the short term, that is, up to 3 months (OR = 1.63; 95% CI = 1.07–2.47) [151]. By contrast, a randomized, placebo-controlled trial by Spiller et al. failed to identify any clinical benefit, including intestinal pain and discomfort, of *S. cerevisiae* I-3856 supplementation at a dose of 1000 mg per day, in comparison to a placebo [152].

Prebiotics are fibers and other non-digestible ingredients that benefit the host by selectively boosting the growth and activity of select microorganisms in the colon, mainly lactobacilli and bifidobacteria. They are considered either as an addition to probiotics or an alternative to them. Several pre-clinical dissertations have emerged underlining the beneficial role of prebiotics in terms of attenuating chronic pain, such as PDX/GOS reducing chronic visceral pain induced by intracolonic zymosan injection in rats [153]. In human studies, a prebiotic galacto-oligosaccharide mixture supplemented for 2 weeks reduced abdominal pain associated with GI disorders in adults. The treatment arm reported significantly lower scores for bloating, flatulence, and pain. However, there was no improvement in quality of life throughout the study [154]. Lastly, a study on the symbiotic containing *Bacillus coagulans* on 88 pediatric patients showed a reduction of abdominal pain that was present after treatment (60% vs. 39.5%, $p = 0.044$) but not after 12 weeks of follow-up [155].

6.2. FODMAP Diet

Recent studies have demonstrated that functional GI symptoms can be induced by colonic gas production in patients with visceral hypersensitivity. In those patients, short-chain fermentable carbohydrates increase small intestinal water volume, resulting in increased colonic gas production. Therefore, dietary restriction of short-chain fermentable carbohydrates (low-FODMAP diet) should theoretically ameliorate the symptoms of IBS. In pre-clinical studies, the low-FODMAP diet (LFD) altered the gut microbial composition, resulting in reduced fecal lipopolysaccharide of Gram-negative bacteria. In contrast to a high-FODMAP diet, there is a significant reduction of *Akkermancia muciniphila* and *Actinobacteria* [156]. Therefore, it could be beneficial in reducing gut mucosal inflammation and restoring the barrier function of the gut, ultimately leading to the alleviation of visceral pain [156].

In a clinical setting, the FODMAP diet has led to a reduction in IBS severity, with decreased frequency of pain episodes ($p < 0.01$) and increased quality of life [157]. In another study by Pedersen et al., LFD resulted in a greater reduction of disease severity but no improvement in quality of life [158]. In a double-blind, placebo-controlled trial on 40 patients with IBS by Hustoft et al., LFD with fructans lowered the severity of nausea, vomiting, and flatulence [159]. Overall, up to 86% of IBS patients improve clinically in terms of GI symptoms, as well as abdominal pain, bloating, and constipation, while following the diet [160].

6.3. Fecal Microbiota Transplantation

Fecal microbiota transplantation (FMT) involves the transfer of microbial flora from a healthy donor stool to the recipient's intestinal tract to normalize the target intestinal microbiota composition and function. One of the most notable examples of the use of FMT in clinical practice is *Clostridium difficile* infection (CDI), which often occurs in patients whose microbiota has been suppressed by prolonged antibiotic therapy. Recent evidence suggests that the gut microbiota composition is linked to the occurrence of abdominal pain and its frequency, duration, and intensity in the general population [161]. Moreover, in an animal model of colitis, FMT administration to control rats resulted in long-lasting visceral hypersensitivity [162]. Several mechanisms have been proposed through which FMT might affect chronic pain, including competition with pathogenic bacteria, protection of the intestinal barrier, or stimulation of the intestinal immune system [163]. An open-label study on FMT in humans with IBS showed marked improvement in abdominal pain that was associated with the abundance of *Akkermansia muciniphila* [164].

Moreover, allogenic FMT resulted in a significant decrease in symptoms of IBS ($p = 0.02$), which was not present in the autologous FMT group ($p = 0.16$) [165]. Furthermore, a metagenomic sequencing study revealed that following FMT the taxonomic profile of the recipient shifts towards a donor-like profile, inducing long-term changes in the gut microbiota, which mirror the clinical effect of the treatment [166].

In order to perform successful FMT, several criteria must be met. Firstly, donor selection should be strict, excluding those at risk of harboring an infectious agent. Moreover, recipients must not receive major immunosuppressive therapy, or suffer from serious comorbidities that would put them at risk [167]. While FMT is relatively safe, some of the studies suggest its potential drawbacks. One study suggested that FMT might be associated with diarrhea, abdominal cramping, belching, and nausea within 3 h post-FMT [168]. Moreover, there exists a possibility of development of long-term adverse effects due to alteration of the gut microbiota. More long-term, follow-up studies are required to address this issue [169].

7. Conclusions

In recent years, numerous studies have provided data on the role of the gut microbiome and its influence on other tissues. It is known that alteration in the microbiome could be one of the factors contributing to the development of cancer and neurological, gastrointestinal, cardiovascular, and metabolic diseases. Lately, many studies have also investigated the role of the human microbiome in the pathogenesis of different types of pain (Table 1). Proper assessment and control of pain are essential for improving quality of life in many patients. Despite the availability of various pain management methods, there is still a great need for research on factors contributing to pain pathogenesis and novel therapies. Recent studies suggest that the human microbiome may be an essential component of the pathogenesis of multiple types of pain. Neuropathic pain could result from the gut microbiome's influence on T-cell immune response, disrupting the regulation of pro- and anti-inflammatory cytokine production. Furthermore, alteration of the immune cell response and cytokine production by the gut microbiome could contribute to the development of inflammatory diseases, such as endometriosis. Chronic visceral pain remains a challenge to efficient treatment. The human microbiome contributes to the still unknown pathogenesis of FGIDs, providing a promising direction for further studies. Additionally, common symptoms such as headaches are influenced by the gut microbiome. An altered gut–brain axis could trigger a migraine. Moreover, the regulation of inflammatory mediators that contributes to migraine is disrupted by dysbiosis. The gut microbiome could also impact the efficacy of pain management, leading to opioid tolerance. The contribution of the human microbiome to the pathogenesis of multiple types of pain leads to its use as a possible target for analgesic therapies. Pro- and prebiotics are already widely used in clinical practice. They are reported to be effective in reducing chronic visceral pain and migraine. However, there is still a great need for further evaluation of their efficacy and influence on patients' quality of life. Another approach assumes the modification of the gut microbiome with a specific diet, such as a low-FODMAP diet, which could be beneficial for patients with IBS, reducing symptoms and pain episodes. The usage of FMT is recommended in the treatment of *Clostridium difficile* infection.

Table 1. Summary of novel studies that investigated the role of the human microbiome in the pathogenesis of different types of pain.

Neuropathic Pain and Central Mechanisms of Pain Regulation	Inflammation and Inflammatory Pain	Visceral Pain, Peripheral Mechanisms of Pain Regulation, and IBS	Headache and Its Association with Drugs	The Gut Microbiota as a Therapeutic Target in Chronic Pain
[46] Yang C, Fang X, Zhan G, et al. Key role of gut microbiota in anhedonia-like phenotype in rodents with neuropathic pain.	[56] Jiang I, Yong PJ, Allaire C, Bedaiwy MA. Intricate Connections between the Microbiota and Endometriosis.	[82] Moloney RD, Johnson AC, O'Mahony SM, Dinan TG, Greenwood-Van Meerveld B, Cryan JF. Stress and the Microbiota–Gut–Brain Axis in Visceral Pain: Relevance to Irritable Bowel Syndrome.	[17] Léa LT, Caula C, Moulding T, Lyles A, Wohrer D, Titomanlio L. Brain to Belly: Abdominal variants of migraine and functional abdominal pain disorders associated with migraine.	[145] Li Y-J, Dai C, Jiang M. Mechanisms of Probiotic VSL#3 in a Rat Model of Visceral Hypersensitivity Involves the Mast Cell-PAR2-TRPV1 Pathway.
[42] Baron R, Binder A, Wasner G. Neuropathic pain: diagnosis, pathophysiological mechanisms, and treatment.	[77] Shoskes DA, Wang H, Polackwich AS, Tucky B, Altemus J, Eng C. Analysis of Gut Microbiome Reveals Significant Differences between Men with Chronic Prostatitis/Chronic Pelvic Pain Syndrome and Controls.	[104] Morreale C, Bresesti I, Bosi A, Baj A, Giaroni C, Agosti M, et al. Microbiota and Pain: Save Your Gut Feeling.	[12] Guo R, Chen LH, Xing C, Liu T. Pain regulation by gut microbiota: molecular mechanisms and therapeutic potential.	[146] Zhao K, Yu L, Wang X, He Y, Lu B. Clostridium butyricum regulates visceral hypersensitivity of irritable bowel syndrome by inhibiting colonic mucous low grade inflammation through its action on NLRP6.
		[25] Santoni M, Miccini F, Battelli N. Gut microbiota, immunity and pain. Immunol		[147] Zhang J, Song L, Wang Y, Liu C, Zhang L, et al. Beneficial effect of butyrate-producing Lachnospiraceae on stress-induced visceral hypersensitivity in rats.
		[136] Bhave S, Gade A, Kang M, Hauser KF, Dewey WL, Akbarali HI. Connexin-purinergic signaling in enteric glia mediates the prolonged effect of morphine on constipation.		

Moreover, FMT is reported to efficiently reduce visceral pain among IBS patients. However, these studies have some limitations. There is a strong need for further evaluation of concepts and previous results. Additional long-term studies are required to assess the potential side effects of gut microbiota alteration. Moreover, the differences in the methodology of the studies impede the precise comparison of the results. Pittayanon et al., in their systematic review, reported concerns about deficiencies in studies' methodology and statistical analysis [95]. The shortcomings, such as lack of data on administrated antibiotics, and differences in the microbiome evaluation methods, are reasons for inconsistency in reviewed papers.

Despite the significant development in the understanding of the human microbiome in the pathogenesis of pain, there are still many areas to be investigated. A detailed evaluation of the influence of the altered microbiome on the gut–brain axis could be a critical factor in understanding the impact of dysbiosis on several tissues and pain development [18]. The detailed characterization of the gut microbiome in chronic, visceral, or headache states and their interaction with the gut–brain axis could deliver novel insight into the pathogenesis of a different type of pain. Further molecular studies could develop novel targets for analgetic treatment that could significantly improve numerous patients' quality of life.

Author Contributions: Conceptualization, K.U. and A.P.; methodology, Ł.U.; formal analysis, J.R.; investigation, B.S.; writing—original draft preparation, A.G. and J.S.; writing—review and editing, F.M. and A.P.; visualization, B.S.; supervision, J.R.; project administration, A.P. All authors have read and agreed to the published version of the manuscript.

Funding: This research received no external funding.

Institutional Review Board Statement: Not applicable.

Informed Consent Statement: Not applicable.

Data Availability Statement: Not applicable.

Acknowledgments: The authors thank Piotr Michalski from the Academy of Art in Szczecin for his assistance in composing the figures.

Conflicts of Interest: The authors declare no conflict of interest.

References

1. Sommer, F.; Bäckhed, F. The Gut Microbiota—Masters of Host Development and Physiology. *Nat. Rev. Microbiol.* **2013**, *11*, 227–238. [CrossRef] [PubMed]
2. Karczewski, J.; Troost, F.J.; Konings, I.; Dekker, J.; Kleerebezem, M.; Brummer, R.J.M.; Wells, J.M. Regulation of Human Epithelial Tight Junction Proteins by *Lactobacillus plantarum* In Vivo and Protective Effects on the Epithelial Barrier. *Am. J. Physiol. Gastrointest. Liver. Physiol.* **2010**, *298*, G851–G859. [CrossRef] [PubMed]
3. Hugon, P.; Dufour, J.C.; Colson, P.; Fournier, P.E.; Sallah, K.; Raoult, D. A Comprehensive Repertoire of Prokaryotic Species Identified in Human Beings. *Lancet Infect. Dis.* **2015**, *15*, 1211–1219. [CrossRef]
4. Sender, R.; Fuchs, S.; Milo, R. Revised Estimates for the Number of Human and Bacteria Cells in the Body. *PLoS Biol.* **2016**, *14*. [CrossRef]
5. Bengmark, S. Ecological Control of the Gastrointestinal Tract. The Role of Probiotic Flora. *Gut* **1998**, *42*, 2–7. [CrossRef]
6. Vuong, H.E.; Yano, J.M.; Fung, T.C.; Hsiao, E.Y. The microbiome and host behavior. *Annu. Rev. Neurosci.* **2017**, *40*, 21–49. [CrossRef]
7. Schmidt, T.S.B.; Raes, J.; Bork, P. The human gut microbiome: From association to modulation. *Cell* **2018**, *172*, 1198–1215. [CrossRef]
8. Dardmeh, F.; Nielsen, H.I.; Alipour, H.; Kjaergaard, B.; Brandsborg, E.; Gazerani, P. Potential nociceptive regulatory effect of probiotic Lactobacillus rhamnosus PB01 (DSM 14870) on mechanical sensitivity in diet-induced obesity model. *Pain Res. Manag.* **2016**, *2016*, 5080438. [CrossRef]
9. Belkaid, Y.; Hand, T.W. Role of the microbiota in immunity and inflammation. *Cell* **2014**, *157*, 121–141. [CrossRef]
10. Russo, R.; Cristiano, C.; Avagliano, C.; De Caro, C.; La Rana, G.; Raso, G.M.; Canani, R.B.; Meli, R.; Calignano, A. Gut–brain axis: Role of lipids in the regulation of inflammation, pain and CNS diseases. *Curr. Med. Chem.* **2018**, *25*, 3930–3952. [CrossRef]
11. Keshavarzian, A.; Green, S.J.; Engen, P.A.; Voigt, R.M.; Naqib, A.; Forsyth, C.B.; Mutlu, E.; Shannon, K.M. Colonic bacterial composition in Parkinson's disease. *Mov. Disord.* **2015**, *30*, 1351–1360. [CrossRef]
12. Guo, R.; Chen, L.H.; Xing, C.; Liu, T. Pain Regulation by Gut Microbiota: Molecular Mechanisms and Therapeutic potential. *Br. J. Anaesth.* **2019**, *123*, 637–654. [CrossRef]
13. O'Mahony, S.M.; Clarke, G.; Borre, Y.E.; Dinan, T.G.; Cryan, J.F. Serotonin, Tryptophan Metabolism and the Brain-Gut-Microbiome Axis. *Behav. Brain Res.* **2015**, *277*, 32–48. [CrossRef]
14. Li, X.; Watanabe, K.; Kimura, I. Gut microbiota dysbiosis drives and implies novel therapeutic strategies for diabetes mellitus and related metabolic diseases. *Front. Immunol.* **2017**, *8*, 1882. [CrossRef]
15. Nicholson, J.K.; Holmes, E.; Kinross, J.; Burcelin, R.; Gibson, G.; Jia, W.; Pettersson, S. Host–gut microbiota metabolic interactions. *Science* **2012**, *336*, 1262–1267. [CrossRef]
16. Heiss, C.N.; Olofsson, L.E. The role of the gut microbiota in development, function and disorders of the central nervous system and the enteric nervous system. *J. Neuroendocrinol.* **2019**, *31*, e12684. [CrossRef]
17. Léa, L.T.; Caula, C.; Moulding, T.; Lyles, A.; Wohrer, D.; Titomanlio, L. Brain to Belly: Abdominal variants of migraine and functional abdominal pain disorders associated with migraine. *J. Neurogastroenterol. Motil.* **2021**, *27*, 482–494.
18. Parada Venegas, D.; De la Fuente, M.K.; Landskron, G.; González, M.J.; Quera, R.; Dijkstra, G.; Harmsen, H.J.M.; Faber, K.N.; Hermoso, M.A. Short Chain Fatty Acids (SCFAs)-Mediated Gut Epithelial and Immune Regulation and Its Relevance for Inflammatory Bowel Diseases. *Front. Immunol.* **2019**, *10*, 277. [CrossRef]

19. Rea, K.; O'Mahony, S.M.; Dinan, T.G.; Cryan, J.F. The role of the gastrointestinal microbiota in visceral pain. *Handb. Exp. Pharmacol.* **2017**, *239*, 269–287.
20. Kolodziejczyk, A.A.; Zheng, D.; Shibolet, O.; Elinav, E. The role of the microbiome in NAFLD and NASH. *EMBO Mol. Med.* **2019**, *11*, e9302. [CrossRef]
21. Wahlstrom, A. Outside the liver box: The gut microbiota as pivotal modulator of liver diseases. *Biochim. Biophys. Acta Mol. Basis Dis.* **2019**, *1865*, 912–919. [CrossRef]
22. Massari, F.; Mollica, V.; di Nunno, V.; Gatto, L.; Santoni, M.; Scarpelli, M.; Cimadamore, A.; Lopez-Beltran, A.; Cheng, L.; Battelli, N.; et al. The Human Microbiota and Prostate Cancer: Friend or Foe? *Cancers* **2019**, *11*, 459. [CrossRef] [PubMed]
23. Cimadamore, A.; Santoni, M.; Massari, F.; Gasparrini, S.; Cheng, L.; López-Beltrán, A.; Montironi, R.; Scarpelli, M. Microbiome and Cancers, with Focus on Genitourinary Tumors. *Front. Oncol.* **2019**, *9*, 178. [CrossRef] [PubMed]
24. Neish, A.S. Microbes in Gastrointestinal Health and Disease. *Gastroenterology* **2009**, *136*, 65–80. [CrossRef]
25. Santoni, M.; Miccini, F.; Battelli, N. Gut Microbiota, Immunity and Pain. *Immunol. Lett.* **2021**, *229*, 44–47. [CrossRef] [PubMed]
26. Corrêa-Oliveira, R.; Fachi, J.L.; Vieira, A.; Sato, F.T.; Vinolo, M.A.R. Regulation of Immune Cell Function by Short-Chain Fatty Acids. *Clin. Transl. Immunol.* **2016**, *5*, e73. [CrossRef]
27. Chey, W.Y.; Jin, H.O.; Lee, M.H.; Sun, S.W.; Lee, K.Y. Colonic Motility Abnormality in Patients with Irritable Bowel Syndrome Exhibiting Abdominal Pain and Diarrhea. *Am. J. Gastroenterol.* **2001**, *96*, 1499–1506. [CrossRef]
28. Psichas, A.; Reimann, F.; Gribble, F.M. Gut Chemosensing Mechanisms. *J. Clin. Invest.* **2015**, *125*, 908–917. [CrossRef]
29. Amirkhanzadeh Barandouzi, Z.; Starkweather, A.R.; Henderson, W.A.; Gyamfi, A.; Cong, X.S. Altered Composition of Gut Microbiota in Depression: A Systematic Review. *Front. Psychiatry* **2020**, *11*, 1–10.
30. Arzani, M.; Jahromi, S.R.; Ghorbani, Z.; Vahabizad, F.; Martelletti, P.; Ghaemi, A.; Sacco, S.; Togha, M.; EHF-SAS. Gut-Brain Axis and Migraine Headache: A Comprehensive review. *J. Headache Pain* **2020**, *21*, 15. [CrossRef]
31. Sudo, N.; Chida, Y.; Aiba, Y.; Sonoda, J.; Oyama, N.; Yu, X.N.; Kubo, C.; Koga, Y. Postnatal Microbial Colonization Programs the Hypothalamic-Pituitary-Adrenal System for Stress Response in Mice. *J. Physiol.* **2004**, *558*, 263–275. [CrossRef]
32. Drożdżal, S.; Rosik, J.; Lechowicz, K.; Machaj, F.; Szostak, B.; Majewski, P.; Rotter, I.; Kotfis, K. COVID-19: Pain Management in Patients with SARS-CoV-2 Infection-Molecular Mechanisms, Challenges, and Perspectives. *Brain Sci.* **2020**, *10*, 465. [CrossRef]
33. Neufeld, K.A.M.; Kang, N.; Bienenstock, J.; Foster, J.A. Effects of Intestinal Microbiota on Anxiety-Like Behavior. *Commun. Integr. Biol.* **2011**, *4*, 492–494. [CrossRef]
34. Bercik, P.; Verdu, E.F.; Foster, J.A.; Macri, J.; Potter, M.; Huang, X.; Malinowski, P.; Jackson, W.; Blennerhassett, P.; Neufeld, K.A.; et al. Chronic Gastrointestinal Inflammation Induces Anxiety-Like Behavior and Alters Central Nervous System Biochemistry in Mice. *Gastroenterology* **2010**, *139*, 2102–2112.e1. [CrossRef]
35. Bercik, P.; Denou, E.; Collins, J.; Jackson, W.; Lu, J.; Jury, J.; Deng, Y.; Blennerhassett, P.; Macri, J.; McCoy, K.D.; et al. The Intestinal Microbiota Affect Central Levels of Brain-Derived Neurotropic Factor and Behavior in Mice. *Gastroenterology* **2011**, *141*, 599–609.e3. [CrossRef] [PubMed]
36. Basbaum, A.I.; Bautista, D.M.; Scherrer, G.; Julius, D. Cellular and molecular mechanisms of pain. *Cell* **2009**, *139*, 267–284. [CrossRef]
37. Julius, D.; Basbaum, A.I. Molecular mechanisms of nociception. *Nature* **2001**, *413*, 203–210. [CrossRef]
38. Braz, J.; Solorzano, C.; Wang, X.; Basbaum, A.I. Transmitting pain and itch messages: A contemporary view of the spinal cord circuits that generate gate control. *Neuron* **2014**, *82*, 522–536. [CrossRef]
39. Ji, R.R.; Chamessian, A.; Zhang, Y.Q. Pain regulation by non-neuronal cells and inflammation. *Science* **2016**, *354*, 572–577. [CrossRef]
40. Ossipov, M.H.; Dussor, G.O.; Porreca, F. Central modulation of pain. *J. Clin. Investig.* **2010**, *120*, 3779–3787. [CrossRef]
41. Scholz, J.; Woolf, C.J. Can we conquer pain? *Nat. Neurosci.* **2002**, *5*, 1062–1067. [CrossRef] [PubMed]
42. Baron, R.; Binder, A.; Wasner, G. Neuropathic Pain: Diagnosis, Pathophysiological Mechanisms, and Treatment. *Lancet Neurol.* **2010**, *9*, 807–819. [CrossRef]
43. Cavaletti, G.; Marmiroli, P. Chemotherapy-induced peripheral neurotoxicity. *Nat. Rev. Neurol.* **2010**, *6*, 657–666. [CrossRef] [PubMed]
44. Hershman, D.L.; Lacchetti, C.; Dworkin, R.H.; Lavoie Smith, E.M.; Bleeker, J.; Cavaletti, G.; Chauhan, C.; Gavin, P.; Lavino, A.; Lustberg, M.B.; et al. Prevention and management of chemotherapy-induced peripheral neuropathy in survivors of adult cancers: American Society of Clinical Oncology clinical practice guideline. *J. Clin. Oncol.* **2014**, *32*, 1941–1967. [CrossRef] [PubMed]
45. Duan, L.; Zhang, X.-D.; Miao, W.-Y.; Sun, Y.-J.; Xiong, G.; Wu, Q.; Li, G.; Yang, P.; Yu, H.; Li, H.; et al. PDGFRβ Cells Rapidly Relay Inflammatory Signal from the Circulatory System to Neurons via Chemokine CCL2. *Neuron* **2018**, *100*, 183–200.e8. [CrossRef]
46. Yang, C.; Fang, X.; Zhan, G.; Huang, N.; Li, S.; Bi, J.; Jiang, R.; Yang, L.; Miao, L.; Zhu, B.; et al. Key role of gut microbiota in anhedonia-like phenotype in rodents with neuropathic pain. *Transl. Psychiatry* **2019**, *9*, 57. [CrossRef]
47. Gao, Y.J.; Ji, R.R. Chemokines, Neuronal-Glial Interactions, and Central Processing of Neuropathic Pain. *Pharmacol. Ther.* **2010**, *126*, 56–68. [CrossRef]
48. Matsuda, M.; Huh, Y.; Ji, R.R. Roles of Inflammation, Neurogenic Inflammation, and Neuroinflammation in Pain. *J. Anesth.* **2019**, *33*, 131–139. [CrossRef]

49. Sampson, T.R.; Debelius, J.W.; Thron, T.; Janssen, S.; Shastri, G.G.; Ilhan, Z.E.; Challis, C.; Schretter, C.E.; Rocha, S.; Gradinaru, V.; et al. Gut Microbiota Regulate Motor Deficits and Neuroinflammation in a Model of Parkinson's Disease. *Cell* **2016**, *167*, 1469–1480.e12. [CrossRef]
50. Ding, W.; You, Z.; Chen, Q.; Yang, L.; Doheny, J.; Zhou, X.; Li, N.; Wang, S.; Hu, K.; Chen, L.; et al. Gut Microbiota Influences Neuropathic Pain through Modulating Proinflammatory and Anti-inflammatory T Cells. *Anesth. Analg.* **2021**, *132*, 1146–1155. [CrossRef]
51. Huang, J.; Zhang, C.; Wang, J.; Guo, Q.; Zou, W. Oral Lactobacillus reuteri LR06 or Bifidobacterium BL5b supplement do not produce analgesic effects on neuropathic and inflammatory pain in rats. *Brain Behav.* **2019**, *9*, e01260. [CrossRef]
52. Mukaida, N. Intestinal microbiota: Unexpected alliance with tumor therapy. *Immunotherapy* **2014**, *6*, 231–233. [CrossRef]
53. Vázquez-Baeza, Y.; Callewaert, C.; Debelius, J.; Hyde, E.; Marotz, C.; Morton, J.T.; Swafford, A.; Vrbanac, A.; Dorrestein, P.C.; Knight, R. Impacts of the Human Gut Microbiome on Therapeutics. *Annu. Rev. Pharmacol. Toxicol.* **2018**, *58*, 253–270. [CrossRef]
54. Shen, S.; Lim, G.; You, Z.; Ding, W.; Huang, P.; Ran, C.; Doheny, J.; Caravan, P.; Tate, S.; Hu, K.; et al. Gut microbiota is critical for the induction of chemotherapy-induced pain. *Nat. Neurosci.* **2017**, *20*, 1213–1216. [CrossRef]
55. Castelli, V.; Palumbo, P.; D'Angelo, M.; Moorthy, N.K.; Antonosante, A.; Catanesi, M.; Lombardi, F.; Iannotta, D.; Cinque, B.; Benedetti, E.; et al. Probiotic DSF counteracts chemotherapy induced neuropathic pain. *Oncotarget* **2018**, *9*, 27998–28008. [CrossRef]
56. Jiang, I.; Yong, P.J.; Allaire, C.; Bedaiwy, M.A. Intricate Connections between the Microbiota and Endometriosis. *Int. J. Mol. Sci.* **2021**, *22*, 5644. [CrossRef]
57. Hooper, L.v.; Littman, D.R.; Macpherson, A.J. Interactions between the Microbiota and the Immune System. *Science* **2012**, *336*, 1268–1273. [CrossRef]
58. Martin, D.H.; Marrazzo, J.M. The Vaginal Microbiome: Current Understanding and Future Directions. *J. Infect. Dis.* **2016**, *214* (Suppl. 1), S36–S41. [CrossRef]
59. Muzny, C.A.; Łaniewski, P.; Schwebke, J.R.; Herbst-Kralovetz, M.M. Host-Vaginal Microbiota Interactions in the Pathogenesis of Bacterial Vaginosis. *Curr. Opin. Infect. Dis.* **2020**, *33*, 59–65. [CrossRef]
60. Blander, J.M.; Longman, R.S.; Iliev, I.D.; Sonnenberg, G.F.; Artis, D. Regulation of Inflammation by Microbiota Interactions with the Host. *Nat. Immunol.* **2017**, *18*, 851–860. [CrossRef]
61. Dols, J.A.M.; Molenaar, D.; van der Helm, J.J.; Caspers, M.P.M.; Angelino-Bart, A.d.K.; Schuren, F.H.J.; Speksnijder, A.G.C.L.; Westerhoff, H.V.; Richardus, J.H.; Boon, M.E.; et al. Molecular Assessment of Bacterial Vaginosis by Lactobacillus Abundance and Species Diversity. *BMC Infect. Dis.* **2016**, *16*, 180. [CrossRef] [PubMed]
62. Baker, J.M.; Chase, D.M.; Herbst-Kralovetz, M.M. Uterine Microbiota: Residents, Tourists, or Invaders? *Front. Immunol.* **2018**, *9*, 208. [CrossRef] [PubMed]
63. Møller, B.R.; Kristiansen, F.v.; Thorsen, P.; Frost, L.; Mogensen, S.C. Sterility of the Uterine Cavity. *Acta Obstet. Gynecol. Scand.* **1995**, *74*, 216–219. [CrossRef] [PubMed]
64. Moreno, I.; Codoñer, F.M.; Vilella, F.; Valbuena, D.; Martinez-Blanch, J.F.; Jimenez-Almazán, J.; Alonso, R.; Alamá, P.; Remohí, J.; Pellicer, A.; et al. Evidence that the Endometrial Microbiota Has an Effect on Implantation Success or Failure. *Am. J. Obstet. Gynecol.* **2016**, *215*, 684–703. [CrossRef] [PubMed]
65. Ata, B.; Yildiz, S.; Turkgeldi, E.; Brocal, V.P.; Dinleyici, E.C.; Moya, A.; Urman, B. The Endobiota Study: Comparison of Vaginal, Cervical and Gut Microbiota Between Women with Stage 3/4 Endometriosis and Healthy Controls. *Sci. Rep.* **2019**, *9*, 2204. [CrossRef]
66. Bourlev, V.; Volkov, N.; Pavlovitch, S.; Lets, N.; Larsson, A.; Olovsson, M. The relationship between microvessel density, proliferative activity and expression of vascular endothelial growth factor-A and its receptors in eutopic endometrium and endometriotic lesions. *Reproduction* **2006**, *132*, 501–509. [CrossRef]
67. Hernandes, C.; Silveira, P.; Rodrigues Sereia, A.F.; Christoff, A.P.; Mendes, H.; Valter de Oliveira, L.F.; Podgaec, S. Microbiome Profile of Deep Endometriosis Patients: Comparison of Vaginal Fluid, Endometrium and Lesion. *Diagnostics* **2020**, *10*, 163. [CrossRef]
68. Akiyama, K.; Nishioka, K.; Khan, K.N.; Tanaka, Y.; Mori, T.; Nakaya, T.; Kitawaki, J. Molecular detection of microbial colonization in cervical mucus of women with and without endometriosis. *Am. J. Reprod. Immunol.* **2019**, *82*, e13147. [CrossRef]
69. Wei, W.; Zhang, X.; Tang, H.; Zeng, L.; Wu, R. Microbiota Composition and Distribution along the Female Reproductive Tract of Women with Endometriosis. *Ann. Clin. Microbiol. Antimicrob.* **2020**, *19*, 15. [CrossRef]
70. Perrotta, A.R.; Borrelli, G.M.; Martins, C.O.; Kallas, E.G.; Sanabani, S.S.; Griffith, L.G.; Alm, E.J.; Abrao, M.S. The Vaginal Microbiome as a Tool to Predict rASRM Stage of Disease in Endometriosis: A Pilot Study. *Reprod. Sci.* **2020**, *27*, 1064–1073. [CrossRef]
71. Deng, T.; Shang, A.; Zheng, Y.; Zhang, L.; Sun, H.; Wang, W. Log (*Lactobacillus crispatus/Gardnerella vaginalis*): A new indicator of diagnosing bacterial vaginosis. *Bioengineered* **2022**, *13*, 2981–2991. [CrossRef]
72. Tohill, B.C.; Heilig, C.M.; Klein, R.S.; Rompalo, A.; Cu-Uvin, S.; Brown, W.; Duerr, A. Vaginal flora morphotypic profiles and assessment of bacterial vaginosis in women at risk for HIV infection. *Infect. Dis. Obstet. Gynecol.* **2004**, *12*, 121–126. [CrossRef]
73. Dols, J.A.; Smit, P.W.; Kort, R.; Reid, G.; Schuren, F.H.; Tempelman, H.; Bontekoe, T.R.; Korporaal, H.; Boon, M.E. Microarray-Based Identification of Clinically Relevant Vaginal Bacteria in Relation to Bacterial Vaginosis. *Am. J. Obstet. Gynecol.* **2011**, *204*, 305.e1–305.e7. [CrossRef]

74. Verstraelen, H.; Verhelst, R. Bacterial vaginosis: An update on Diagnosis and Treatment. *Expert Rev. Anti Infect. Ther.* **2009**, *7*, 1109–1124. [CrossRef]
75. James, S.L.; Abate, D.; Abate, K.H.; Abay, S.M.; Abbafati, C.; Abbasi, N.; Abbastar, H.; Abd-Allah, F.; Abdela, J.; Abdelalim, A.; et al. Global, Regional, and National Incidence, Prevalence, and Years Lived with Disability for 354 Diseases and Injuries for 195 Countries and Territories, 1990–2017: A Systematic Analysis for the Global Burden of Disease Study 2017. *Lancet* **2018**, *392*, 1789–1858. [CrossRef]
76. Gaskin, D.J.; Richard, P. The Economic Costs of Pain in the United States. *J. Pain* **2012**, *13*, 715–724. [CrossRef]
77. Shoskes, D.A.; Wang, H.; Polackwich, A.S.; Tucky, B.; Altemus, J.; Eng, C. Analysis of Gut Microbiome Reveals Significant Differences between Men with Chronic Prostatitis/Chronic Pelvic Pain Syndrome and Controls. *J. Urol.* **2016**, *196*, 435–441. [CrossRef]
78. Du, H.X.; Yue, S.Y.; Niu, D.; Liu, C.; Zhang, L.G.; Chen, J.; Chen, Y.; Guan, Y.; Xiao-Liang, H.; Chun, L.; et al. Gut Microflora Modulates Th17/Treg Cell Differentiation in Experimental Autoimmune Prostatitis via the Short-Chain Fatty Acid Propionate. *Front. Immunol.* **2022**, *13*, 1. [CrossRef]
79. Ohadian Moghadam, S.; Momeni, S.A. Human Microbiome and Prostate Cancer Development: Current Insights into the Prevention and Treatment. *Front. Med.* **2021**, *15*, 11–32. [CrossRef]
80. Crocetto, F.; Boccellino, M.; Barone, B.; di Zazzo, E.; Sciarra, A.; Galasso, G.; Settembre, G.; Quagliuolo, L.; Imbimbo, C.; Boffo, S.; et al. The Crosstalk between Prostate Cancer and Microbiota Inflammation: Nutraceutical Products Are Useful to Balance This Interplay? *Nutrients* **2020**, *12*, 2648. [CrossRef]
81. Rahman-Enyart, A.; Yaggie, R.E.; Bollinger, J.L.; Arvanitis, C.; Winter, D.R.; Schaeffer, A.J.; Klumpp, D.J. Acyloxyacyl Hydrolase Regulates Microglia-Mediated Pelvic Pain. Streicher JM, Editor. *PLoS ONE* **2022**, *17*, e0269140. [CrossRef] [PubMed]
82. Moloney, R.D.; Johnson, A.C.; O'Mahony, S.M.; Dinan, T.G.; Greenwood-Van Meerveld, B.; Cryan, J.F. Stress and the Microbiota–Gut–Brain Axis in Visceral Pain: Relevance to Irritable Bowel Syndrome. *CNS Neurosci. Ther.* **2016**, *22*, 102. [CrossRef] [PubMed]
83. McLean, M.H.; Dieguez, D.; Miller, L.M.; Young, H.A. Does the Microbiota Play a Role in the Pathogenesis of Autoimmune Diseases? *Gut* **2015**, *64*, 332–341. [CrossRef] [PubMed]
84. Sheehan, D.; Moran, C.; Shanahan, F. The Microbiota in Inflammatory Bowel Disease. *J. Gastroenterol.* **2015**, *50*, 495–507. [CrossRef] [PubMed]
85. Valitutti, F.; Cucchiara, S.; Fasano, A. Celiac disease and the microbiome. *Nutrients* **2019**, *11*, 2403. [CrossRef]
86. Vicentini, F.A.; Keenan, C.M.; Wallace, L.E.; Woods, C.; Cavin, J.-B.; Flockton, A.R.; Macklin, W.B.; Belkind-Gerson, J.; Hirota, S.A.; Sharkey, K.A. Intestinal Microbiota Shapes Gut Physiology and Regulates Enteric Neurons and Glia. *Microbiome* **2021**, *9*, 210. [CrossRef]
87. De Palma, G.; Lynch, M.D.J.; Lu, J.; Dang, V.T.; Deng, Y.; Jury, J.; Umeh, G.; Miranda, P.M.; Pastor, M.P.; Sidani, S.; et al. Transplantation of Fecal Microbiota from Patients with Irritable Bowel Syndrome Alters Gut Function and Behavior in Recipient Mice. *Sci. Transl. Med.* **2017**, *9*, eaaf6397. [CrossRef]
88. Crouzet, L.; Gaultier, E.; Del'Homme, C.; Cartier, C.; Delmas, E.; Dapoigny, M.; Fioramonti, J.; Bernalier-Donadille, A. The Hypersensitivity to Colonic Distension of IBS Patients Can Be Transferred to Rats through Their Fecal Microbiota. *Neurogastroenterol. Motil.* **2013**, *25*, e272–e282. [CrossRef]
89. Malinen, E.; Rinttilä, T.; Kajander, K.; Mättö, J.; Kassinen, A.; Krogius, L.; Saarela, M.; Korpela, R.; Palva, A. Analysis of the Fecal Microbiota of Irritable Bowel Syndrome Patients and Healthy Controls with Real-Time PCR. *Am. J. Gastroenterol.* **2005**, *100*, 373–382. [CrossRef]
90. Lyra, A.; Rinttilä, T.; Nikkilä, J.; Krogius-Kurikka, L.; Kajander, K.; Malinen, E.; Mättö, J.; Mäkelä, L.; Palva, A. 'Diarrhoea-Predominant Irritable Bowel Syndrome Distinguishable by 16S rRNA Gene Phylotype Quantification. *World J Gastroenterol.* **2009**, *15*, 5936–5945. [CrossRef]
91. Tana, C.; Umesaki, Y.; Imaoka, A.; Handa, T.; Kanazawa, M.; Fukudo, S. Altered Profiles of Intestinal Microbiota and Organic Acids May be the Origin of Symptoms in Irritable Bowel Syndrome. *Neurogastroenterol. Motil.* **2010**, *22*, 512-e115. [CrossRef]
92. Mayer, E.A.; Savidge, T.; Shulman, R.J. Brain-Gut Microbiome Interactions and Functional Bowel Disorders. *Gastroenterology* **2014**, *146*, 1500–1512. [CrossRef]
93. Maccaferri, S.; Candela, M.; Turroni, S.; Centanni, M.; Severgnini, M.; Consolandi, C.; Cavina, P.; Brigidi, P. IBS-Associated Phylogenetic Unbalances of the Intestinal Microbiota Are Not Reverted by Probiotic Supplementation. *Gut Microbes* **2012**, *3*, 406–413. [CrossRef]
94. Noor, S.O.; Ridgway, K.; Scovell, L.; Kemsley, E.K.; Lund, E.K.; Jamieson, C.; Johnson, I.T.; Narbad, A. Ulcerative Colitis and Irritable Bowel Patients Exhibit Distinct Abnormalities of the Gut Microbiota. *BMC Gastroenterol.* **2010**, *10*, 134. [CrossRef]
95. Pittayanon, R.; Lau, J.T.; Yuan, Y.; Leontiadis, G.I.; Tse, F.; Surette, M.; Moayyedi, P. Gut Microbiota in Patients with Irritable Bowel Syndrome-A Systematic Review. *Gastroenterology* **2019**, *157*, 97–108. [CrossRef]
96. Sisson, G.; Ayis, S.; Sherwood, R.A.; Bjarnason, I. Randomised Clinical Trial: A Liquid Multi-Strain Probiotic vs. Placebo in the Irritable Bowel Syndrome—A 12 Week Double-Blind Study. *Aliment. Pharmacol. Ther.* **2014**, *40*, 51–62. [CrossRef]
97. Guglielmetti, S.; Mora, D.; Gschwender, M.; Popp, K. Randomised Clinical Trial: Bifidobacterium bifidum MIMBb75 Significantly Alleviates Irritable Bowel Syndrome and Improves Quality of Life—A Double-Blind, Placebo-Controlled Study. *Aliment. Pharmacol. Ther.* **2011**, *33*, 1123–1132. [CrossRef]

98. Yoon, J.S.; Sohn, W.; Lee, O.Y.; Lee, S.P.; Lee, K.N.; Jun, D.W.; Lee, H.L.; Yoon, B.C.; Choi, H.S.; Chung, W.S.; et al. Effect of Multispecies Probiotics on Irritable Bowel Syndrome: A Randomized, Double-Blind, Placebo-Controlled Trial. *J. Gastroenterol. Hepatol.* **2014**, *29*, 52–59. [CrossRef]
99. Lopez-Siles, M.; Duncan, S.H.; Garcia-Gil, L.J.; Martinez-Medina, M. *Faecalibacterium prausnitzii*: From Microbiology to Diagnostics and Prognostics. *ISME J.* **2017**, *11*, 841–852. [CrossRef]
100. Sessenwein, J.L.; Baker, C.C.; Pradhananga, S.; Maitland, M.E.; Petrof, E.O.; Allen-Vercoe, E.; Noordhof, C.; Reed, D.E.; Vanner, S.J.; Lomax, A.E. Protease-Mediated Suppression of DRG Neuron Excitability by Commensal Bacteria. *J. Neurosci.* **2017**, *37*, 11758–11768. [CrossRef]
101. Lomax, A.E.; Pradhananga, S.; Sessenwein, J.L.; O'Malley, D. Bacterial modulation of visceral sensation: Mediators and mechanisms. *Am. J. Physiol. Gastrointest. Liver Physiol.* **2019**, *317*, G363–G372. [CrossRef] [PubMed]
102. Pradhananga, S.; Tashtush, A.A.; Allen-Vercoe, E.; Petrof, E.O.; Lomax, A.E. Protease-dependent excitation of nodose ganglion neurons by commensal gut bacteria. *J. Physiol.* **2020**, *598*, 2137–2151. [CrossRef] [PubMed]
103. Pinto-Sanchez, M.I.; Hall, G.B.; Ghajar, K.; Nardelli, A.; Bolino, C.; Lau, J.T.; Martin, F.-P.; Cominetti, O.; Welsh, C.; Rieder, A.; et al. Probiotic Bifidobacterium longum NCC3001 Reduces Depression Scores and Alters Brain Activity: A Pilot Study in Patients with Irritable Bowel Syndrome. *Gastroenterology* **2017**, *153*, 448–459.e8. [CrossRef] [PubMed]
104. Morreale, C.; Bresesti, I.; Bosi, A.; Baj, A.; Giaroni, C.; Agosti, M.; Salvatore, S. Microbiota and Pain: Save Your Gut Feeling. *Cells* **2022**, *11*, 971. [CrossRef] [PubMed]
105. Mawe, G.M.; Hoffman, J.M. Serotonin Signalling in the Gut-Functions, Dysfunctions and Therapeutic Targets. *Nat. Rev. Gastroenterol. Hepatol.* **2013**, *10*, 473–486. [CrossRef] [PubMed]
106. Gershon, M.D. Review Article: Serotonin Receptors and Transporters—Roles in Normal and Abnormal Gastrointestinal Motility. *Aliment. Pharmacol. Ther. Supplement.* **2004**, *20*, 3–14. [CrossRef]
107. Costedio, M.M.; Hyman, N.; Mawe, G.M. Serotonin and its role in colonic function and in gastrointestinal disorders. *Dis. Colon. Rectum.* **2007**, *50*, 376–388. [CrossRef]
108. Bistoletti, M.; Bosi, A.; Banfi, D.; Giaroni, C.; Baj, A. The Microbiota-Gut-Brain Axis: Focus on the Fundamental Communication Pathways. *Prog. Mol. Biol. Transl. Sci.* **2020**, *176*, 43–110.
109. Kuwahara, A.; Matsuda, K.; Kuwahara, Y.; Asano, S.; Inui, T.; Marunaka, Y. Microbiota-gut-brain axis: Enteroendocrine cells and the enteric nervous system form an interface between the microbiota and the central nervous system. *Biomed. Res.* **2020**, *41*, 199–216. [CrossRef]
110. Baj, A.; Moro, E.; Bistoletti, M.; Orlandi, V.; Crema, F.; Giaroni, C. Glutamatergic Signaling Along the Microbiota-Gut-Brain Axis. *Int. J. Mol. Sci.* **2019**, *20*, 1482. [CrossRef]
111. Bosi, A.; Banfi, D.; Bistoletti, M.; Giaroni, C.; Baj, A. Tryptophan Metabolites Along the Microbiota-Gut-Brain Axis: An Interkingdom Communication System Influencing the Gut in Health and Disease. *Int. J. Tryptophan. Res.* **2020**, *13*, 1178646920928984. [CrossRef]
112. Varela, R.B.; Valvassori, S.S.; Lopes-Borges, J.; Mariot, E.; Dal-Pont, G.C.; Amboni, R.T.; Bianchini, G.; Quevedo, J. Sodium butyrate and Mood Stabilizers Block Ouabain-Induced Hyperlocomotion and Increase BDNF, NGF and GDNF Levels in Brain of Wistar Rats. *J. Psychiatr. Res.* **2015**, *61*, 114–121. [CrossRef]
113. Jornada, L.K.; Moretti, M.; Valvassori, S.S.; Ferreira, C.L.; Padilha, P.T.; Arent, C.O.; Fries, G.R.; Kapczinski, F.; Quevedo, J. Effects of mood stabilizers on hippocampus and amygdala BDNF levels in an animal model of mania induced by ouabain. *J. Psychiatr. Res.* **2010**, *44*, 506–510. [CrossRef]
114. Guo, C.; Huo, Y.J.; Li, Y.; Han, Y.; Zhou, D. Gut-Brain Axis: Focus on Gut Metabolites Short-Chain Fatty Acids. *World J. Clin. Cases* **2022**, *10*, 1754–1763. [CrossRef]
115. Agus, A.; Planchais, J.; Sokol, H. Gut Microbiota Regulation of Tryptophan Metabolism in Health and Disease. *Cell Host Microbe* **2018**, *23*, 716–724. [CrossRef]
116. Sanchez, S.; Rodríguez-Sanoja, R.; Ramos, A.; Demain, A.L. Our Microbes Not Only Produce Antibiotics, They Also Overproduce Amino Acids. *J. Antibiot.* **2017**, *71*, 26–36. [CrossRef]
117. Wendisch, V.F.; Jorge, J.M.P.; Pérez-García, F.; Sgobba, E. Updates on industrial production of amino acids using Corynebacterium glutamicum. *World J. Microbiol. Biotechnol.* **2016**, *32*, 105. [CrossRef]
118. Nakayama, Y.; Hashimoto, K.-i.; Sawada, Y.; Sokabe, M.; Kawasaki, H.; Martinac, B. *Corynebacterium glutamicum* Mechanosensitive Channels: Towards Unpuzzling "Glutamate Efflux" for Amino Acid Production. *Biophys. Rev.* **2018**, *10*, 1359–1369. [CrossRef]
119. Zareian, M.; Ebrahimpour, A.; Bakar, F.A.; Mohamed, A.K.S.; Forghani, B.; Ab-Kadir, M.S.B.; Saari, M. A Glutamic Acid-Producing Lactic Acid Bacteria Isolated from Malaysian Fermented Foods. *Int. J. Mol. Sci.* **2012**, *13*, 5482–5497. [CrossRef]
120. Zhang, L.; Wang, R.; Bai, T.; Xiang, X.; Qian, W.; Song, J.; Hou, X. EphrinB2/ephB2-Mediated Myenteric Synaptic Plasticity: Mechanisms Underlying the Persistent Muscle Hypercontractility and Pain in Postinfectious IBS. *FASEB J.* **2019**, *33*, 13644–13659. [CrossRef]
121. Neunlist, M.; Michel, K.; Reiche, D.; Dobreva, G.; Huber, K.; Schemann, M. Glycine Activates Myenteric Neurones in Adult Guinea-Pigs. *J. Physiol.* **2001**, *536*, 727–739. [CrossRef] [PubMed]
122. Caputi, V.; Marsilio, I.; Filpa, V.; Cerantola, S.; Orso, G.; Bistoletti, M.; Paccagnella, N.; De Martin, S.; Montopoli, M.; Dall'Acqua, S.; et al. Antibiotic-Induced Dysbiosis of the Microbiota Impairs Gut Neuromuscular Function in Juvenile Mice. *Br. J. Pharmacol.* **2017**, *174*, 3623–3639. [CrossRef] [PubMed]

123. Gronier, B.; Savignac, H.M.; Di Miceli, M.; Idriss, S.M.; Tzortzis, G.; Anthony, D.; Burnet, P.W. Increased Cortical Neuronal Responses to NMDA and Improved Attentional Set-Shifting Performance in Rats following Prebiotic (B-GOS ®) Ingestion. *Eur. Neuropsychopharmacol.* **2018**, *28*, 211–224. [CrossRef] [PubMed]
124. Jiang, C.; Lin, W.J.; Salton, S.R. Role of a VGF/BDNF/TrkB Autoregulatory Feedback Loop in Rapid-Acting Antidepressant Efficacy. *J. Mol. Neurosci.* **2019**, *68*, 504–509. [CrossRef] [PubMed]
125. Bravo, J.A.; Forsythe, P.; Chew, M.V.; Escaravage, E.; Savignac, H.M.; Dinan, T.G.; Bienenstock, J.; Cryan, J.F. Ingestion of *Lactobacillus* Strain Regulates Emotional Behavior and Central GABA Receptor Expression in a Mouse Via the Vagus Nerve. *Proc. Natl. Acad. Sci. USA* **2011**, *108*, 16050–16055. [CrossRef] [PubMed]
126. Perez-Berezo, T.; Pujo, J.; Martin, P.; Le Faouder, P.; Galano, J.-M.; Guy, A.; Knauf, C.; Tabet, J.C.; Tronnet, S.; Barreau, F.; et al. Identification of an Analgesic Lipopeptide Produced by the Probiotic *Escherichia coli* Strain Nissle 1917. *Nat. Commun.* **2017**, *8*, 1314. [CrossRef]
127. May, A. Hints on Diagnosing and Treating Headache. *Dtsch. Arztebl. Int.* **2018**, *115*, 299–308. [CrossRef]
128. Aurora, S.K.; Shrewsbury, S.B.; Ray, S.; Hindiyeh, N.; Nguyen, L. A Link between Gastrointestinal Disorders and Migraine: Insights into the Gut–Brain Connection. *Headache J. Head Face Pain* **2021**, *61*, 576–589. [CrossRef]
129. Dodick, D.W. Migraine. *Lancet* **2018**, *391*, 1315–1330. [CrossRef]
130. Amaral, F.A.; Sachs, D.; Costa, V.V.; Fagundes, C.T.; Cisalpino, D.; Cunha, T.M.; Ferreira, S.H.; Cunha, F.Q.; Silva, T.A.; Nicoli, J.R.; et al. Commensal microbiota is fundamental for the development of inflammatory pain. *Proc. Natl. Acad. Sci. USA* **2008**, *105*, 2193–2197. [CrossRef]
131. Sensenig, J.; Marrongelle, J.; Johnson, M.; Staverosky, T. Permission Treatment of Migraine with Targeted Nutrition Focused on Improved Assimilation and Elimination. *Altern. Med. Rev.* **2001**, *6*, 488–494.
132. De Roos, N.M.; van Hemert, S.; Rovers, J.M.P.; Smits, M.G.; Witteman, B.J.M. The effects of a multispecies probiotic on migraine and markers of intestinal permeability–results of a randomized placebo-controlled study. *Eur. J. Clin. Nutr.* **2017**, *71*, 1455–1462. [CrossRef]
133. Smith, H.S. Opioid Metabolism. *Mayo Clin. Proc.* **2009**, *84*, 613–624. [CrossRef]
134. Pappagallo, M. Incidence, Prevalence, and Management of Opioid Bowel Dysfunction. *Am. J. Surg.* **2001**, *182*, S11–S18. [CrossRef]
135. Acharya, C.; Betrapally, N.S.; Gillevet, P.M.; Sterling, R.K.; Akbarali, H.; White, M.B.; Ganapathy, D.; Fagan, A.; Sikaroodi, M.; Bajaj, J.S. Chronic opioid use is associated with altered gut microbiota and predicts readmissions in patients with cirrhosis. *Aliment. Pharmacol. Ther.* **2017**, *45*, 319–331. [CrossRef]
136. Bhave, S.; Gade, A.; Kang, M.; Hauser, K.F.; Dewey, W.L.; Akbarali, H.I. Connexin-Purinergic Signaling in Enteric Glia Mediates the Prolonged Effect of Morphine on Constipation. *FASEB J.* **2017**, *31*, 2649–2660. [CrossRef]
137. Kang, M.; Mischel, R.A.; Bhave, S.; Komla, E.; Cho, A.; Huang, C.; Dewey, W.L.; Akbarali, H.I. The Effect of Gut Microbiome on Tolerance to Morphine Mediated Antinociception in Mice. *Sci. Rep.* **2017**, *7*, 42658. [CrossRef]
138. Zhang, L.; Meng, J.; Ban, Y.; Jalodia, R.; Chupikova, I.; Fernandez, I.; Brito, N.; Sharma, U.; Abreu, M.T.; Ramakrishnan, S.; et al. Morphine Tolerance is Attenuated in Germfree Mice and Reversed by Probiotics, Implicating the Role of Gut Microbiome. *Proc. Natl. Acad. Sci. USA* **2019**, *116*, 13523–13532. [CrossRef]
139. Mischel, R.A.; Dewey, W.L.; Akbarali, H.I. Tolerance to Morphine-Induced Inhibition of TTX-R Sodium Channels in Dorsal Root Ganglia Neurons Is Modulated by Gut-Derived Mediators. *iScience* **2018**, *2*, 193–209. [CrossRef]
140. Williams, N.T. Probiotics. *Am. J. Health Pharm.* **2010**, *67*, 449–458. [CrossRef]
141. Arora, T.; Singh, S.; Sharma, R.K. Probiotics: Interaction with gut microbiome and antiobesity potential. *Nutrition* **2013**, *29*, 591–596. [CrossRef] [PubMed]
142. Ng, S.C.; Hart, A.L.; Kamm, M.A.; Stagg, A.J.; Knight, S.C. Mechanisms of action of probiotics: Recent advances. *Inflamm. Bowel Dis.* **2009**, *15*, 300–310. [CrossRef] [PubMed]
143. Abd El-Gawad, I.A.; El-Sayed, E.M.; Hafez, S.A.; El-Zeini, H.M.; Saleh, F.A. The hypocholesterolaemic effect of milk yoghurt and soy-yoghurt containing bifidobacteria in rats fed on a cholesterol-enriched diet. *Int. Dairy J.* **2005**, *15*, 37–44. [CrossRef]
144. Ohland, C.L.; MacNaughton, W.K. Probiotic bacteria and intestinal epithelial barrier function. *Am. J. Physiol. Liver Physiol.* **2010**, *298*, G807–G819. [CrossRef] [PubMed]
145. Li, Y.-J.; Dai, C.; Jiang, M. Mechanisms of Probiotic VSL#3 in a Rat Model of Visceral Hypersensitivity Involves the Mast Cell-PAR2-TRPV1 Pathway. *Dig. Dis. Sci.* **2019**, *64*, 1182–1192. [CrossRef]
146. Zhao, K.; Yu, L.; Wang, X.; He, Y.; Lu, B. Clostridium butyricum regulates visceral hypersensitivity of irritable bowel syndrome by inhibiting colonic mucous low grade inflammation through its action on NLRP6. *Acta Biochim. Biophys. Sin.* **2018**, *50*, 216–223. [CrossRef]
147. Zhang, J.; Song, L.; Wang, Y.; Liu, C.; Zhang, L.; Zhu, S.; Liu, S.; Duan, L. Beneficial effect of butyrate-producing Lachnospiraceae on stress-induced visceral hypersensitivity in rats. *J. Gastroenterol. Hepatol.* **2019**, *34*, 1368–1376. [CrossRef]
148. Mckernan, D.P.; Fitzgerald, P.; Dinan, T.G.; Cryan, J.F. The probiotic Bifidobacterium infantis 35624 displays visceral antinociceptive effects in the rat. *Neurogastroenterol. Motil.* **2010**, *22*, 1029-e268. [CrossRef]
149. Weizman, Z.; Abu-Abed, J.; Binsztok, M. Lactobacillus reuteri DSM 17938 for the Management of Functional Abdominal Pain in Childhood: A Randomized, Double-Blind, Placebo-Controlled Trial. *J. Pediatr.* **2016**, *174*, 160–164.e1. [CrossRef]

150. Giannetti, E.; Maglione, M.; Alessandrella, A.; Strisciuglio, C.; De Giovanni, D.; Campanozzi, A.; Miele, E.; Staiano, A. A mixture of 3 bifidobacteria decreases abdominal pain and improves the quality of life in children with irritable bowel syndrome. *J. Clin. Gastroenterol.* **2017**, *51*, e5–e10. [CrossRef]
151. Newlove-Delgado, T.; Abbott, R.A.; Martin, A.E. Probiotics for Children with Recurrent Abdominal Pain. *JAMA Pediatr.* **2019**, *173*, 183–184. [CrossRef]
152. Spiller, R.; Pélerin, F.; Decherf, A.C.; Maudet, C.; Housez, B.; Cazaubiel, M.; Jüsten, P. Randomized double blind placebo-controlled trial of Saccharomyces cerevisiae CNCM I-3856 in irritable bowel syndrome: Improvement in abdominal pain and bloating in those with predominant constipation. *United Eur. Gastroenterol. J.* **2015**, *4*, 353–362. [CrossRef]
153. Kannampalli, P.; Pochiraju, S.; Chichlowski, M.; Berg, B.M.; Rudolph, C.; Bruckert, M.; Miranda, A.; Sengupta, J.N. Probiotic Lactobacillus rhamnosus GG (LGG) and prebiotic prevent neonatal inflammation-induced visceral hypersensitivity in adult rats. *Neurogastroenterol. Motil.* **2014**, *26*, 1694–1704. [CrossRef]
154. Vulevic, J.; Tzortzis, G.; Juric, A.; Gibson, G.R. Effect of a prebiotic galactooligosaccharide mixture (B-GOS®) on gastrointestinal symptoms in adults selected from a general population who suffer with bloating, abdominal pain, or flatulence. *Neurogastroenterol. Motil.* **2018**, *30*, e13440. [CrossRef]
155. Saneian, H.; Pourmoghaddas, Z.; Roohafza, H.; Gholamrezaei, A. Synbiotic containing *Bacillus coagulans* and fructo-oligosaccharides for functional abdominal pain in children. *Gastroenterol. Hepatol. Bed Bench* **2015**, *8*, 56–65.
156. Zhou, S.-Y.; Gilliland, M.; Wu, X.; Leelasinjaroen, P.; Zhang, G.; Zhou, H.; Ye, B.; Lu, Y.; Owyang, C. FODMAP diet modulates visceral nociception by lipopolysaccharide-mediated intestinal inflammation and barrier dysfunction. *J. Clin. Investig.* **2018**, *128*, 267–280. [CrossRef]
157. Harvie, R. A Reduction in FODMAP Intake Correlates Strongly with a Reduction in IBS Symptoms—The FIBS Study. Ph.D. Thesis, University of Otago, Dunedin, New Zealand, 2014.
158. Pedersen, N.; Andersen, N.N.; Végh, Z.; Jensen, L.; Ankersen, D.V.; Felding, M.; Simonsen, M.H.; Burisch, J.; Munkholm, P. Ehealth: Low FODMAP diet vs Lactobacillus rhamnosus GG in irritable bowel syndrome. *World J. Gastroenterol.* **2014**, *20*, 16215. [CrossRef]
159. Hustoft, T.N.; Hausken, T.; Ystad, S.O.; Valeur, J.; Brokstad, K.; Hatlebakk, J.G.; Lied, G.A. Effects of varying dietary content of fermentable short-chain carbohydrates on symptoms, fecal microenvironment, and cytokine profiles in patients with irritable bowel syndrome. *Neurogastroenterol. Motil.* **2017**, *29*, e12969. [CrossRef]
160. Nanayakkara, W.S.; Skidmore, P.M.; O'Brien, L.; Wilkinson, T.J.; Gearry, R.B. Efficacy of the low FODMAP diet for treating irritable bowel syndrome: The evidence to date. *Clin. Exp. Gastroenterol.* **2016**, *9*, 131–142. [CrossRef]
161. Hadizadeh, F.; Bonfiglio, F.; Belheouane, M.; Vallier, M.; Sauer, S.; Bang, C.; Bujanda, L.; Andreasson, A.; Agreus, L.; Engstrand, L.; et al. Faecal microbiota composition associates with abdominal pain in the general population. *Gut* **2018**, *67*, 778–779. [CrossRef]
162. Lucarini, E.; Di Pilato, V.; Parisio, C.; Micheli, L.; Toti, A.; Pacini, A.; Bartolucci, G.; Baldi, S.; Niccolai, E.; Amedei, A.; et al. Visceral sensitivity modulation by faecal microbiota transplantation: The active role of gut bacteria in pain persistence. *Pain* **2022**, *163*, 861–877. [CrossRef] [PubMed]
163. Khoruts, A.; Sadowsky, M.J. Understanding the mechanisms of faecal microbiota transplantation. *Nat. Rev. Gastroenterol. Hepatol.* **2016**, *13*, 508–516. [CrossRef] [PubMed]
164. Cruz-Aguilar, R.M.; Wantia, N.; Clavel, T.; Vehreschild, M.J.G.T.; Buch, T.; Bajbouj, M.; Haller, D.; Busch, D.; Schmid, R.M.; Stein-Thoeringer, C.K. An Open-Labeled Study on Fecal Microbiota Transfer in Irritable Bowel Syndrome Patients Reveals Improvement in Abdominal Pain Associated with the Relative Abundance of Akkermansia Muciniphila. *Digestion* **2019**, *100*, 127–138. [CrossRef] [PubMed]
165. Holster, S.; Lindqvist, C.M.; Repsilber, D.; Salonen, A.; de Vos, W.M.; König, J.; Brummer, R.J. The Effect of Allogenic Versus Autologous Fecal Microbiota Transfer on Symptoms, Visceral Perception and Fecal and Mucosal Microbiota in Irritable Bowel Syndrome: A Randomized Controlled Study. *Clin. Transl. Gastroenterol.* **2019**, *10*, e00034. [CrossRef]
166. Goll, R.; Johnsen, P.H.; Hjerde, E.; Diab, J.; Valle, P.C.; Hilpusch, F.; Cavanagh, J.P. Effects of fecal microbiota transplantation in subjects with irritable bowel syndrome are mirrored by changes in gut microbiome. *Gut Microbes* **2020**, *12*, 1794263. [CrossRef]
167. Borody, T.J.; Khoruts, A. Fecal microbiota transplantation and emerging applications. *Nat. Rev. Gastroenterol. Hepatol.* **2011**, *20*, 88–96. [CrossRef]
168. Van Nood, E.; Vrieze, A.; Nieuwdorp, M.; Fuentes, S.; Zoetendal, E.G.; De Vos, W.M.; Visser, C.E.; Kuijper, E.J.; Bartelsman, J.F.W.M.; Tijssen, J.G.P.; et al. Duodenal Infusion of Donor Feces for Recurrent Clostridium difficile. *N. Engl. J. Med.* **2013**, *368*, 407–415. [CrossRef]
169. Gupta, S.; Allen-Vercoe, E.; Petrof, E.O. Fecal microbiota transplantation: In perspective. *Therap. Adv. Gastroenterol.* **2016**, *9*, 229–239. [CrossRef]

MDPI
St. Alban-Anlage 66
4052 Basel
Switzerland
www.mdpi.com

International Journal of Molecular Sciences Editorial Office
E-mail: ijms@mdpi.com
www.mdpi.com/journal/ijms

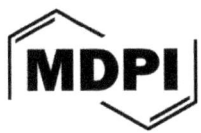

Disclaimer/Publisher's Note: The statements, opinions and data contained in all publications are solely those of the individual author(s) and contributor(s) and not of MDPI and/or the editor(s). MDPI and/or the editor(s) disclaim responsibility for any injury to people or property resulting from any ideas, methods, instructions or products referred to in the content.

www.ingramcontent.com/pod-product-compliance
Lightning Source LLC
LaVergne TN
LVHW070738100526
838202LV00013B/1262